RADIOLOGY
CASE REVIEW SERIES | Spine Imaging

RADIOLOGY

CASE REVIEW SERIES | Spine Imaging

Allison Grayev, MD

Department of Radiology
University of Wisconsin
Madison, Wisconsin

Sayed Ali, MD

Associate Professor of Clinical Radiology
Temple University School of Medicine
Philadelphia, Pennsylvania

Reuben Grech, MD

Neuroradiologist
Medical Imaging Department
Mater Dei Hospital
Malta

SERIES EDITOR

Roland Talanow, MD, PhD

President
Department of Radiology Education
Radiopolis, a subdivision of InnoMed, LLC
Stateline, Nevada

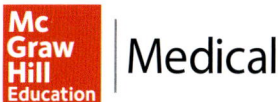

New York   Chicago   San Francisco   Athens   London
Madrid   Mexico City   Milan   New Delhi   Singapore
Sydney   Toronto

Radiology Case Review Series: Spine Imaging

1 2 3 4 5 6 7 8 9 0   CTP/CTP   19 18 17 16 15

ISBN 978-0-07-179808-2
MHID 0-07-179808-0

This book was set in Times LT Std. by Thomson Digital.
The editors were Michael Weitz and Regina Y. Brown.
The production supervisor was Richard Ruzycka.
Project management was provided by Sarita Yadav, Thomson Digital.
China Translation & Printing Services, Ltd., was printer and binder.

This book is printed on acid-free paper.

Library of Congress Cataloging-in-Publication Data
Grayev, Allison, author.
  Spine imaging / Allison Grayev, Sayed Ali, Reuben Grech.
    p. ; cm. — (Radiology case review series)
  Includes bibliographical references and indexes.
  ISBN 978-0-07-179808-2 (pbk. : alk. paper) — ISBN 0-07-179808-0 (pbk. : alk. paper)
  I. Ali, Sayed, author. II. Grech, Reuben, author. III. Title. IV. Series: Radiology case review series.
  [DNLM: 1. Spinal Diseases—radiography—Case Reports. 2. Spinal Diseases—radiography—Problems and Exercises. 3. Radiology—methods—Case Reports.
4. Radiology—methods—Problems and Exercises. 5. Spinal Diseases—diagnosis—Case Reports. 6. Spinal Diseases—diagnosis—Problems and Exercises. 7. Spine—radiography—Case Reports. 8. Spine—radiography—Problems and Exercises. WE 18.2]
  RC402.2.R33
  616.7'307572—dc23
                                                        2014039103

McGraw-Hill Education books are available at special quantity discounts to use as premiums and sales promotions or for use in corporate training programs. To contact a representative, please visit the Contact Us pages at www.mhprofessional.com.

For my wonderful family and colleagues without
whom this would not have been possible.
— Allison Grayev, MD

To my parents, siblings, Chandra and my incredible sons
Rayhan and Kian, for your support in all that I do.
— Sayed Ali, MD

To my loved ones. Your continuous support was invaluable.
— Reuben Grech, MD

Contents

Series Preface

Maybe I have an obsession for cases, but when I was a radiology resident I loved to learn especially from cases, not only because they are short, exciting, and fun—similar to a detective story in which the aim is to get to "the bottom" of the case—but also because, in the end, that's what radiologists are faced with during their daily work. Since medical school, I have been fascinated with learning, not only for my own benefit but also for the sake of teaching others, and I have enjoyed combining my IT skills with my growing knowledge to develop programs that help others in their learning process. Later, during my radiology residency, my passion for case-based learning grew to a level where the idea was born to create a case-based journal: integrating new concepts and technologies that aid in the traditional learning process. Only a few years later, the *Journal of Radiology Case Reports* became an internationally popular and PubMed indexed radiology journal—popular not only because of the interactive features but also because of the case-based approach. This led me to the next step: why not tackle something that I especially admired during my residency but that could be improved—creating a new interactive case-based review series? I imagined a book series that would take into account new developments in teaching and technology and changes in the examination process.

As did most other radiology residents, I loved the traditional case review books, especially for preparation for the boards. These books are quick and fun to read and focus in a condensed way on material that will be examined in the final boards. However, nothing is perfect and these traditional case review books had their own intrinsic flaws. The authors and I have tried to learn from our experience by putting the good things into this new book series but omitting the bad parts and exchanging them with innovative features.

What are the features that distinguish this series from traditional series of review books?

To save space, traditional review books provide two cases on one page. This requires the reader to turn the page to read the answer for the first case but could lead to unintentional "cheating" by seeing also the answer of the second case. Doesn't this defeat the purpose of a review book? From my own authoring experience on the *USMLE Help* book series, it was well appreciated that we avoided such accidental cheating by separating one case from the other. Taking the positive experience from that book series, we decided that each case in this series should consist of two pages: page 1

with images and questions and page 2 with the answers and explanations. This approach avoids unintentional peeking at the answers before deciding on the correct answers yourself. We keep it strict: one case per page! This way it remains up to your own knowledge to figure out the right answer.

Another example that residents (including me) did miss in traditional case review books is that these books did not highlight the pertinent findings on the images: sometimes, even looking at the images as a group of residents, we could not find the abnormality. This is not only frustrating but also time-consuming. When you prepare for the boards, you want to use your time as efficiently as possible. Why not show annotated images? We tackled that challenge by providing, on the second page of each case, the same images with annotations or additional images that highlight the findings.

When you are preparing for the boards and managing your clinical duties, time is a luxury that becomes even more precious. Does the resident preparing for the boards truly need lengthy discussions as in a typical textbook? Or does the resident rather want a "rapid fire" mode in which he or she can "fly" through as many cases as possible in the shortest possible time? This is the reality when you start your work after the boards! Part of our concept with the new series is providing short "pearls" instead of lengthy discussions. The reader can easily read and memorize these "pearls."

Another challenge in traditional books is that questions are asked on the first page and no direct answer is provided, only a lengthy block of discussion. Again, this might become time-consuming to find the right spot where the answer is located if you have doubts about one of several answer choices. Remember: time is money—and life! Therefore, we decided to provide explanations to *each* individual question, so that the reader knows exactly where to find the right answer to the right question. Questions are phrased in an intuitive way so that they fit not only the print version but also the multiple-choice questions for that particular case in our online version. This system enables you to move back and forth between the print version and the online version.

In addition, we have provided up to 3 references for each case. This case review is not intended to replace traditional textbooks. Instead, it is intended to reiterate and strengthen your already existing knowledge (from your training) and to fill potential gaps in your knowledge.

However, in a collaborative effort with the *Journal of Radiology Case Reports* and the international radiology community Radiolopolis, we have developed an online repository with more comprehensive information for each case, such as demographics, discussions, more image examples, interactive image stacks with scroll, a window/level feature, and other interactive features that almost resemble a workstation. In addition, we are planning ahead toward the new Radiology Boards format and are providing rapid fire online sessions and mock examinations that use the cases in the print version. Each case in the print version is crosslinked to the online version using a case ID. The case ID number appears to the right of the diagnosis heading at the top of the second page of each case. Each case can be accessed using the case ID number at the following web site: www.radiologycasereviews.com/case/ID, in which "ID" represents the case ID number. If you have any questions regarding this web site, please e-mail the series editor directly at roland@talanow.info.

I am particularly proud of such a symbiotic endeavor of print and interactive online education and I am grateful to McGraw-Hill for giving me and the authors the opportunity to provide such a unique and innovative method of radiology education, which, in my opinion, may be a trendsetter.

The primary audience of this book series is the radiology resident, particularly the resident in the final year who is preparing for the radiology boards. However, each book in

this series is structured on difficulty levels so that the series also becomes useful to an audience with limited experience in radiology (nonradiologist physicians or medical students) up to subspecialty-trained radiologists who are preparing for their CAQs or who just want to refresh their knowledge and use this series as a reference.

I am delighted to have such an excellent team of US and international educators as authors on this innovative book series. These authors have been thoroughly evaluated and selected based on their excellent contributions to the *Journal of Radiology Case Reports*, the Radiolopolis community, and other academic and scientific accomplishments.

It brings especially personal satisfaction to me that this project has enabled each author to be involved in the overall decision-making process and improvements regarding the print and online content. This makes each participant not only an author but also part of a great radiology product that will appeal to many readers.

Finally, I hope you will experience this case review book as it is intended to be: a quick, pertinent, "get to the point" radiology case review that provides essential information for the radiology boards in the shortest time available, which, in the end, is crucial for preparation for the boards.

Roland Talanow, MD, PhD

Preface

Spine imaging has always appealed to me as it crosses several different subspecialties and imaging modalities, combining biomechanical and neurological reasoning to aid in patient imaging. This compilation of spine cases is designed to both review common entities and challenge you to stretch your diagnostic abilities. It is my hope that this will not only enable you to prepare for examinations, but also prepare you for your career and aid you in appreciating the value that a well-trained radiologist can add in spinal imaging.

Allison Grayev, MD
Sayed Ali, MD
Reuben Grech, MD

RADIOLOGY

CASE REVIEW SERIES | Spine Imaging

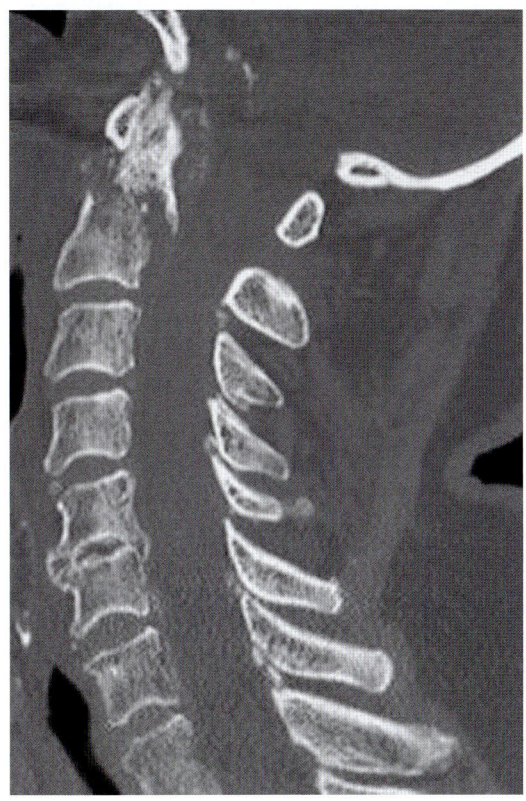 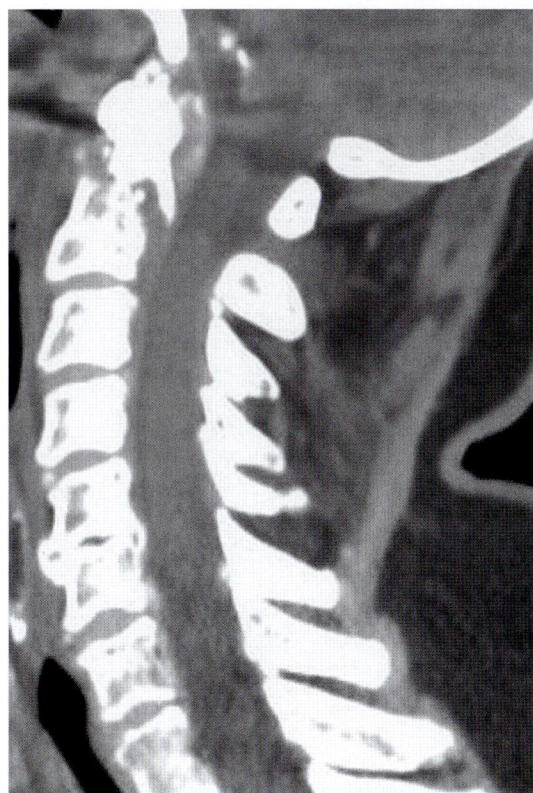

1. What should be included in the differential diagnosis?

2. What structures are involved?

3. What type of odontoid fracture is associated with the highest degree of nonunion?

4. What are the mechanisms of injury?

5. What are treatment options?

Case ranking/difficulty:

Category: Vertebral body

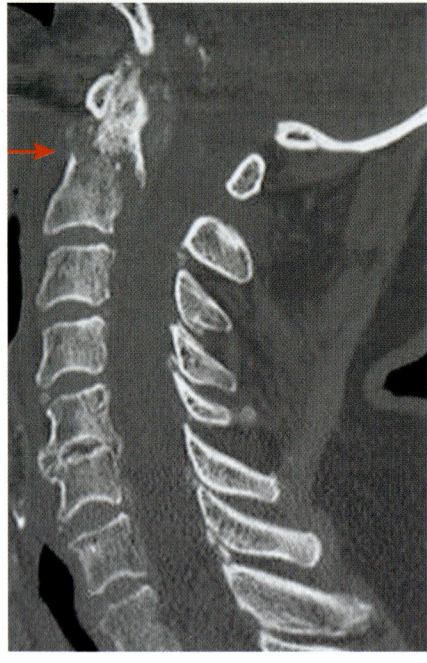

Sagittal reconstructed CT image at bone windows demonstrates lucency through the base of the odontoid with associated displacement and angulation.

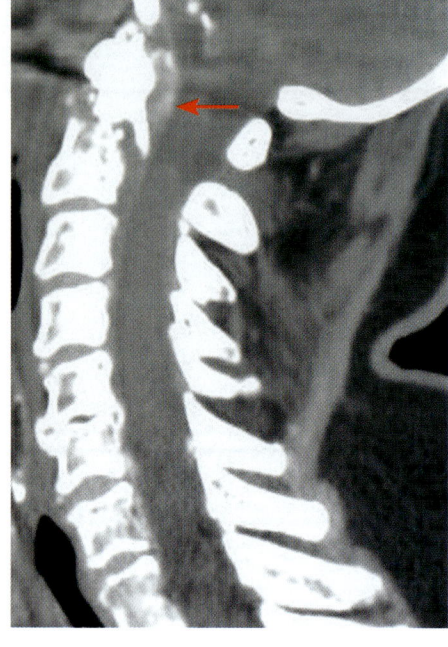

Sagittal reconstructed CT image at soft tissue windows demonstrates epidural hematoma associated with odontoid fracture.

Answers

1. C2 fractures (all subtypes) and os odontoideum need to be considered in the setting of lucency within the C2 vertebral body.

2. Type 2 fractures traverse the base of the dens.

3. Type 2 fractures have the highest incidence of nonunion. The prevalence of nonunion in type 2 fractures approaches 50%.

4. Flexion loading is the most common mechanism, followed by extension loading.

5. Analgesia and halo fixation are appropriate first-line treatment methods; however, if the patient is older or there is a greater degree of displacement (5 mm anterior or 2 mm posterior), these patients often require surgical fixation.

- The fracture is usually the result of a hyperflexion or hyperextension injury, and may occur in the setting of high-speed trauma (motor vehicle accident) or lower-velocity trauma (fall from a standing height, particularly in the elderly).
- Type 2 odontoid fractures are most at risk for nonunion.
- Features associated with nonunion include increased displacement (>5 mm anterior or >2 mm posterior), advanced patient age, comminution, and delay in diagnosis.
- Classification of dens fractures:
  - Type 1—through the odontoid tip
  - Type 2—through the odontoid base
  - Type 3—involvement of the vertebral body

Pearls

- Type 2 odontoid fractures are the most common subtype of odontoid fractures and odontoid fractures are the most common cervical spine fracture, accounting for up to 15% of all cervical spine fractures.

Suggested Readings

Greene KA, Dickman CA, Marciano FF, Drabier JB, Hadley MN, Sonntag VKH. Acute axis fractures: analysis of management and outcome in 340 consecutive cases. *Spine.* 1997;22:1843-1852.

Rao SK, Wasyliw C, Nunez DB. Spectrum of imaging findings in hyperextension injuries of the neck. *Radiographics.* 2005;25:1239-1254.

Neck pain

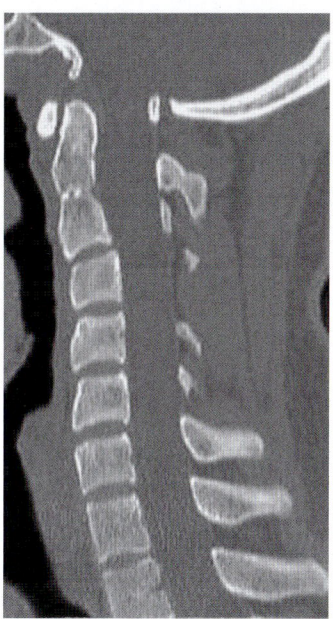

1. What should be included in the differential diagnosis?

2. What are common presenting symptoms?

3. What measurement is used to assess this abnormality?

4. What is the etiology?

5. What are treatment options?

Case ranking/difficulty:

Category: Vertebral body

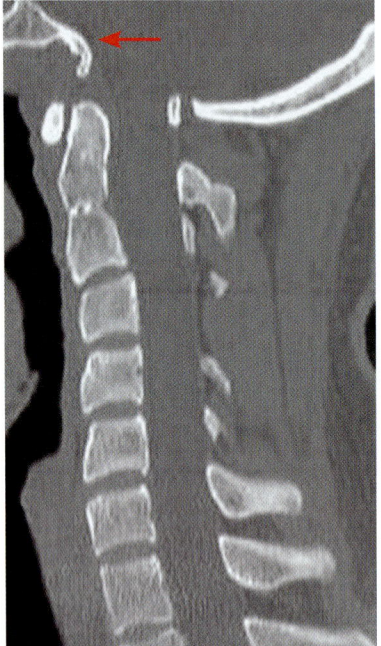

Sagittal CT image demonstrates a short hypoplastic clivus with associated platybasia. Incidentally noted is congenital fusion of C2 and C3.

Answers

1. Abnormalities of the craniocervical junction should be considered, including basilar impression, basilar invagination, clival hypoplasia, occipital condyle hypoplasia, and atlantooccipital assimilation.

2. Platybasia unto itself is generally asymptomatic; however, pain, syrinx, and myelopathy can be seen in association with basilar invagination.

3. Platybasia is assessed using the Welcher basal angle, which is formed at the intersection of tangents drawn from the clivus and sphenoid bone.

4. Many etiologies can cause platybasia, including rickets, osteomalacia, trauma, osteogenesis imperfecta, cleidocranial dysostosis, and Paget disease.

5. Conservative management is most appropriate for isolated platybasia; however, if basilar invagination is present, surgery may be indicated to reduce complications.

Pearls

- Platybasia is defined as a Welcher basal angle of greater than 143°. The Welcher basal angle is the angle formed when tangents from the clivus and sphenoid bone intersect. The normal angle is between 125° and 143°.
- While platybasia may be an isolated finding, there is a strong association with basilar invagination.
- Platybasia can be seen with cleidocranial dysostosis, osteogenesis imperfecta, Paget disease, trauma, or rickets/osteomalacia.
- Platybasia unto itself is asymptomatic; however, there is an association with basilar invagination.
- Basilar invagination refers to acquired cephalad displacement of the dens above the foramen magnum.
- Basilar impression refers to congenital cephalad displacement of the dens above the foramen magnum.

Suggested Readings

Cronin CG, Lohan DG, Mhuircheartigh JN, Meehan CP, Murphy J, Roche C. "CT evaluation of Chamberlain's, McGregor's and McRae's skull-base lines." *Clin Radiol.* 2009;64:64-69.

Smoker WRK. "Craniovertebral junction: normal anatomy, craniometry, and congenital anomalies. *Radiographics.* 1994;14:255-277.

Smoker WRK, Khanna G. Imaging the craniocervical junction. *Childs Nerv Syst.* 2008;24:1123-1145.

Back pain

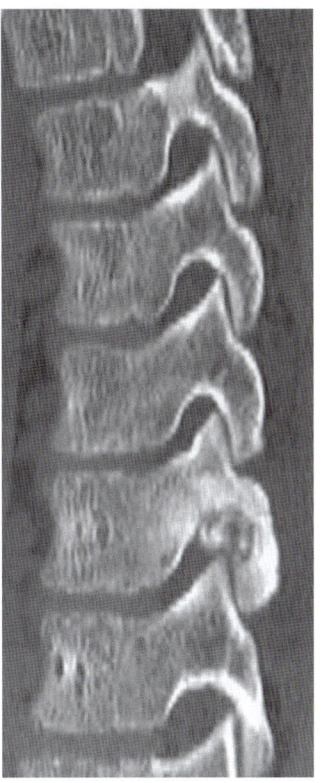

1. What should be included in the differential diagnosis?

2. What are common presenting symptoms?

3. What are components of the classification system?

4. Which portions of the spine are affected?

5. What are treatment options?

Case ranking/difficulty:

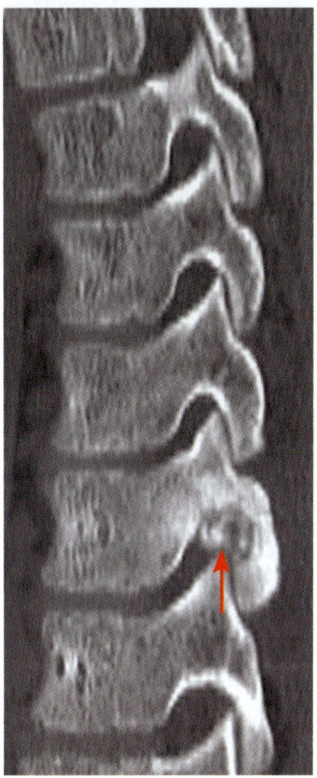

Sagittal reconstructed CT image at bone windows demonstrates well-circumscribed lesion in the inferior left pedicle of T10 with extension to the superior articulating facet, and with associated sclerotic changes.

Answers

1. Numerous entities may present as sclerotic foci within the posterior elements, including osteoblastoma, osteomyelitis, sclerotic metastasis, lymphoma, and osteoid osteoma.

2. The classic presentation is scoliosis and nighttime pain, relieved by nonsteroidal anti-inflammatory medications.

3. The most commonly used classification scheme (Kransdorf et al) separates osteoid osteomas into medullary, cortical, and subperiosteal in location.

4. Osteoid osteoma can affect any portion of the spine, but is most often seen in the mobile spine, split evenly between cervical, thoracic, and lumbar regions.

5. Conservative management, surgical resection, and/or percutaneous radiofrequency ablation are all treatment options. Depending on the instability associated with surgical resection, fixation may be needed. Percutaneous ethanol ablation is contraindicated given the close proximity to spinal cord and nerve roots. Also, given the natural tendency of osteoid osteomas to heal spontaneously, conservative management on long term NSAIDS has been successful.

Pearls

- Osteoid osteoma is a benign primary bone tumor that is most commonly seen in boys and young men.
- The lesion is characterized by a cortical location, a mineralized nidus, and surrounding reactive sclerosis.
- These lesions most commonly occur in long bones, with only approximately 10% within the spine. When they do occur in the spine, the posterior elements are most commonly involved.
- If lesions are greater than 1.5 cm, they are categorized as osteoblastomas. Some argue that osteoblastomas are different lesions as they are associated with a small risk of malignant degeneration.
- Patients often present with scoliosis related to pain and muscle spasm.
- Treatment traditionally consists of surgical resection; however, there is a growing body of literature looking at the use of percutaneous cryotherapy and radioablation.

Suggested Readings

Chai JW, Hong SH, Choi JY, et al. Radiologic diagnosis of osteoid osteoma: from simple to challenging findings. *Radiographics*. 2010;30:737-749.

Gasbarrini A, Cappuccio M, Bandiera S, Amendola L, van Urk P, Boriani S. Osteoid osteoma of the mobile spine. *Spine*. 2011;36:2089-2093.

Goto T1, Shinoda Y, Okuma T, et al. Administration of nonsteroidal anti-inflammatory drugs accelerates spontaneous healing of osteoid osteoma. *Arch Orthop Trauma Surg*. 2011;131(5):619-625.

Kransdorf MJ, Stull MA, Gilkey FW, Moser RP. Osteoid osteoma. *Radiographics*. 1991;11:671-696.

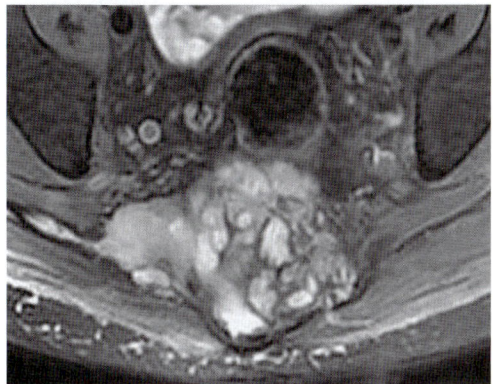 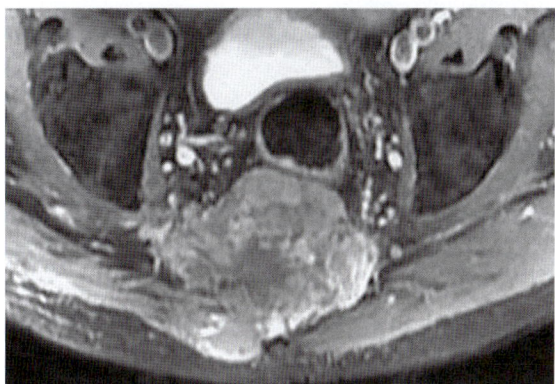

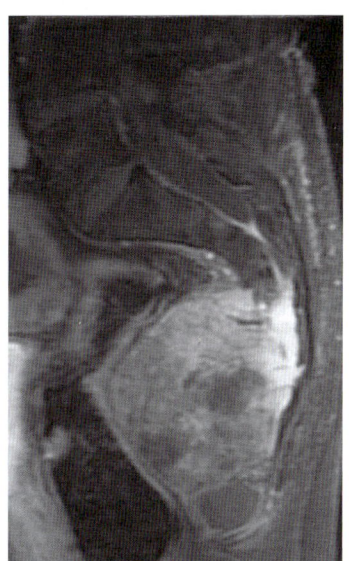

1. What should be included in the differential diagnosis?

2. What is the classic imaging appearance?

3. What are common presenting symptoms?

4. What is the etiology?

5. What are treatment options?

Case ranking/difficulty:

Category: Vertebral body

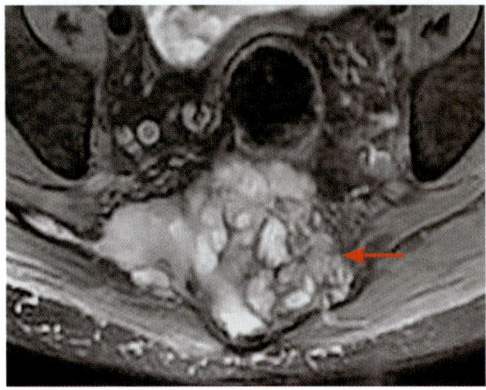

Axial T2 image demonstrates multilobulated T2 hyperintense mass.

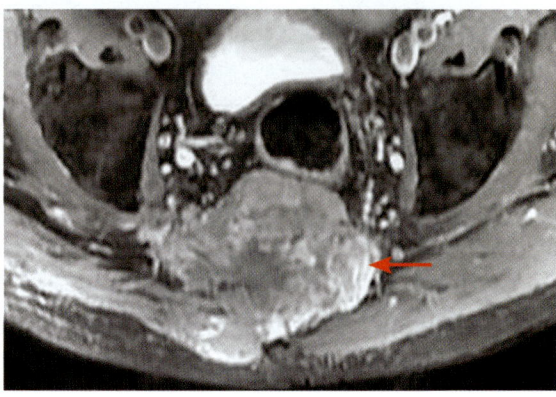

Axial T1 image following gadolinium administration demonstrates irregular enhancement of the expansile sacral mass.

4. Chordomas arise secondary to notochordal remnant degeneration.

5. Treatment includes surgical resection—gross total resection increases overall survival—with adjuvant radiotherapy. There is no role for chemotherapy or plasmapheresis. Biopsy can increase disease recurrence by seeding the tract.

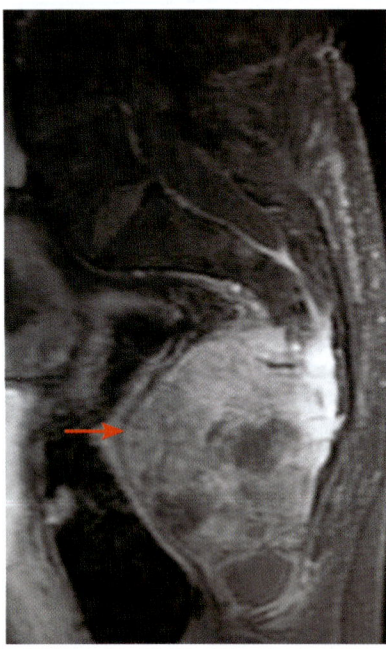

Sagittal T1 image following gadolinium administration demonstrates irregular enhancement of the expansile sacrococcygeal mass.

Answers

1. Many lesions can present as an expansile T2 hyperintense destructive osseous lesion, including metastasis, plasmacytoma, chordoma, lymphoma, chondrosarcoma and giant cell tumor.

2. Chordomas often present as a destructive osseous lesion with an associated soft tissue mass, which demonstrates T2 hyperintensity and irregular septal enhancement.

3. Sacral chordomas can grow to a large size before diagnosis and often present with slowly progressive symptoms over months to years, including back pain, constipation, radicular symptoms, and incontinence.

Pearls

- Chordoma is a rare tumor arising from notochordal remnants.
- The sacrum is the most common site (30-50%), followed by the skull base, and finally the remainder of the spine.
- They generally present as a T2 hyperintense, lobulated mass with extensive osseous destruction.
- Symptoms at presentation are based on location; however, sacral lesions often grow rather large before becoming symptomatic.
- Prognosis is based on size at diagnosis and pathologic findings, including necrosis.
- Treatment is surgical resection with adjuvant radiotherapy, and total resection increases survival.

Suggested Readings

deBruine FT, Kroon HM. Spinal chordoma: radiologic features in 14 cases. *AJR.* 1988;150:861-863.

Rich TA, Schiller A, Suit HD, Mankin HJ. Clinical and pathologic review of 48 cases of chordoma. *Cancer.* 1985;56:182-187.

Snowmobile accident

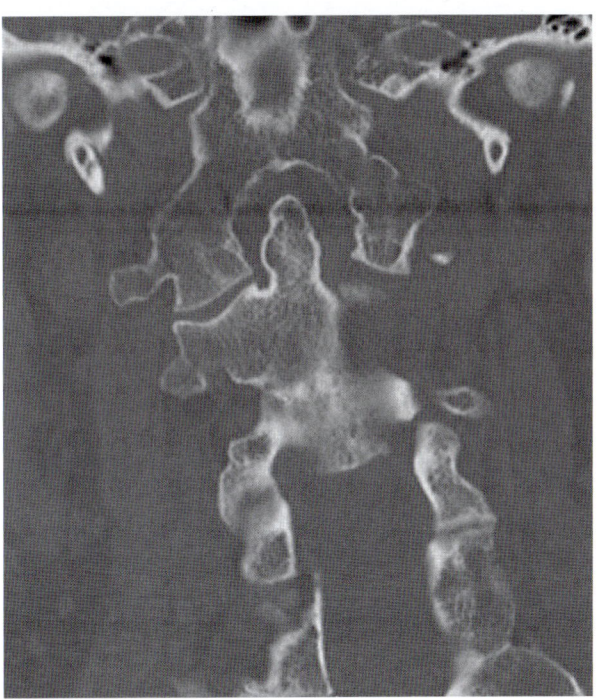

1. What should be included in the differential diagnosis?

2. What is the etiology?

3. What are the presenting symptoms?

4. What is the next step in evaluation?

5. What are treatment options?

Case ranking/difficulty:

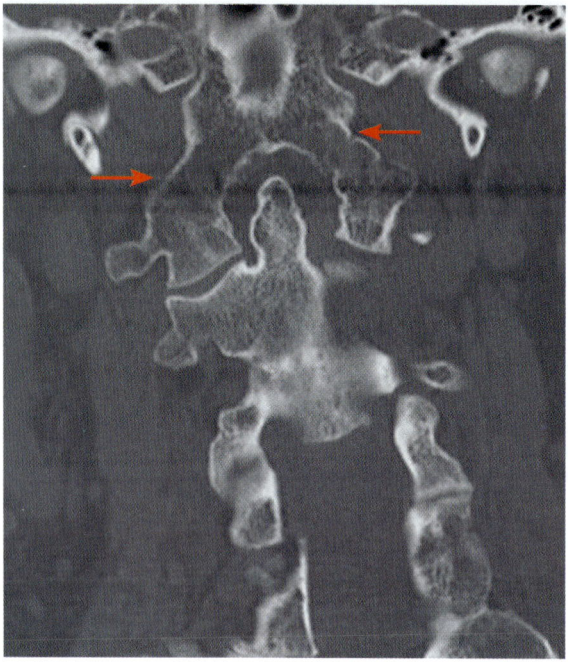

Coronal reconstructed image from a cervical spine CT demonstrates complete fusion of the occipital condyles and C1 arch.

Answers

1. Atlantooccipital assimilation is an abnormality of vertebral fusion along the Klippel Feil spectrum. Basilar invagination is a complication of atlantooccipital assimilation.

2. Atlantooccipital assimilation arises secondary to a segmentation failure between the fourth occipital sclerotome and the first spinal sclerotome.

3. Headaches, particularly occipital or those exacerbated by cervical spine movement, myelopathic symptoms, and cranial nerve or brainstem deficits, can be seen in atlantooccipital assimilation. However, this is usually an asymptomatic abnormality.

4. Flexion/extension radiographs allow for identification of unstable craniocervical junction anomalies, which should be referred for surgical fixation.

5. While observation and activity restriction are appropriate for asymptomatic lesions, symptomatic lesions require more aggressive management, including traction, surgical decompression, and/or surgical fusion.

Pearls

- Anomalies of the craniocervical junction are not uncommon in clinical practice. It is important to be able to differentiate those that require surgical fixation from those that do not.
- Atlantooccipital fusion is one of the more common malformations, and while it is often asymptomatic, there are reports of associated myelopathic symptoms as basilar invagination develops.
- There is a risk of instability, and evaluation with flexion/extension radiographs may be indicated.
- If one fusion anomaly is noted during evaluation of the spine, have a higher index of suspicion to look for an additional abnormality.

Suggested Readings

Rande AV, Rai R, Prabhu LV, Kumaran M, Pai MM. Atlas assimilation: a case report. *Neuroanatomy*. 2007;6:32-33.

Smoker WRK. Craniovertebral junction: normal anatomy, craniometry, and congenital anomalies. *Radiographics*. 1994;14:255-277.

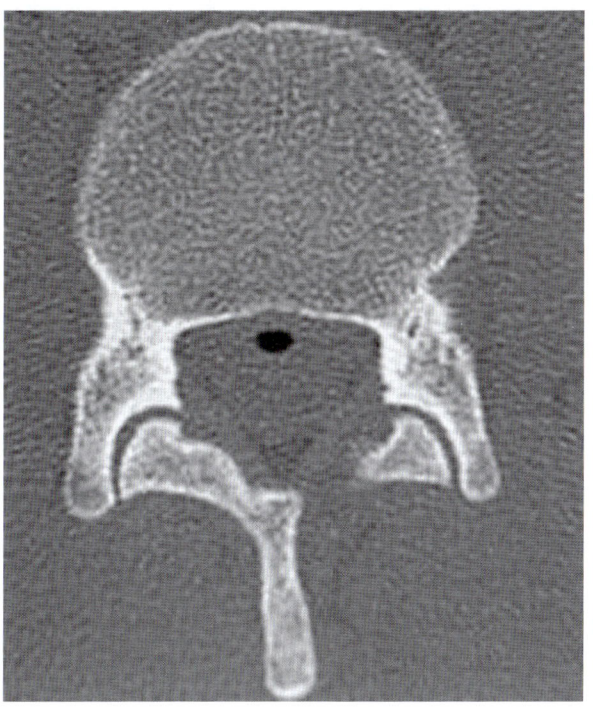
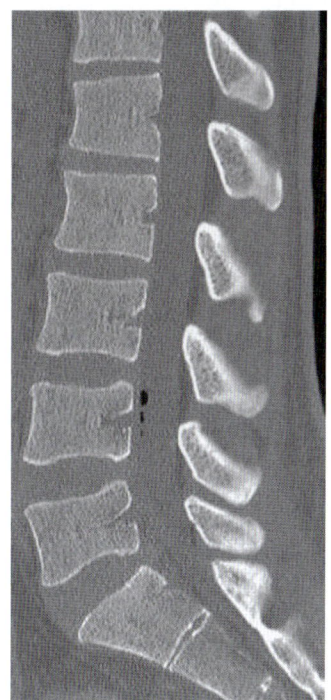

1. What patient information should be considered prior to planning a lumbar puncture?

2. What are the preferred levels for performing lumbar puncture?

3. What complications may lead to the development of lower extremity paresthesias during a lumbar puncture?

4. What are the indications for fluoroscopic guidance for lumbar puncture?

5. What are the treatment options?

Case ranking/difficulty: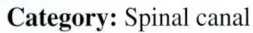

Category: Spinal canal

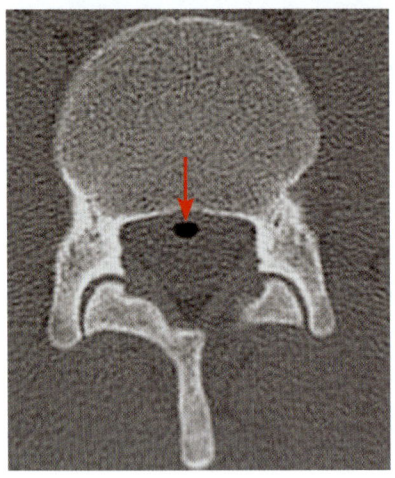

Axial CT image demonstrates focal gas in the anterior epidural space.

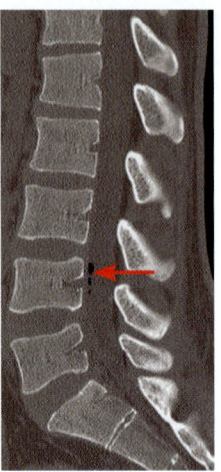

Sagittal CT image demonstrates focal gas in the anterior epidural space.

Answers

1. Laboratory evaluation for coagulopathy, evaluation for increased intracranial pressure, review of patient history for recent lumbar surgery, prior lumbar imaging studies, and the patient ability to give consent should be considered in planning a lumbar puncture.

2. L2-L3 and L3-L4 are the preferred levels; they are generally below the level of the cord but the spinal canal remains largest at these levels.

3. Inadvertent administration of anesthetic may result in lower extremity paresthesia; however, consideration of epidural hematoma is important, particularly in a patient with borderline coagulation values.

4. Fluoroscopic guidance may be of benefit in the obese patient or postoperative patient, where landmarks may not be readily apparent. Additionally, if attempts without guidance are unsuccessful, fluoroscopy may increase the success rate.

5. Even if there is a small component of epidural hematoma, conservative management with spontaneous resolution of symptoms is the rule. In the particularly coagulopathic patient, alerting neurosurgery may be indicated in case of rapidly enlarging hematoma.

Pearls

- It is imperative to maintain excellent technique when performing lumbar punctures to avoid complication.
- Anesthetizing the soft tissues should be performed only after placing negative pressure on the syringe to avoid intra-arterial injection.
- Epidural injection is more difficult to exclude as by definition there should not be return with negative pressure.
- In the case of probable epidural injection of anesthetic, imaging may need to be performed, particularly in the coagulopathic patient to exclude epidural hematoma.

Suggested Readings

ACR-ASNR Practice guideline for the performance of myelography and cisternography. Revised (2008).

Ruff RL, Dougherty JH. Complications of lumbar puncture followed by anticoagulation. *Stroke*. 1981;12:879-881.

Yu SD, Chen MY, Johnson AJ. Factors associated with traumatic fluoroscopy-guided lumbar punctures: a retrospective review. *AJNR*. 2009;30:512-515.

Radicular pain

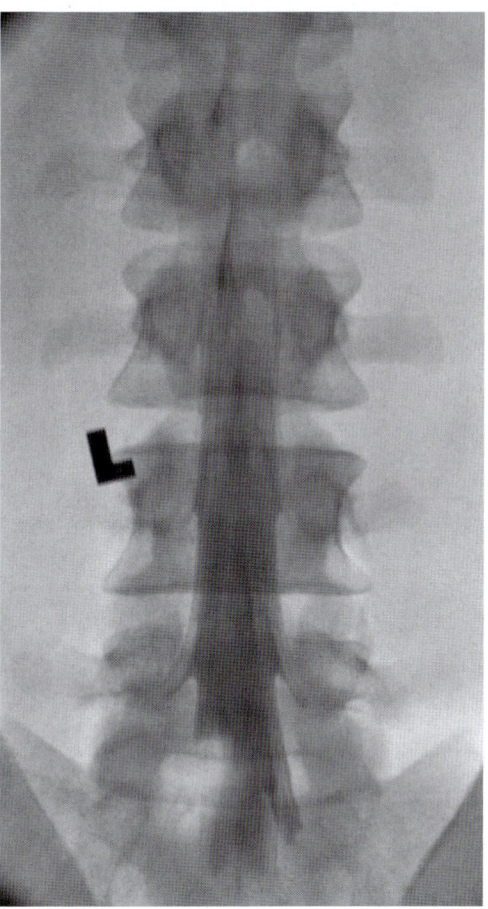

1. What should be included in the differential diagnosis?

2. What are common presenting symptoms?

3. What are the components of the intervertebral disc?

4. What is the natural history?

5. What are the treatment options?

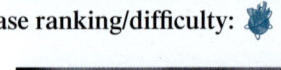

Case ranking/difficulty:

Category: Nerve roots/Nerve plexus/Peripheral nerves

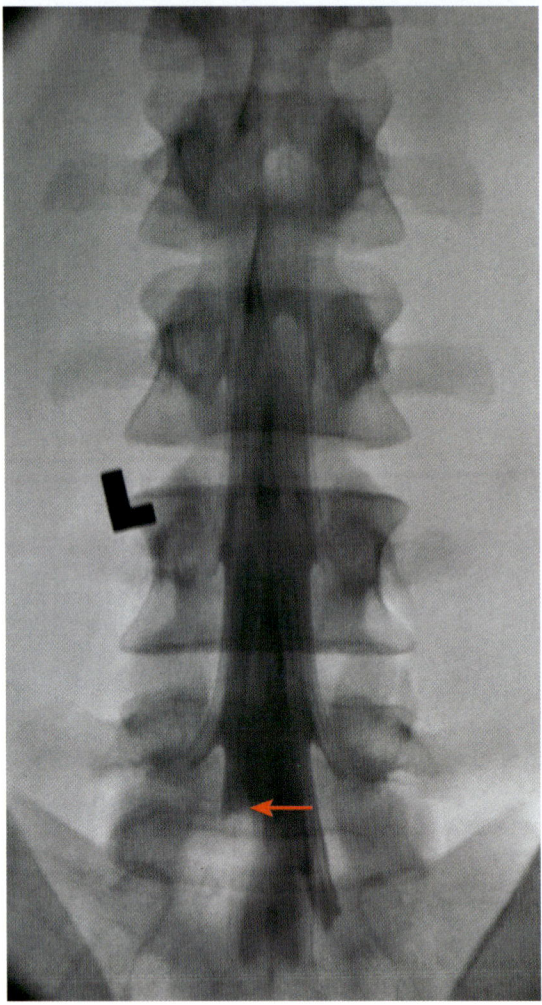

AP radiograph following intrathecal administration of contrast demonstrates a left-sided filling defect.

Answers

1. Extradural space-occupying lesions include epidural abscess, epidural hematoma, disc herniation, epidural fibrosis, and nerve sheath tumor.

2. Radiculopathy and back pain are the most common presenting symptoms. Patients will manifest normal to decreased reflexes and may have lower extremity weakness.

3. The central nucleus pulposus is surrounded by the transitional zone and the peripheral annulus fibrosis.

4. Most patients will have spontaneous resorption with conservative management; however, there is potential for worsening disease and development of diskogenic endplate changes or sequestered fragments.

5. Most patients will have resolution of symptoms with conservative management/physical therapy. Chemonucleolysis and diskectomy can be performed in refractory cases.

Pearls

- Disc herniations are one of the most common etiologies of lumbar radiculopathy seen in an average radiology practice.
- During the evaluation of disc herniations, it is important to evaluate compression of the thecal sac, the lateral recesses, and the neural foramina.
- A protrusion is a herniation of less than 50% of the circumference of the disc—this can be divided into focal (<25%) or broad based (25%-50%).
- A herniation of >50% is termed a bulge.
- Protrusions can be defined as extrusions if the base of the herniation is narrower than the remainder of the herniated disc.
- If there is a piece of herniated disc that is not continuous with the underlying disc, this can be termed a sequestered disc fragment. This is important to report as the surgeons may need to explore to find a sequestered fragment.
- There are eight cervical nerve roots but only seven cervical vertebrae; thus, at the C7-T1 level, the C8 nerve roots are exiting.
- At the level of this disc protrusion (L5-S1), the disc could impact the exiting L5 nerve root in the foramen or the traversing S1 nerve root in the lateral recess.

Suggested Readings

Weber H. Lumbar disk herniation: a controlled, prospective study with 10 years of observation. *Spine.* 1983;8:131-140.

Weinstein JN, Tosteson TS, Lurie JD, et al. Surgical vs nonoperative treatment for lumbar disk herniation. *JAMA.* 2006;296:2441-2450.

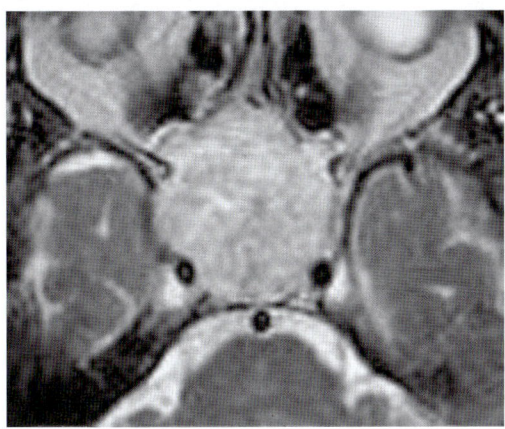 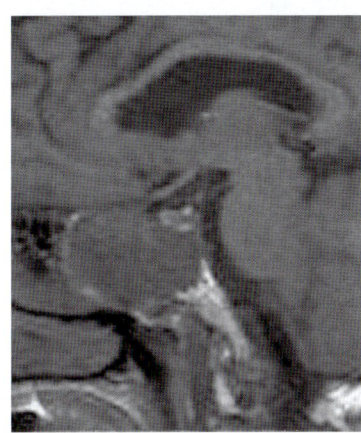

1. What is the most likely etiology of this lesion?

2. What is the common imaging appearance?

3. Where do these lesions commonly occur?

4. What are common presenting symptoms?

5. What are the treatment options?

Case ranking/difficulty: 🌑

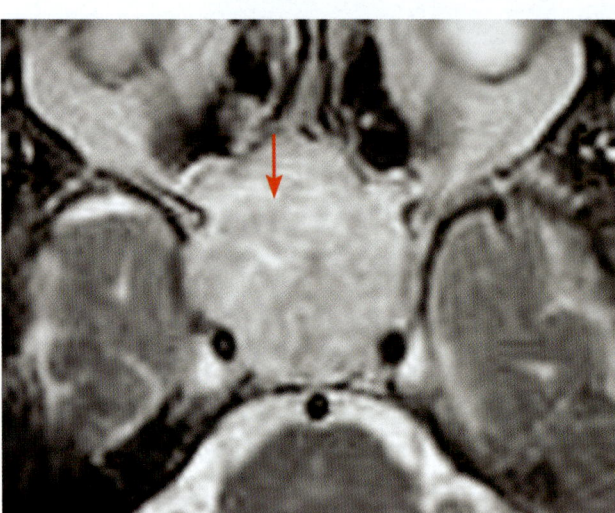

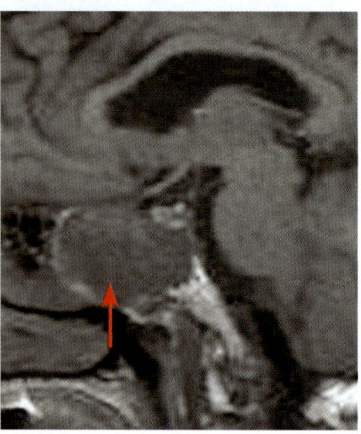

Sagittal T2 image demonstrates expansile T1 hypointense clival lesion.

Axial T2 image demonstrates expansile T2 hyperintense mass involving the clivus and sphenoid sinuses with extension into the posterior orbits.

Answers

1. Expansile T2 hyperintense destructive osseous lesions include chondrosarcoma, metastasis, chordoma, plasmacytoma, and lymphoma. Destructive lesions of the clivus also include nasopharyngeal carcinoma, pituitary adenoma, pituitary carcinoma, and intraosseous meningioma.

2. While chordomas are typically T2 hyperintense and T1 hypointense with avid enhancement, there can be foci of T1 hyperintensity, representing foci of hemorrhage or mineralization.

3. While these lesions can occur at any location within the spine, the sacrum and coccyx are most common, followed by the clivus.

4. Clival chordomas generally present with headaches and occasionally associated cranial neuropathies, including diplopia and facial pain. There is potential to develop vertebrobasilar insufficiency with posterior extension of tumor.

5. Treatment includes surgical resection—gross total resection increases overall survival—with adjuvant chemotherapy. There is no role for chemotherapy. Biopsy can increase disease recurrence by seeding the tract.

Pearls

- Chordoma is a rare tumor arising from notochordal remnants.
- The skull base is the second most common location, after the sacrum.
- Chordomas are classically T2 hyperintense lobulated masses with extensive osseous destruction.
- Presentation of clival chordomas often include headache and cranial nerve dysfunction, particularly palsy of the sixth cranial nerve leading to diplopia.
- Skull base tumors are notoriously difficult to resect, and adjuvant radiotherapy plays an important role in management.
- These tumors tend to spread primarily through direct spread, with distant hematogenous spread less likely.

Suggested Readings

Erdem E, Angtuaco EC, Van Hemert R, Park JS, Al-Mefty O. Comprehensive review of intracranial chordoma. *Radiographics*. 2003;23:995-1009.

Rich TA, Schiller A, Suit HD, Mankin HJ. Clinical and pathologic review of 48 cases of chordoma. *Cancer*. 1985;56:182-187.

Sickle cell anemia, back pain

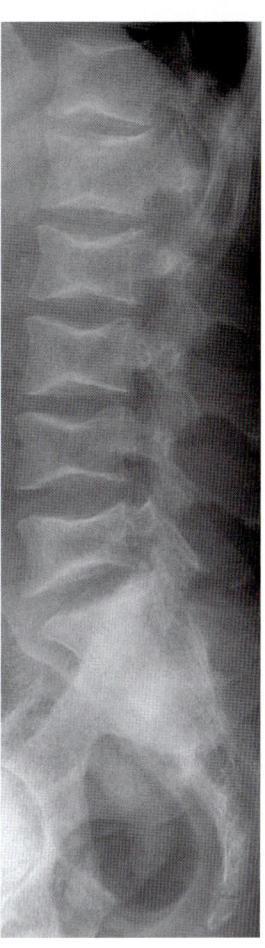

1. What should be included in the differential diagnosis?

2. What should be included in the differential diagnosis of vertebral body abnormalities in sickle cell anemia?

3. What is the pathophysiology leading to this abnormality?

4. What are additional osseous manifestations of this disease?

5. What are the treatment options?

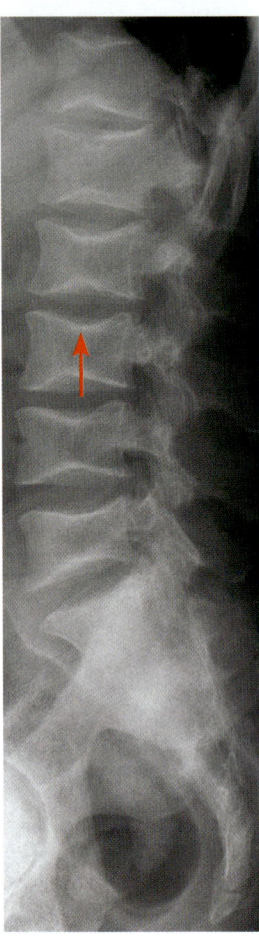

Lateral radiograph demonstrates biconcave deformity of the vertebral bodies.

Answers

1. Etiologies of hypointense marrow and vertebral body malformations include osteopetrosis, leukemia, pyknodysostosis, osteopathia striata, and sickle cell anemia.

2. Sickle cell anemia can produce osseous infarction, pathologic fracture, fish mouth deformity, and secondary osteomyelitis.

3. Reactivation of red marrow leads to marrow expansion, which thins the cortex and leaves it vulnerable to compression from the adjacent disc.

4. Additional osseous manifestations of sickle cell disease include bone-in-bone vertebra, avascular necrosis, and hair-on-end calvarium.

5. For asymptomatic concave vertebral bodies, no treatment is required. If a patient presents in sickle cell crisis, the key components of treatment are hydration, supplemental oxygenation, and pain control.

Pearls

- The fish mouth (Lincoln log or H shaped) vertebra is formed secondary to weakening of the endplates from marrow activation and associated medullary expansion.
- As the medullary cavity expands, the endplates become weakened and collapse.
- It is important to differentiate this from pathologic fracture, which is a recognized complication.
- Associated findings may include T1 and T2 marrow hypointensity, secondary to reactivation, and superimposed bone infarcts.

Suggested Readings

Ejindu VC, Hine AL, Mashayekhi M, Shorvon PJ, Misra RR. Musculoskeletal manifestations of sickle cell disease. *Radiographics*. 2007;27:1005-1021.

Ganguly A, Boswell W, Aniq H. Musculoskeletal manifestations of sickle cell anaemia: a pictorial review. *Anemia*. 2011:9.

New onset seizures

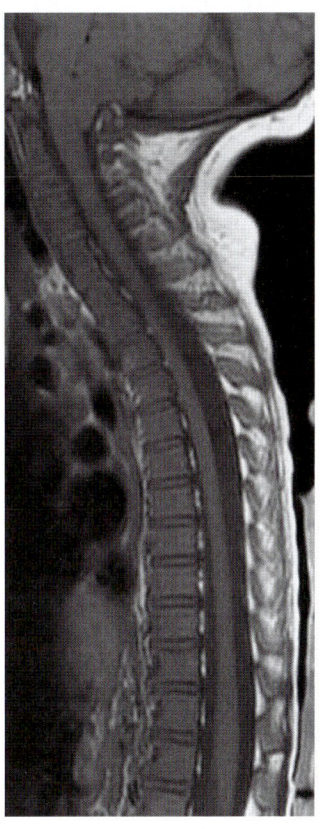

1. Which are associated abnormalities?

2. What are the presenting symptoms?

3. What should be included in the imaging evaluation?

4. What are associated syndromes?

5. What are the treatment options?

Case ranking/difficulty:

Category: Spinal cord

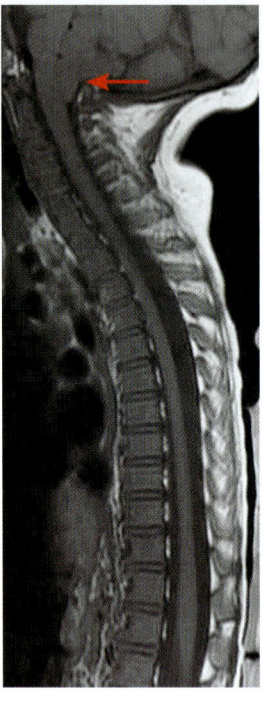

Sagittal T1 image demonstrates cerebellar tonsils extending through foramen magnum; no syringomyelia.

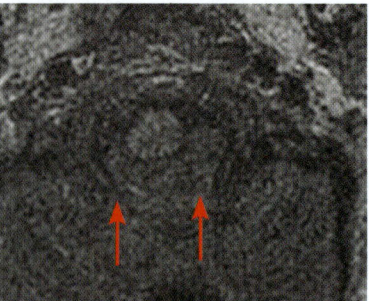

Axial T1 image demonstrates cerebellar tonsils crowding the posterior foramen magnum.

Answers

1. Chiari I malformation is associated with abnormalities of the skull base, skeleton, and fourth occipital sclerotome, including scoliosis, retroflexed dens, kyphosis, platybasia, and short clivus.

2. Headache, gait disturbance, and myelopathy are the most common presenting symptoms. Additionally, Chiari patients can develop cranial nerve palsy and ocular disturbances.

3. MRI of the brain can be useful in the evaluation of hydrocephalus while spine imaging can be used to evaluate for the presence of syrinx. Cerebrospinal fluid flow studies at the foramen magnum can be helpful in the quantification of flow both preoperatively and postoperatively.

4. There are multiple syndromes associated with Chiari I malformation, including Williams syndrome, achondroplasia, and Klippel Feil syndrome.

5. Asymptomatic patients can often be followed with imaging studies, while symptomatic patients often require suboccipital craniectomy. Resection of the posterior elements of C1 can be required depending on the caudal extension of the cerebellar tonsils. Tonsillar resection can be performed if needed.

Pearls

- Chiari I malformation is a heterogeneous group of disorders.
- Chiari I is characterized by caudal extension of the cerebellar tonsils more than 5 mm below the foramen magnum. Some argue that up to 6 mm can be normal, particularly in children.
- The tonsils develop a peg configuration, instead of the normal rounded configuration.
- The causative etiologies are variable, including both autosomal dominant and autosomal recessive genetics, syndrome-associated malformations, and Chiari malformations associated with malformation of the skull base.
- If the tonsils extend greater than 12 mm below the foramen magnum, the patients are more likely to be symptomatic.

Suggested Readings

Elster AD, Chen MY. Chiari I malformations: clinical and radiologic reapparaisal. *Radiology*. 1992;183:347-353.

Milhorat T, Chou MW, Trinidad EM, et al. Chiari I malformation redefined: clinical and radiographic findings for 364 symptomatic patients. *Neurosurgery*. 1999;44:1005-1017.

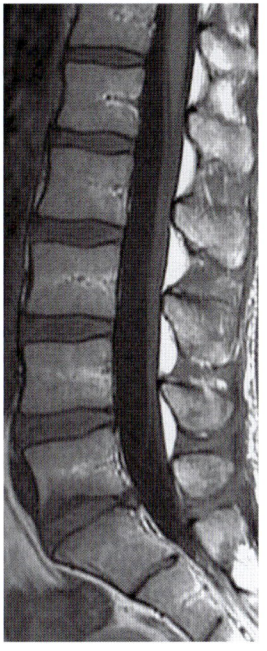 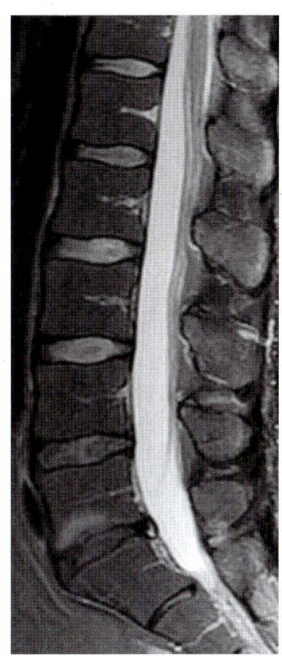

1. What should be included in the differential
   diagnosis?

2. Why is it important to identify degenerative
   endplate changes?

3. What is the staging system?

4. What is the most common phase?

5. What are the treatment options?

Case ranking/difficulty:

Category: Vertebral body

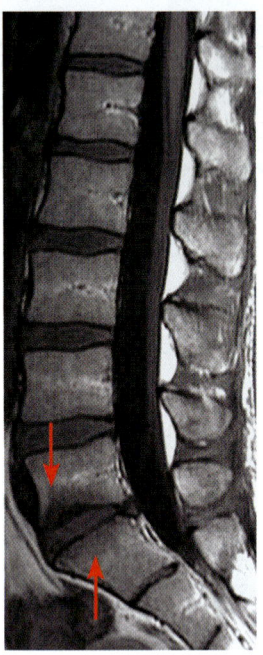

Sagittal T1 image demonstrates hypointensity along the inferior endplate of L5 and superior endplate of S1 with adjacent disc degeneration.

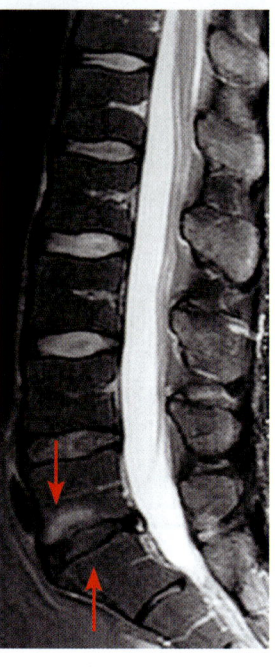

Sagittal T2 image demonstrates hyperintensity along the inferior endplate of L5 and hypointensity along the superior endplate of S1 with adjacent disc degeneration.

Answers

1. Differential considerations include diskogenic endplate changes and diskitis/osteomyelitis.

2. It is important to find differentiate diskogenic endplate changes from metastasis or infection. While these changes could serve as a potential source of back pain, there are no findings that are sufficient to predict positive diskography results.

3. Type 1 changes are T1 hypointense and T2 hyperintense secondary to edema. Type 2 changes are T1 and T2 hyperintense secondary to fatty infiltration. Type 3 changes are T1 and T2 hypointense secondary to sclerosis.

4. In patients undergoing MRI for degenerative disc disease, approximately 15% will have Type 2 changes (5% Type 1 and 1% Type 3).

5. Conservative management is usually indicated; spinal fusion may be considered for refractory pain.

Pearls

- Degenerative endplate changes most commonly occur in the lumbar spine adjacent to degenerative changes within the intervertebral disc.
- There are three recognized phases:
  - Phase I (edema/vascular marrow)—T1 hypointense, T2 hyperintense
  - Phase II (fatty infiltration)—T1 hyperintense, T2 iso-to hyperintense
  - Phase III (fibrosis)—T1 hypointense, T2 hypointense
- Phase I changes may also demonstrate contrast enhancement.
- It is important to recognize the characteristic imaging appearance of these degenerative changes in order to exclude either osseous lesion or infection.

Suggested Readings

Albert HB, Manniche C. Modic changes following lumbar disc herniation. *Eur Spine J*. 2007;16:977-982.

Thompson KR, Dagher AP, Eckel TS, Clark M, Reinig JW. Modic changes on MR images as studied with provocative diskography. *Radiology*. 2009;250:849-855.

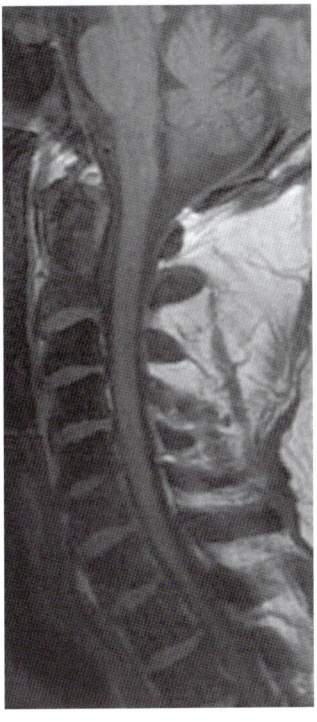 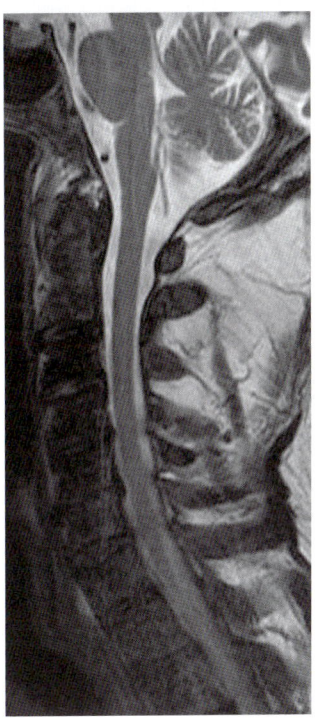

1. What should be included in the differential diagnosis?

2. What are common presenting symptoms?

3. What additional imaging studies should be considered?

4. Which primary malignancies tend to have sclerotic metastatic lesions?

5. What are the treatment options?

Case ranking/difficulty:

Category: Vertebral body

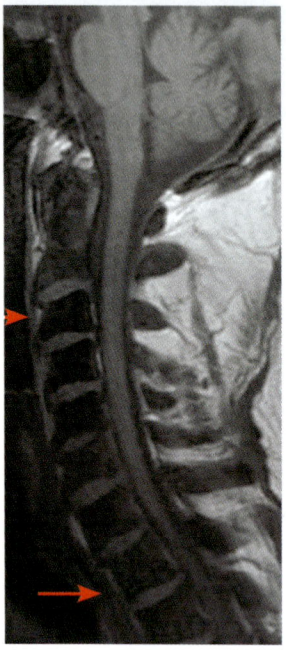

Sagittal T1 image demonstrates diffuse marrow hypointensity.

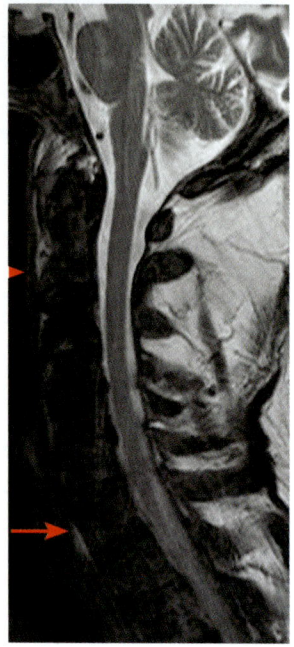

Sagittal T2 image demonstrates diffuse marrow hypointensity.

Answers

1. Etiologies of hypointense marrow include myelofibrosis, reactivation of red marrow, leukemia, osteopetrosis, and metastatic marrow infiltration.

2. Potential presenting symptoms of axial skeletal metastasis include pain, pathologic fracture, cord compression, and radicular symptoms.

3. CT or FDG-PET scan may be indicated for assessing extraosseous disease. Bone scan can be helpful for identifying appendicular sites of involvement.

4. Renal cell and thyroid cancers often present with lytic lesions.

5. Analgesia and treatment of the primary malignancy, including chemotherapy and radiation, are the mainstays of treatment of diffuse metastatic disease. Vertebroplasty may be indicated in the setting of superimposed compression fracture.

Pearls

- Diffuse marrow infiltration is a less common pattern of osseous metastatic disease than focal osseous metastatic lesions.

- However, it is an important entity to recognize as it can be associated with malignancy-associated anemia secondary to marrow replacement.
- Look for an intervertebral disc that is brighter than the vertebral body marrow on T1 images.
- Treatment is aimed at the primary malignancy.
- Advanced imaging techniques, including diffusion-weighted imaging, have been explored to evaluate the presence of marrow infiltration.

Suggested Readings

Padhani AR, van Ree K, Collins DJ, D'Sa S, Makris A. Assessing the relation between bone marrow signal intensity and apparent diffusion coefficient in diffusion-weighted MRI. *AJR*. 2013; 200:163-170.

Schmidt GP, Reiser MF, Baur-Melnyk A. Whole-body MRI for the staging and follow-up of patients with metastasis. *Eur J Radiol*. 2009;70:393-400.

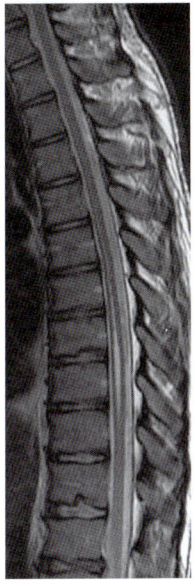 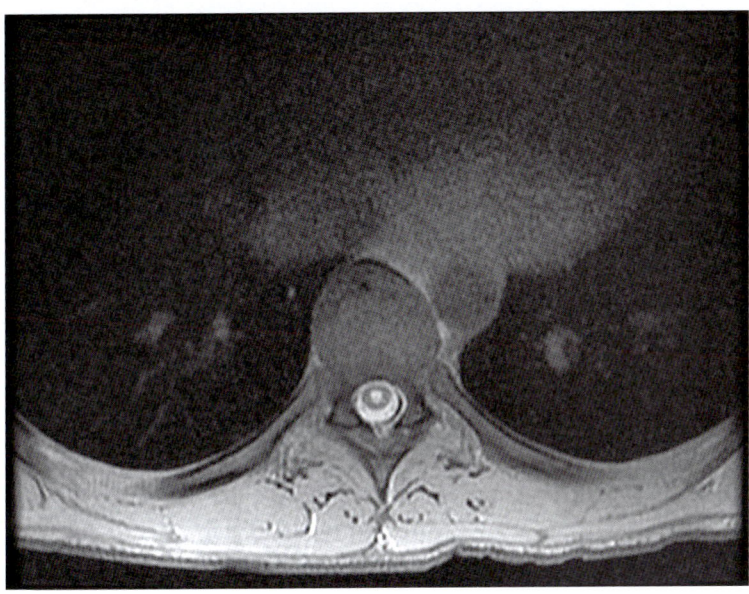

1. What should be included in the differential diagnosis?

2. What are common presenting symptoms?

3. What is the classic clinical presentation?

4. What is the prognosis if untreated?

5. What are the treatment options?

Case ranking/difficulty: 🌼

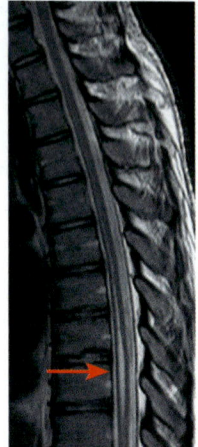

Sagittal T2 image demonstrates anterior T2 hyperintensity within the cord.

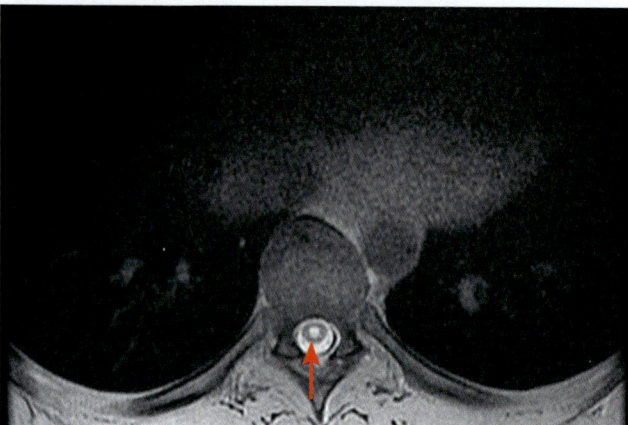

Axial T2 image demonstrates anterior T2 hyperintensity within the cord.

Answers

1. Intramedullary T2 hyperintense lesions include cystic intramedullary tumor, hydromyelia, myelomalacia, and syringomyelia.

2. Distal weakness and gait ataxia are the most common presenting symptoms; other symptoms include back pain, radiculopathy, and sphincter dysfunction.

3. The classic presentation is "cloak" distribution of pain and loss of temperature sensation.

4. Primary syringomyelia generally has a slowly progressive course without resolution. Treatment may halt progression, but improves symptoms in less than half of patients.

5. For patients with Chiari I malformation, suboccipital craniectomy is the treatment of choice to improve cerebrospinal fluid flow dynamics. Syringosubarachnoid shunt placement may be considered for patients with idiopathic syringomyelia.

Pearls

- Syringomyelia refers to cystic dilation within the spinal cord, which is not contiguous with the central canal.
- Dilation of the central canal is referred to as hydromyelia. It can be difficult to differentiate hydromyelia from syringomyelia on imaging; pathologically, the former is lined by ependymal cells.
- If there is extension of syringomyelia to the brain stem, it can be termed syringobulbia.
- Syringomyelia can be seen as a complication of trauma; however, it can be a primary diagnosis that generally affects adolescents/young adults. In those cases, it is important to rule out obstruction to cerebrospinal fluid flow, such as Chiari I malformation, or congenital abnormality, such as Chiari II or tethered cord.
- Presenting symptoms are generally myelopathic with ataxia and distal weakness.
- The classic presentation consists of "cloak" distribution loss of pain and temperature sensation.
- Treatment is aimed at resolution of the underlying disruption to flow; however, in patients with idiopathic syringomyelia, placement of a syringosubarachnoid shunt may be necessary.

Suggested Readings

Klekamp J. Treatment of syringomyelia related to nontraumatic arachnoid pathologies of the spinal canal. *Neurosurgery*. 2013;72:376-389.

Williams B. On the pathogenesis of syringomyelia: a review. *J Royal Soc Med*. 1980;73:798-806.

Chiari I malformation

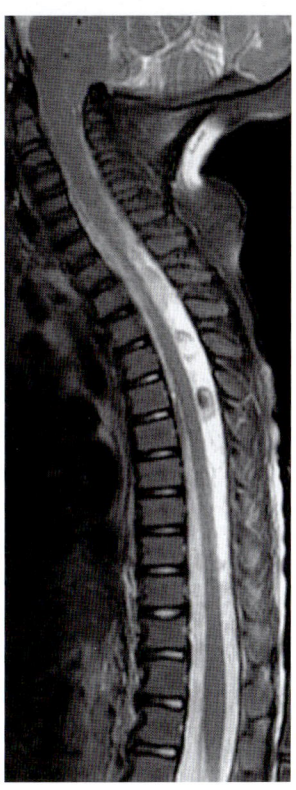

1. What should be included in the differential diagnosis?

2. Why are T2 gradient echo sequences less susceptible to cerebrospinal fluid pulsation artifact?

3. What are common artifacts encountered in spine imaging?

4. How can cardiac gating be used to reduce cerebrospinal fluid pulsation artifact?

5. What are potential solutions when faced with cerebrospinal fluid pulsation artifact?

Case ranking/difficulty:

Category: Thecal sac

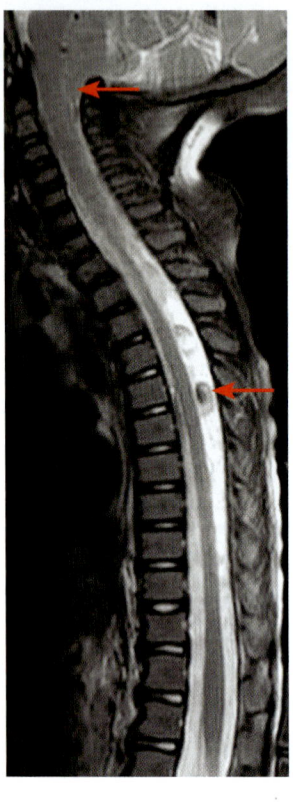

Sagittal T2 image demonstrates T2 hypointense signal dorsal to the cord. Note Chiari I malformation without syrinx.

Answers

1. T2 hypointense signal could represent a flow void, calcified mass, or various stages of hemorrhage. Pulsatility artifact can be confirmed by the lack of findings on additional sequences.

2. Shorter echo time, gradient refocusing pulse applied on the read out gradient, and shorter repetition time make the sequence less susceptible to pulsation artifact while maintaining T2 weighting.

3. Common artifacts encountered in spine imaging include Gibb truncation artifact, cerebrospinal fluid pulsation artifact, respiratory motion artifact, cardiac motion artifact, and bowel peristalsis motion artifact. Artifacts are important to recognize and be able to correct. For example, motion artifact from adjacent organs can often be eliminated by applying strategic saturation bands and swapping phase and frequency encoding directions.

4. Cardiac gating reduces temporal phase-shift effects, both cardiac dependent and unmasked, as well as decreasing time-of-flight effects.

5. Cerebrospinal fluid pulsation artifact can usually be diagnosed based on reviewing all sequences; however, additional T2 gradient echo sequences or peripheral cardiac gating may be necessary in the challenging patient.

Pearls

- Cerebrospinal fluid pulsation artifact is common in children who tend to have hyperdynamic cerebrospinal fluid flow.
- It commonly occurs on T2 fast spin echo (FSE) images, but resolves on other sequences.
- Using T2 gradient echo sequences can help minimize the artifact.
- T2 gradient echo sequences are often preferred in imaging of the cervicothoracic spine where this artifact is most likely to occur.

Suggested Readings

Kwon JW, Yoon YC, Choi S-H. Three-dimensional isotropic T2-weighted cervical MRI at 3T: comparison with two-dimensional T2-weighted sequences. *Clin Radiol.* 2012;67:106-113.

Low RN, Austin MJ, Ma J. Fast spin-echo triple echo dixon: initial clinical experience with a novel pulse sequence for simultaneous fat-suppressed and nonfat-suppressed T2-weighted spine magnetic resonance imaging. *JMRI.* 2011;33:390-400.

Rubin JB, Enzmann DR, Wright A. CSF-gated MR imaging of the spine: theory and clinical implementation. *Radiology.* 1987;163:784-792.

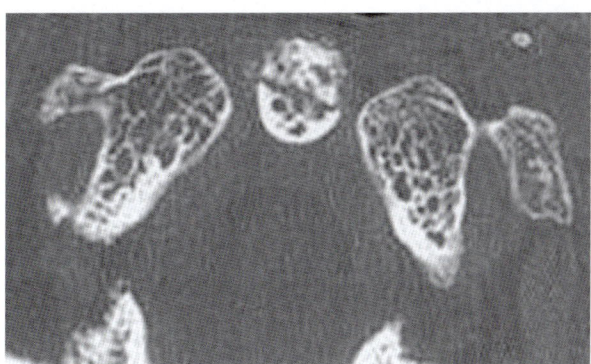

1. What should be included in the differential diagnosis?

2. What structures are involved?

3. What are associated abnormalities?

4. What are the mechanisms of injury?

5. What are the treatment options?

Case ranking/difficulty: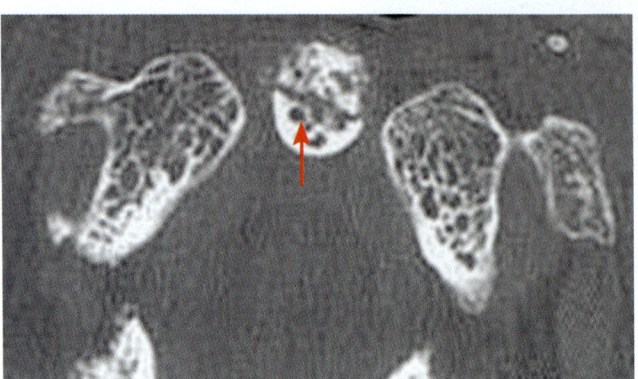

Axial CT image demonstrates lucency through the anterior odontoid tip.

Answers

1. Etiologies of an odontoid lucency include fracture and os odontoideum. Os odontoideum results from a congenital non-union of the cephalad odontoid apophysis. These lesions can be differentiated by their sclerotic border and are usually fixed to the anterior arch of C1.

2. Type 1 fracture traverses the odontoid tip.

3. Type 1 fractures can be seen in conjunction with occipital condyle fractures and atlantooccipital dislocation.

4. This fracture originates from axial loading and hyperextension.

5. This fracture is often managed by cervical immobilization, either through cervical collar or halo fixation.

Pearls

- Type 1 odontoid fractures are the most rare type of dens fracture, consisting of a fracture isolated to the cephalad portion of the dens without involvement of the base or body.
- This type of dens fracture is thought to result from an avulsion injury of the alar ligament.
- These fractures may be treated conservatively using a cervical collar.
- Dynamic flexion and extension views of the spine should be obtained to exclude associated ligamentous or osseous instability.

Suggested Readings

Greene KA, Dickman CA, Marciano FF, Drabier JB, Hadley MN, Sonntag VKH. Acute axis fractures: analysis of management and outcome in 340 consecutive cases. *Spine*. 1997;22:1843-1852.

Rao SK, Wasyliw C, Nunez DB. Spectrum of imaging findings in hyperextension injuries of the neck. *Radiographics*. 2005;25:1239-1254.

Lumbar cutaneous hemangioma

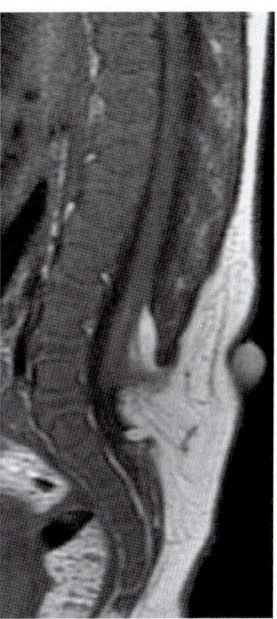

1. What should be included in the differential diagnosis?

2. What are the open spinal dysraphisms?

3. What are common presenting symptoms?

4. What need to be evaluated for the classification of congenital spinal dysraphism?

5. What are the treatment options?

Case ranking/difficulty:

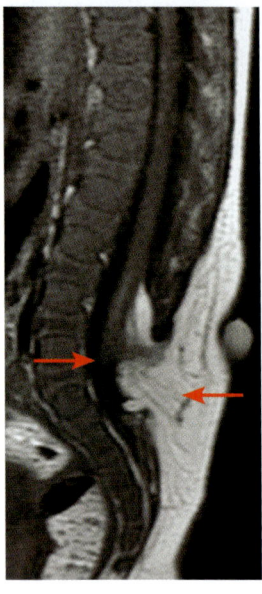

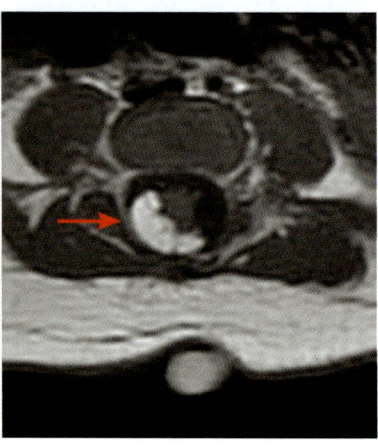

Axial T1 image demonstrates fat containing mass in the dorsal spinal canal, in direct contact with the distal spinal cord. Marker was placed over cutaneous hemangioma (external to patient).

Sagittal image demonstrates dorsal dysraphic defect extending caudally from L3 to L4 with herniation of neural elements, extending caudally to the L5 level, where it terminates in a fatty mass.

Answers

1. Closed spinal dysraphisms include lipomyelocele, lipomyelomeningocele, filum lipoma, diastematomyelia, and spina bifida occulta.

2. Open spinal dysraphisms include meningocele, myelomeningocele, myeloschisis, hemimyelocele, and myelocele.

3. Common presenting symptoms include cutaneous hemangioma, bowel incontinence/constipation, and lower extremity spasticity.

4. Factors that need to be evaluated include location of the neural placode, presence of associated dysraphism, presence of a cutaneous lesion, and documentation of the conus position. A number of vertebral bodies are variable and not included in the evaluation of congenital spinal dysraphisms.

5. Lipoma resection and cord untethering are performed with potential duraplasty to reduce the incidence of cord retethering. Resection of the conus is contraindicated; the goal is preservation of as much neural tissue as possible. Unless there is superimposed instability, there is no indication for surgical fusion.

Pearls

- Lipomyelocele is a subtype of closed spinal dysraphism, suspected by the presence of an overlying cutaneous lesion (hemangioma, hairy patch, skin dimple/pit).
- It is important to document the location of the placode–lipoma interface.
- When the placode–lipoma interface is within the spinal canal, the anomaly is a lipomyelocele; if it lies outside of the spinal canal, the anomaly is a lipomyelomeningocele.
- Patients can present with lower extremity weakness, spasticity, neurogenic bladder, or bowel incontinence/constipation.
- Many patients are diagnosed in the neonatal period during evaluation of the cutaneous lesion.
- Treatment consists of resection of the lipomatous portion of the mass with release of the filum and conus as needed.

Suggested Readings

Rufener SL, Ibrahim M, Raybaud CA, Parmar HA. Congenital spine and spinal cord malformations—pictorial review. *AJR*. 2010;194:S26-S37.

Sarris CE, Tomei KL, Carmel PW, Gandhi CD. Lipomyelomeningocele: pathology, treatment and outcomes. *Neurosurg Focus*. 2012;33:E3.

Low back pain

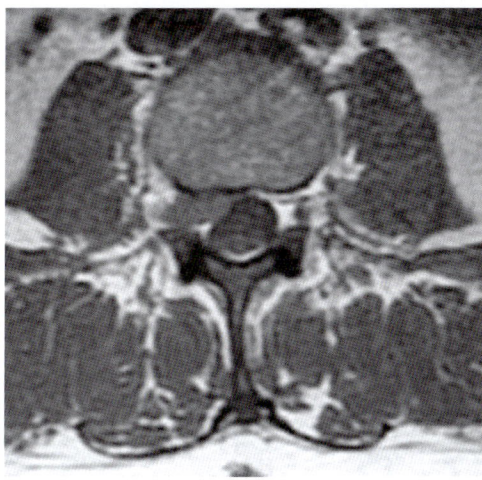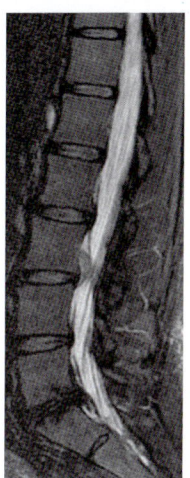

1. What should be included in the differential diagnosis?

2. What are common presenting symptoms?

3. What associated abnormalities are seen?

4. What are the most common levels for this abnormality?

5. What are the treatment options?

Case ranking/difficulty: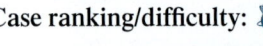

Category: Disc

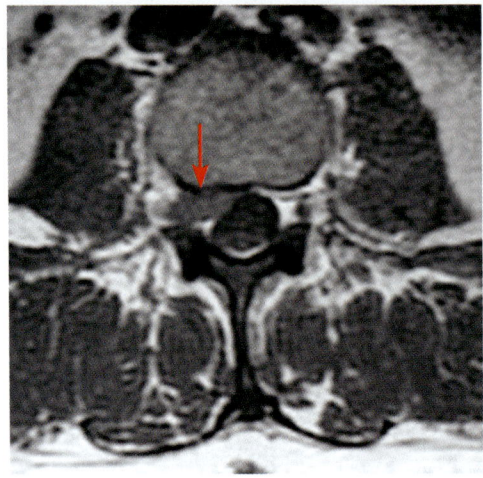

Axial T1 image demonstrates isointense soft tissue within the right lateral recess, consistent with L3-L4 disc extrusion.

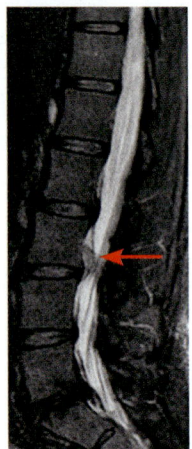

Sagittal T2 image demonstrates L3-L4 disc extrusion with superior migration and sequestration.

Answers

1. Degenerative disc lesions include annular tear, disc bulge, disc herniation, disc protrusion, and disc sequestration.

2. Pain increased with sitting/bending/coughing, radiculopathy, and sphincter dysfunction are all common presenting symptoms.

3. Associated abnormalities include diskogenic endplate changes, enhancement of nerve roots, epidural hematoma, and T2 hypointensity within the intervertebral disc.

4. L4-L5 and L5-S1 account for nearly 90% of all herniations.

5. Conservative management is successful in most patients with surgery reserved for patients with recalcitrant symptoms.

Pearls

- Up to one in three patients has an asymptomatic disc herniation. Terminology is very important in the discussion of degenerative disc disease.
- Disc bulge: >50% disc circumference.
- Disc herniation: <50% disc circumference.
- Disc extrusion: Herniation where the base of the protrusion is narrower than the herniated disc material.
- Disc protrusion: Herniation where the base of the protrusion is wider than the herniated disc material.
- Disc sequestration: Free fragment of disc material.
- Treatment of disc disease is generally conservative—only 10% of patients require surgical intervention secondary to persistent symptoms.

Suggested Readings

Chen CY, Chuang YL, Yao MS, Chiu WT, Chen CL, Chan WP. Posterior epidural migration of a sequestered lumbar disk fragment: MR imaging findings. *AJNR*. 2006;1592-1594.

Schellinger D, Manz HJ, Vidic B, et al. Disk fragment migration. *Radiology*. 1990;175:831-836.

Neck pain

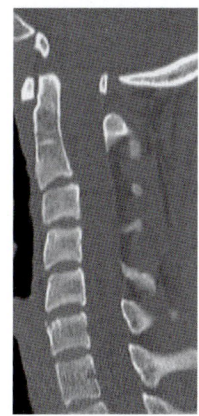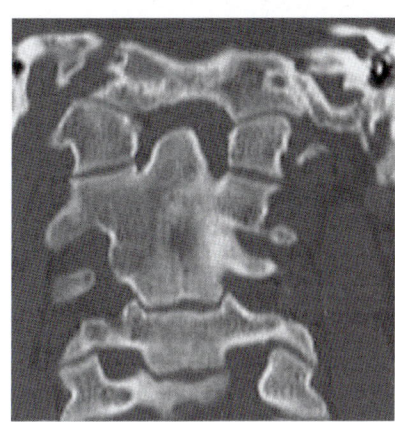

1. What should be included in the differential diagnosis?

2. What are common presenting symptoms?

3. What are the components of the classic triad?

4. What are associated abnormalities?

5. What are the treatment options?

Case ranking/difficulty:

Category: Vertebral body

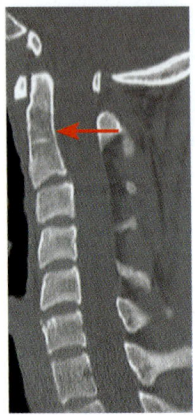

Sagittal CT image demonstrates fusion of the C2 and C3 vertebral bodies.

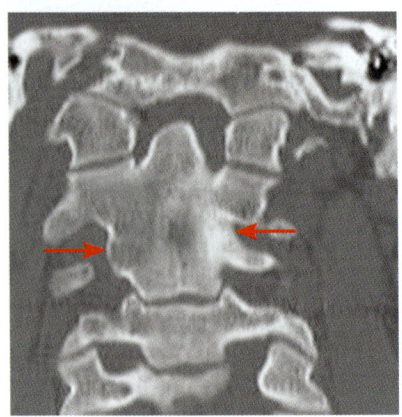

Coronal CT image demonstrates fusion of the C2 and C3 vertebral bodies.

Answers

1. Klippel-Feil syndrome, postoperative fusion, ankylosing spondylitis, and postinfectious fusion could all be considered.

2. Presenting symptoms include pain, alterations of cervical movement, myelopathy, radiculopathy, and neurological deficits in the setting of minor trauma.

3. The components are low hairline, short neck, and abnormal cervical motion.

4. Associated abnormalities include Sprengel deformity, cardiovascular abnormalities, hearing loss, and renal abnormalities.

5. Generally activity restriction is the first step in management followed by bracing and traction as needed. Surgical fusion with decompression may be performed if needed for neurological symptoms.

Pearls

- Klippel Feil refers to congenital fusion of vertebral bodies.
- Unto itself it is harmless; however, there are alterations of biomechanics that place the patient at higher risk of injury in the setting of trauma.

- In addition, there are accelerated degenerative changes at the levels adjacent to the fused vertebrae.
- The classic triad has been described as limited cervical motion, short neck, and low hairline; however, this is present in less than half of patients with vertebral fusions.
- Klippel Feil can be associated with Sprengel deformity, a rare congenital disorder manifested by a high riding scapula, secondary to abnormal migration.
- If the patient has Sprengel deformity, evaluation should be performed for the presence of an omovertebral bone (os omovertebrale), which is present in up to 3/4 of patients, and extends from the superomedial scapula to the transverse process, spinous process, or lamina of C4 through C7.

Suggested Readings

Pizzutillo PD, Woods M, Nicholson L, MacEwen GD. Risk factors in Klippel-Feil syndrome. *Spine.* 1994;19:2110-2116.

Ulmer JL, Elster AD, Ginsberg LE, Williams DW. Klippel-Feil syndrome: CT and MR of acquired and congenital abnormalities of the cervical spine and cord. *J Comp Asst Tomog.* 1993;17:215-224.

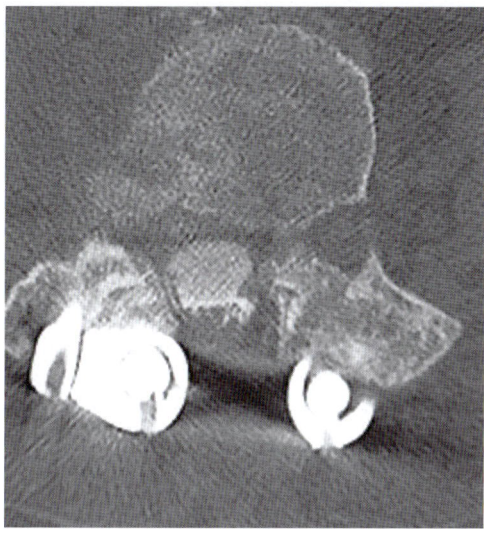 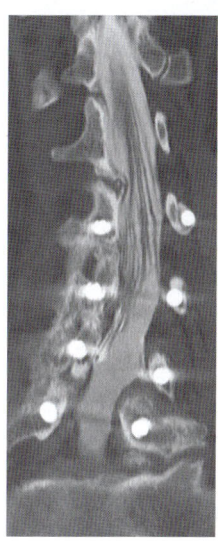

1. What should be included in the differential diagnosis?

2. What are the presenting symptoms?

3. What imaging patterns have been described in this abnormality?

4. What are the etiologies of this abnormality?

5. What are the treatment options?

Case ranking/difficulty:

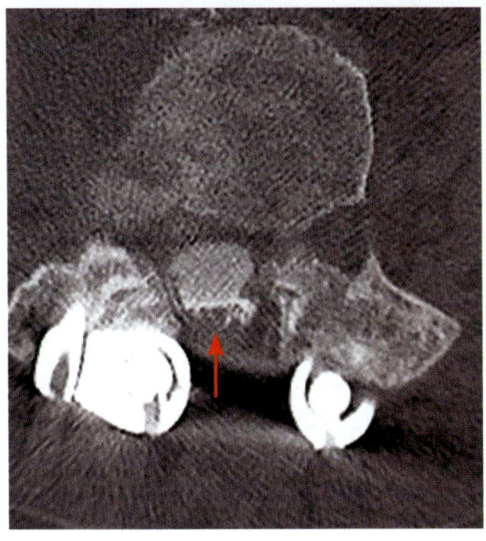

Axial postmyelography CT image demonstrates "empty" appearance of thecal sac with dorsal displacement of nerve roots. Note postoperative changes of laminectomy and bilateral pedicle screw placement.

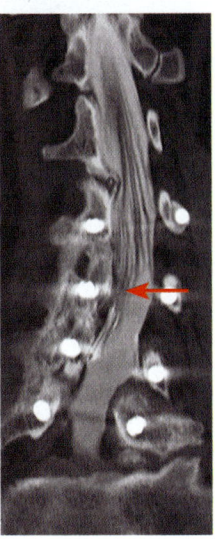

Coronal postmyelography CT image demonstrates lateral displacement and clumping of nerve roots. Note postoperative changes of laminectomy and bilateral pedicle screw placements.

Answers

1. Arachnoiditis can have nodular and linear enhancement of nerve roots, simulating carcinomatous meningitis, or intradural extramedullary tumors (including nerve sheath tumors and metastatic disease). Spinal stenosis can lead to focal clumping of nerve roots at the level of stenosis.

2. Pain and radicular symptoms are most common; others include bowel and bladder dysfunction, paresis, and hypoesthesis.

3. Arachnoiditis can present with an empty thecal sac, secondary to peripheral adhesions of nerve roots, distortion of the thecal sac, clumped nerve roots, and an intrathecal soft tissue mass. The intrathecal soft tissue mass arises from clumping and matting of nerve roots.

4. Potential causes for sterile arachnoiditis include surgery, subarachnoid hemorrhage, intrathecal chemotherapy, myelography, and lumbar puncture; however, postmyelography arachnoiditis rates have dropped following the introduction of water-based contrast.

5. Treatment options include intrathecal steroid injection, laminectomy and lysis of adhesions, and placement of a spinal cord stimulator. Prognosis is dismal despite treatment. Over 50% of patients experience continued pain.

Pearls

- Arachnoiditis is now most commonly seen in the postoperative patient population.
- It can be seen in conjunction with prior meningitis, intrathecal chemotherapy, lumbar puncture, or subarachnoid hemorrhage.
- Arachnoiditis can demonstrate post-gadolinium enhancement in different patterns, which can make the correct diagnosis challenging.
- Patient history is critical in differentiating causes of arachnoiditis.
- Arachnoiditis symptoms tend to be stable over time without significant progression.

Suggested Readings

Van Goethem JWM, Parizel PM, Jinkins JR. Review article: MRI of the postoperative lumbar spine. *Neuroradiology.* 2002;44:723-729.

Young PM, Berquist TH, Bancroft LW, Peterson JJ. Complications of spinal instrumentation. 2007;27:775-789.

Four-story fall onto wet grass

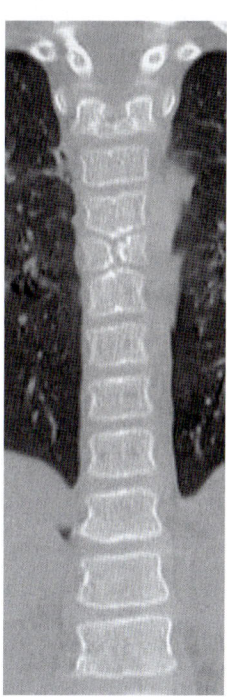

1. When does the anomaly leading to this occur?

2. Which radiograph is most helpful in differentiating this abnormality from wedge fracture?

3. Where does this most commonly occur?

4. What is the etiology?

5. What are the treatment options?

Case ranking/difficulty:

Category: Vertebral body

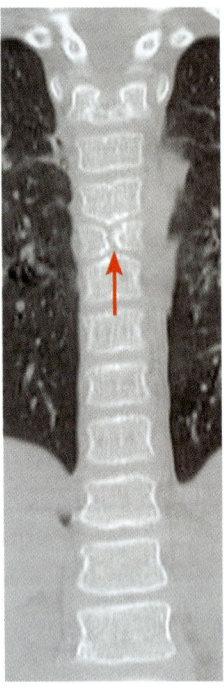

Coronal CT image demonstrates vertically oriented clefting of the midportion of the T6 vertebral body.

Answers

1. The two lateral ossification centers of the vertebral bodies usually fuse between the third and sixth weeks of gestation.

2. AP radiographs are most helpful for evaluation. A butterfly vertebra should demonstrate a lack of midline fusion; however, the two halves of the vertebral body may be different sizes if there is an associated unilateral arterial malformation.

3. The thoracolumbar junction is the most common location of butterfly vertebra.

4. Butterfly vertebrae arise secondary to persistence of the notochord.

5. While some postulate that butterfly vertebra can alter spinal biomechanics and lead to advanced degenerative changes, they are not unstable and do not generally require any treatment.

Pearls

- Butterfly vertebrae are unusual fusion anomalies of the vertebral bodies thought to be secondary to persistence of the notochord.
- There are often additional osseous abnormalities involving the ribs or spine.
- There is an association with genetic syndromes, including Crouzon and Alagille syndromes.
- No treatment is necessary as this is not an unstable finding, but care should be taken not to confuse it with an acute fracture.

Suggested Readings

Garcia F, Florez MT, Conejero JA. A butterfly vertebra or a wedge fracture? *Int Orthop.* 1993;17:7-10.

Sonel B, Yalcin P, Ozturk E, Bokesoy I. Butterfly vertebra: a case report. *Clin Imaging.* 2001;25:206-208.

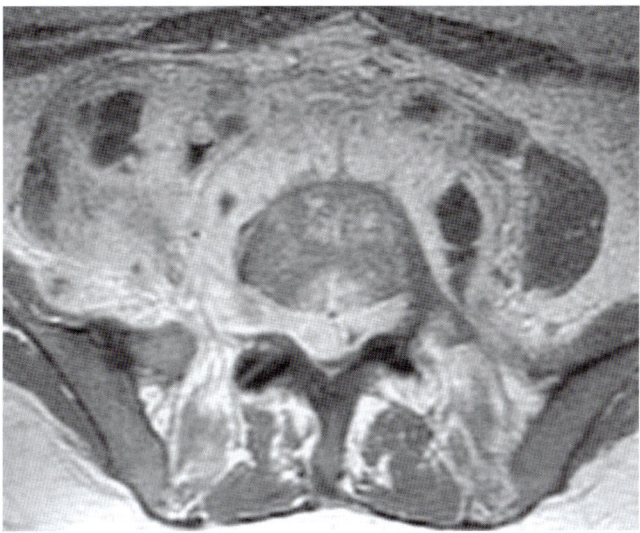 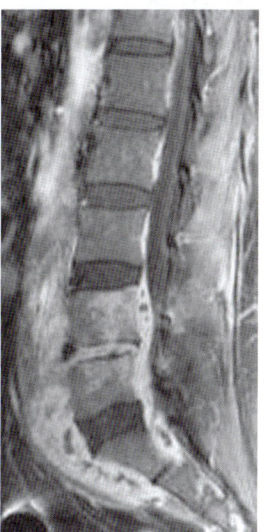

1. What are presenting symptoms?

2. What patient populations are most likely to present with this abnormality?

3. What are the imaging findings within the vertebral bodies?

4. What are the four types of this abnormality that affect humans?

5. What are the associated abnormalities?

Case ranking/difficulty:

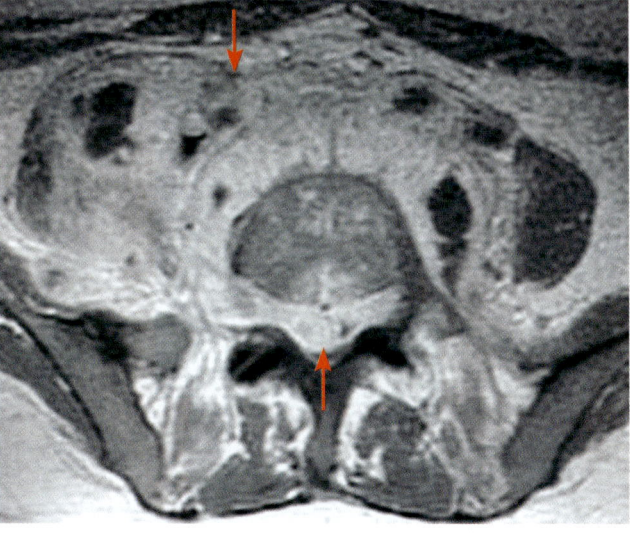

Axial T1 image following gadolinium administration demonstrates right psoas and anterior epidural enhancing fluid collections, consistent with abscesses.

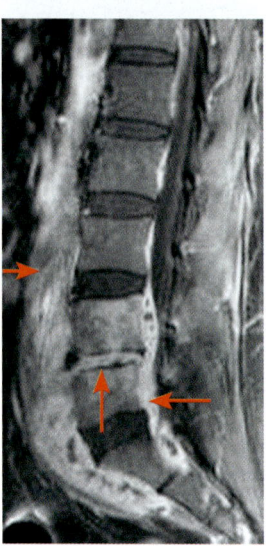

Sagittal T1 image following gadolinium administration demonstrates abnormal enhancement within the L4 and L5 vertebral bodies and intervening disc, as well as the anterior epidural space and prevertebral space.

Answers

1. The presentation is nonspecific and includes fever, malaise, night sweats, weight loss, and polyarthralgia.

2. Brucellosis is a widespread zoonosis seen most commonly in veterinarians and farmers.

3. Classic findings of spondylitis include low T1 signal, high T2 signal, and enhancement.

4. There are six species of *Brucella* but *B abortus*, *B melitensis*, *B suis*, and *B canis* are the four species that infect humans.

5. Associated abnormalities that can be seen in spinal brucellosis include paraspinal abscess, diskitis, epidural abscess, nerve root enhancement, and vertebral body destruction.

Pearls

- Brucellosis is a relatively rare cause of spondylodiskitis; however, it can have an indolent course and mimic tubercular disease.
- Brucellosis is most commonly seen in zoo keepers and farmers.
- Diagnosis can be made by documenting positive Brucella serology, in either serum or cerebrospinal fluid.
- Treatment generally consists of long-term combination antimicrobial therapy, including rifampin, doxycycline, and trimoxazole.

Suggested Readings

Namiduru M, Karaoglan I, Gursoy S, Bayazit N, Sirikei A. Brucellosis of the spine: evaluation of the clinical, laboratory, and radiological findings of 4 patients. *Rheumatol Int*. 2004;24:125-129.

Tekkok IH, Berker M, Ozcan O, Ozgen T, Akalin E. Brucellosis of the spine. *Neurosurgery*. 1993;33:838-844.

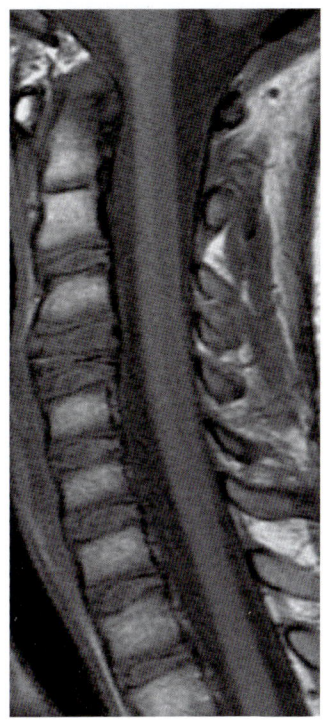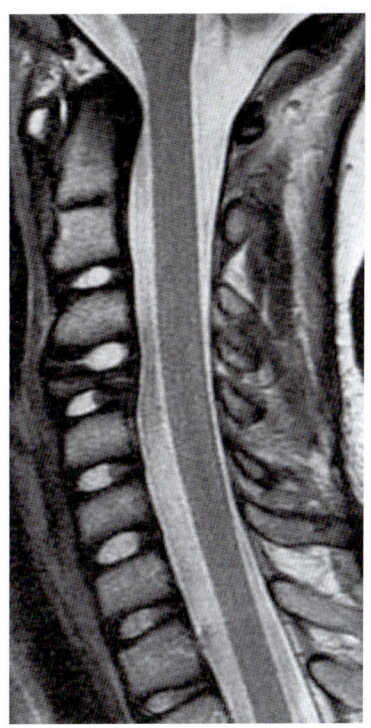

1. What should be included in the differential diagnosis?

2. What are common presenting symptoms?

3. What are associated abnormalities?

4. What portion of the spine is most commonly affected?

5. What are the treatment options?

Case ranking/difficulty:

Category: Vertebral body

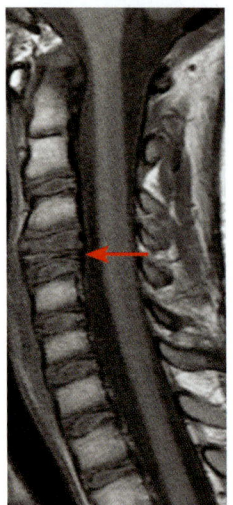

Sagittal T1 image demonstrates loss of vertebral body height and hypointensity of the C4 vertebral body.

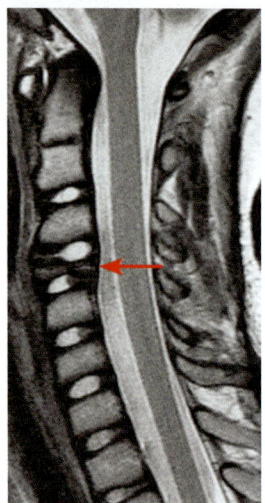

Sagittal T2 image demonstrates loss of vertebral body height and hypointensity of the C4 vertebral body.

Answers

1. Vertebral body collapse can be seen in compression fracture, metastasis, osteomyelitis, and primary bone tumor.

2. Potential presenting symptoms include fever, pain, pathologic fracture, and radiculopathy. Additionally, myelopathy can be seen if the spinal canal is compromised.

3. Potential associated abnormalities in Langerhans cell histiocytosis include cutaneous lesions, lymphadenopathy, gastrointestinal bleeding, proptosis, and diabetes insipidus. Diabetes insipidus arises from involvement of the pituitary infundibulum.

4. Half of cases occur in the thoracic spine with a third within the lumbar spine.

5. Potential treatment modalities depend on the severity of disease and secondary complications and include conservative management, chemotherapy, radiation, surgical resection, and stem cell transplant.

Pearls

- EG represents almost three-quarters of Langerhans cell histiocytosis (LCH) cases and is the most benign subtype.

- EG is limited to osseous lesions.
- Hand-Schüller-Christian disease is an intermediate form of LCH with osseous and visceral lesions.
- Letterer-Siwe disease is the most severe form with extensive visceral involvement.
- EG generally presents before adolescence with multiple lytic lesions, which can be complicated by collapse or pathologic fracture leading to pain.
- The spine is one of the less common sites of osseous involvement, but when involved it often manifests as vertebra plana.
- EG is generally treated conservatively, and there are even reports of spontaneous resolution of vertebra plana.
- More severe variants of LCH are treated with multiagent chemotherapy with radiation and stem cell transplant reserved for recalcitrant lesions.

Suggested Readings

Denaro L, Longo UG, Papalia R, DiMartino A, Maffulli N, Denaro V. Eosinophilic granuloma of the pediatric cervical spine. *Spine*. 2008;33:E936-E941.

Ropper AE, Cahill KS, Hanna JW, McCarthy EF, Gokaslan ZL, Chi JH. Primary vertberal tumors: A review of epidemiologic, histological, and imaging findings, part I: benign tumors. *Neurosurgery*. 2011;69:1171-1180.

Back pain in patient with chronic steroid use

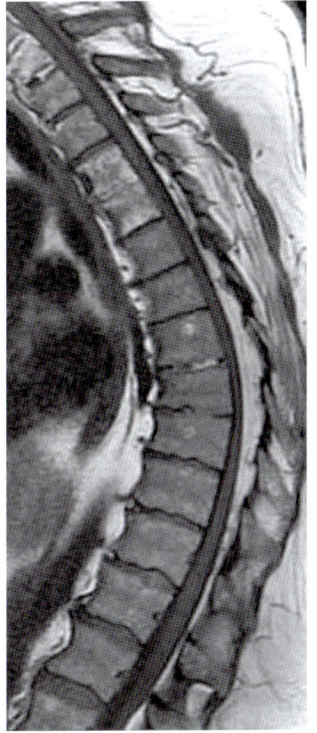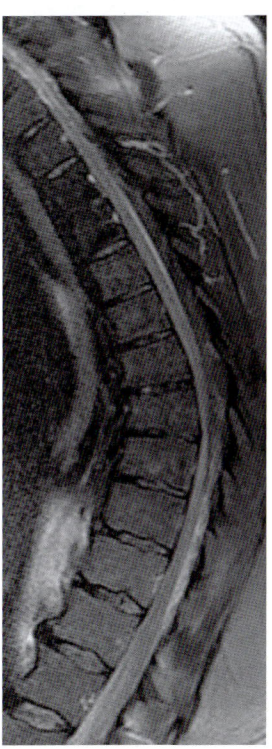

1. What should be included in the differential diagnosis?

2. What are common presenting symptoms?

3. What imaging findings can be helpful in differentiating epidural processes?

4. What part of the spine is most commonly involved?

5. What are the treatment options?

Case ranking/difficulty: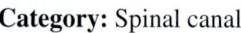

Category: Spinal canal

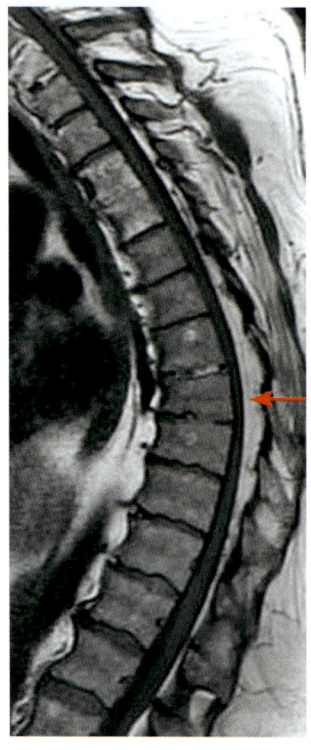

Sagittal T1 image demonstrates dorsal T1 hyperintensity with anterior displacement of the dura.

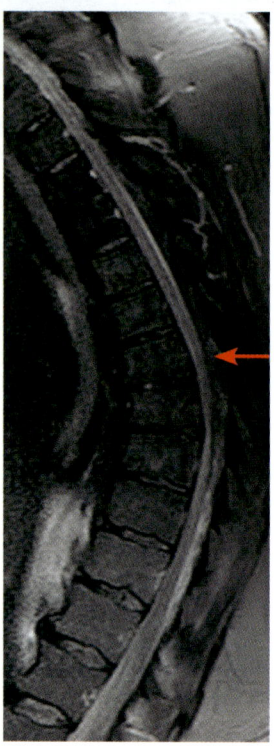

Sagittal T2 image with fat suppression demonstrates dorsal hypointensity with anterior displacement of the dura.

Answers

1. Processes of the epidural space, which may show varying amounts of T1 hyperintensity, include lymphoma, metastasis, hemorrhage, abscess, and lipomatosis.

2. Usually this abnormality is asymptomatic; however, presenting symptoms include back pain, sensory deficits, and myelopathic symptoms.

3. Fat will maintain hyperintensity on T1 and T2 sequences, but should demonstrate decreased signal with the application of fat suppression.

4. The thoracic spine is most commonly involved.

5. As most patients are asymptomatic or have symptoms only vaguely referable to the epidural lipomatosis, conservative management is an appropriate choice. Noninvasive options such as weight loss and tapering of steroids are also good choices with decompression reserved for refractory cases.

Pearls

- Epidural lipomatosis is becoming more common as the population becomes more obese; the most common cause remains exogenous steroid use.
- Epidural lipomatosis should be differentiated from other causes of T1 hyperintensity within the epidural space.
- Fat suppressed images can be helpful in evaluation.
- This is often an asymptomatic process; however, some patients develop radicular or myelopathic symptoms.
- In these cases, surgical decompression should be considered if tapering of steroids or weight loss is not possible.

Suggested Readings

Fassett DR, Schmidt MH. Spinal epidural lipomatosis: a review of its causes and recommendations for treatment. *Neurosurg Focus*. 2004;16:1-3.

Quint DJ, Boulos RS, Sanders WP, Mehta BA, Patel SC, Tiel RL. Epidural lipomatosis. *Radiology*. 1988;169:485-490.

Left leg numbness

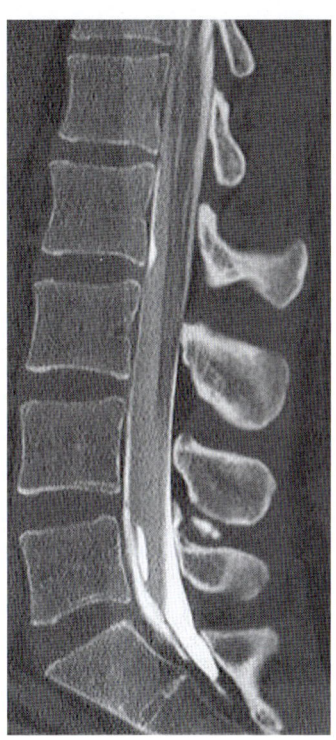

1. What should be included in the differential diagnosis?

2. What are important items to review prior to performing myelography?

3. What are the keys to recognizing extrathecal contrast injection?

4. What are the optimal lumbar levels to gain access for myelography?

5. What are the treatment options?

Case ranking/difficulty:

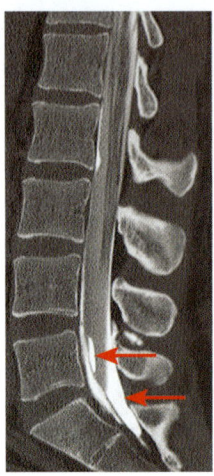

Sagittal CT image following myelogram demonstrates contrast within the subdural, epidural, and intrathecal spaces.

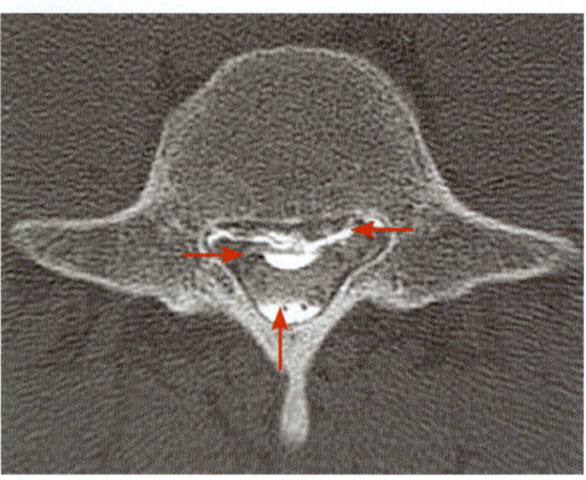

Axial CT image following myelogram demonstrates contrast within the epidural (*ventral right arrow*), subdural (*middle left arrow*), and intrathecal spaces (*dorsal arrow*).

Answers

1. Extradural hyperdensity seen on CT myelography could be caused by subdural or epidural hematoma, epidural metastasis, or posterior longitudinal ligament ossification.

2. Important items to review include coagulation laboratory values, current medications, allergies, and prior imaging studies.

3. The best way to delineate early extrathecal contrast injection is to evaluate for focal pooling of contrast at the site of injection.

4. L2-L3 and L3-L4 are the most optimal levels as they should be below the level of the conus, yet in an area where the thecal sac is still fairly large.

5. Conservative management is indicated. Epidural blood patches are performed for cerebrospinal fluid leaks.

Pearls

- Mixed injections on myelography should be recognized at the time of the procedure.
- If the contrast fails to distribute around the nerve roots of the filum, this is indicative of subdural injection; however, it can sometimes be difficult to discern.
- A mixed injection is less troublesome than a completely extrathecal injection.
- CT following myelography is routinely done, which can delineate the compartments that contain contrast.

Suggested Readings

Harreld JH, McMenamy JM, Toomay SM, Chason DP. Myelography: a primer. *Curr Probl Diagn Radiol.* 2011;4:149-157.

Ozdoba C, Gralla J, Rieke A, Binggeli R, Schroth G. Myelography in the age of MRI: why we do it, and how we do it. *Radiol Res Pract.* 2011;329017:6.

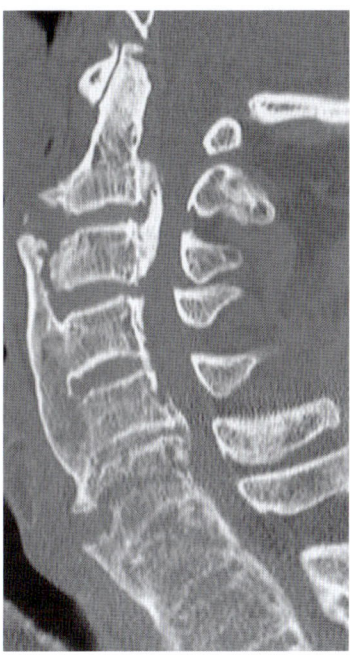

1. What should be included in the differential diagnosis?

2. What is the classification of fractures in this disorder?

3. What underlying disorders are associated with this abnormality?

4. What disorders can lead to axial skeletal osseous overproduction?

5. What are the treatment options?

Case ranking/difficulty: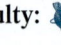

Category: More than one category

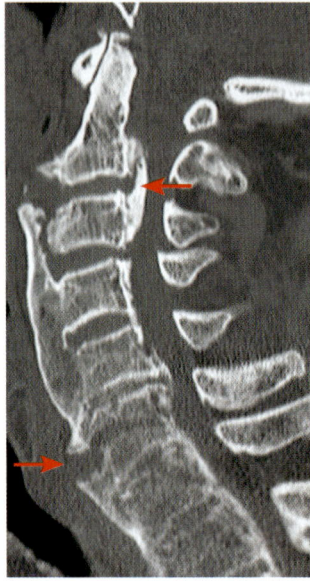

Sagittal image demonstrates flowing anterior osteophytes with lucency extending into the C6 vertebral body. Note associated ossification of the posterior longitudinal ligament.

Answers

1. The differential includes ankylosing spondylitis, psoriatic arthritis, and diffuse idiopathic skeletal hyperostosis.

2. Fractures are classified into four types:

   Type 1—disc injury

   Type 2—body injury

   Type 3—anterior body or posterior disc injury

   Type 4—anterior disc or posterior body injury

   Type 1 fractures are most common in DISH.

3. Type 2 diabetes, cholelithiasis, hypertension, and hypercholesterolemia are all associated with DISH.

4. Seronegative spondyloarthritis, acromegaly, ochronosis, fluorosis, and trauma are additional causes of osseous overproduction in the spine.

5. Patients with fractures superimposed on DISH generally benefit from multilevel fusion given the inherently altered biomechanics.

Pearls

- Diffuse idiopathic skeletal hyperostosis (DISH) is a degenerative disorder characterized by ligamentous and tendinous ossification.
- It is diagnosed when flowing osteophytes bridge four or more adjacent vertebral bodies.
- It also affects the sacroiliac joints and has extraspinal manifestations.
- It affects men twice as often as women and usually older patients (>40 years old).
- The etiology is uncertain but there is a familial pattern.
- The abnormal ossification leads to altered biomechanics and increased risk of fracture at levels of adjacent osseous fusion.
- Careful evaluation of spinal imaging is imperative in patients with DISH as they may suffer an atypical fracture, even in the setting of only minor trauma.
- In addition, patients with DISH often have increased morbidity and mortality in the setting of superimposed fractures in comparison to patients without an ankylosing spinal disorder.

Suggested Readings

Cammisa M, DeSerio A, Guglielmi G. Diffuse idiopathic skeletal hyperostosis. *Eur J Radiol.* 1998;27:S7-S11.

Caron T, Bransford R, Nguyen Q, Agel J, Chapman J, Bellabarba C. Spine fractures in patients with ankylosing spinal disorders. *Spine.* 2010;35:E458-E464.

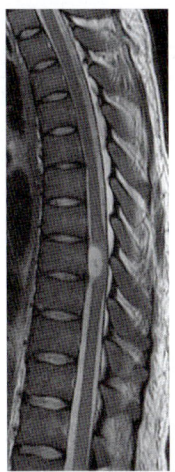 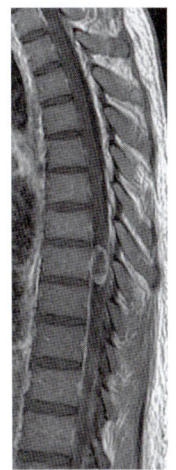 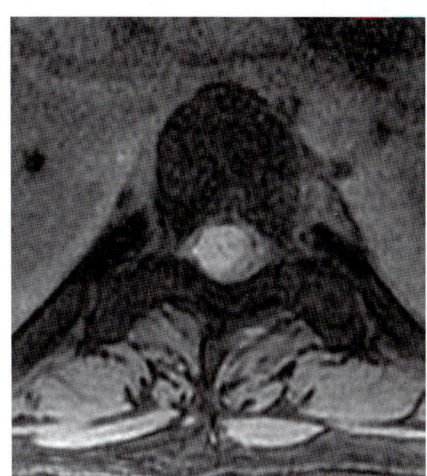

1. What should be included in the differential diagnosis?

2. Which spinal compartment is most commonly affected?

3. What portion of the spine is most commonly affected?

4. What signal characteristics would favor nerve sheath tumor over neurofibroma?

5. What are the treatment options?

Case ranking/difficulty:

Category: Meninges/Nerve sheath

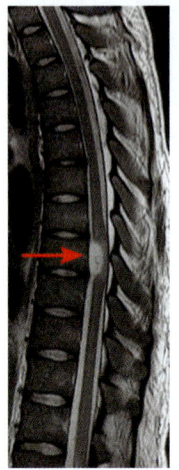

Sagittal T2 image demonstrates a fluid intensity mass in the ventral spinal canal with associated cord displacement and compression.

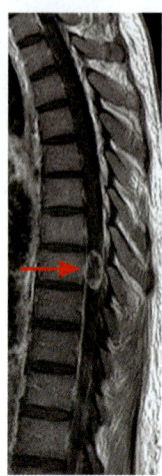

Sagittal T1 image following gadolinium administration demonstrates a peripherally enhancing mass in the ventral spinal canal with associated cord displacement and compression.

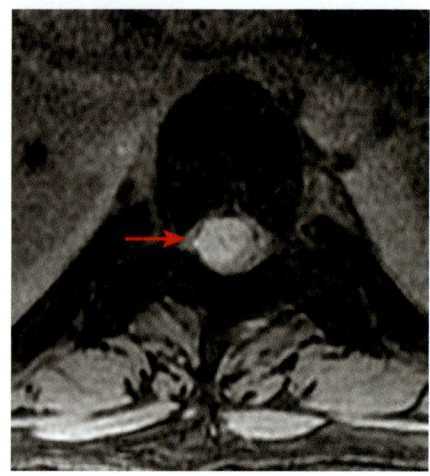

Axial T2 image demonstrates a fluid intensity mass in the ventral spinal canal with associated cord displacement and compression.

Answers

1. Epidermoid and schwannoma are the most common intradural extramedullary lesions to demonstrate cystic signal characteristics. Meningioma and neurofibroma also occur within the intradural extramedullary compartment and should be considered within the differential.

2. 70% are intradural extramedullary in location with the remainder equally divided between extradural and combined intradural and extradural locations.

3. Thoracic spine is most common with equal prevalence in the cervical and lumbar spine.

4. Cystic degeneration, hemorrhage, and lobulated appearance are common imaging findings in schwannoma. Neurofibroma often demonstrates more fusiform enlargement. Calcification is more commonly seen in meningioma.

5. Surgical resection is the treatment of choice for symptomatic lesions or pathologic diagnosis. This may necessitate sacrifice of the associated nerve.

Pearls

- Schwannomas are the most common intradural extramedullary mass in the spine.

- 70% of schwannomas occur in the intradural extramedullary compartment. The remainder are divided equally between the extradural and combined intradural–extradural compartment.
- Imaging characteristics that favor schwannoma include cystic degeneration, hemorrhage, and focal lobulation.
- Neurofibromas tend to be more fusiform in appearance.
- Meningiomas do not usually demonstrate cystic change and are more likely to have calcifications and an enhancing dural tail.
- Schwannomas can be multiple, particularly in association with neurofibromatosis type 2, schwannomatosis, and Carney complex.
- Patients generally present with focal pain; however, myelopathic symptoms may occur in the setting of cord compression.
- Treatment requires complete surgical resection, often associated with sacrifice of the associated nerve.

Suggested Readings

Friedman DP, Tartaglino LM, Flanders AE. Intradural schwannomas of the spine: MR findings with emphasis on contrast-enhancement characteristics. *AJR*. 1992;158: 1347-1350.

Parmar H, Patkar D, Gadani S, Shah J. Cystic lumbar nerve sheath tumours: MRI features in five patients. *Australas Radiol*. 2001;45:123-127.

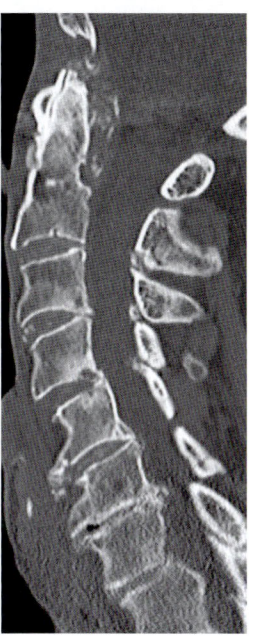

1. In which parts of the spine does this disorder occur?

2. What are synonyms for this abnormality?

3. What are inciting factors in this abnormality?

4. What are classic imaging features?

5. What are the treatment options?

Case ranking/difficulty:

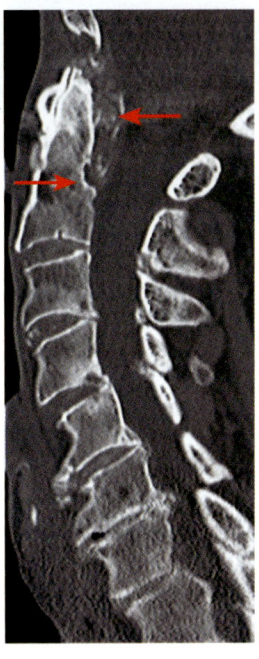

Sagittal CT image demonstrates calcium deposition posterior to the dens with early erosive changes.

enhancement on MRI are imaging features of calcium pyrophosphate deposition; however, the appearance is variable depending on where the crystals are deposited.

5. If patients are symptomatic, treatment is geared at the inciting cause. Surgical resection and fusion can be considered depending on severity of symptomatology and site of involvement.

Answers

1. Deposition occurs in the intervertebral disc, ligamentum flavum, transverse ligament, and apophyseal joints with different symptomatology depending on amount.

2. CPPD is also called pseudogout or articular chondrocalcinosis.

3. Mechanical trauma and inflammation are felt to be inciting factors in deposition of calcium pyrophosphate.

4. Soft tissue and intervertebral disc calcification, osseous erosion, heterogeneous T2 signal, and peripheral

Pearls

- The incidence of calcium pyrophosphate deposition (CPPD) increases with age and may occur in association with other conditions (trauma, surgery, hypophosphatasia, hyperparathyroidism, hypomagnesemia).
- CPPD can also be seen in association with gout and hydroxyapatite deposition.
- Involvement of the dens may become symptomatic, either through compression at the foramen magnum secondary to deposition or instability secondary to dens erosion.
- On microscopic inspection, calcium pyrophosphate crystals are rhomboidal in shape and demonstrate weak positive birefringence under polarized light.

Suggested Readings

Bouvet JP, Le Parc JM, Michalski B, Benlahrache C, Auquier L. Acute neck pain due to calcifications surrounding the odontoid process: the crowded dens syndrome. *Arthritis*. 1985;28:1417-1420.

Salcman M, Khan A, Symonds D. Calcium pyrophosphate arthropathy of the spine: case report and review of the literature. *Neurosurgery*. 1994;34:915-918.

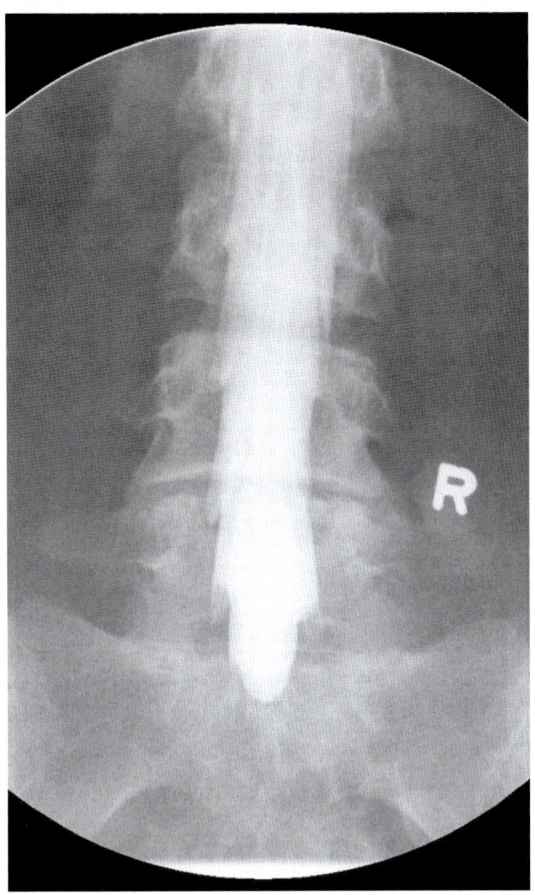
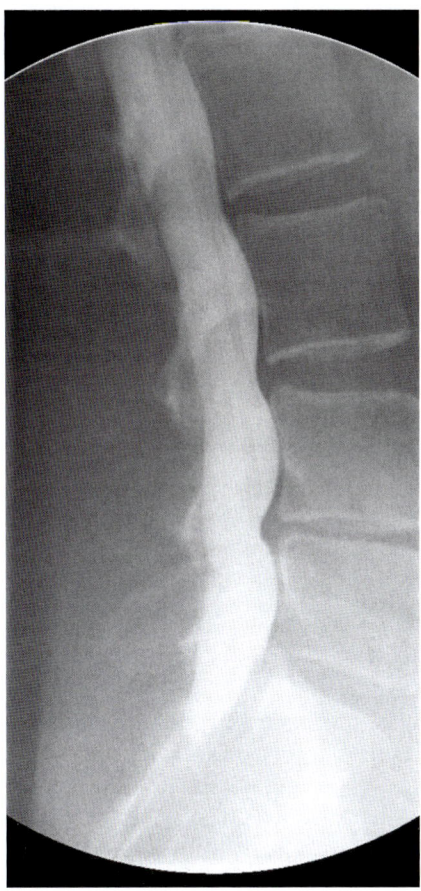

1. What is this procedure called?

2. When is this procedure indicated?

3. Name the two common approaches used.

4. Name some recognized complications of this procedure.

5. Describe the typical postprocedure headache.

Case ranking/difficulty:

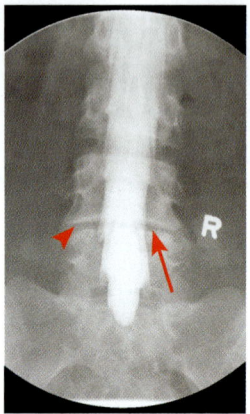

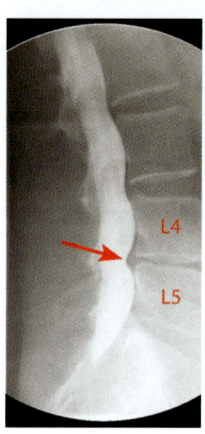

AP film of the lumbar spine following the injection of 12 mL of Iohexol (300 mgL/mL) in the lumbar subarachnoid space via a 22 G spinal needle. Myelography demonstrates disc space narrowing (*arrowhead*) at L4-5 level associated with amputation of the right L4 nerve root sheath (*arrow*).

Lateral projection confirms narrowing of L4-5 intervertebral disc space and a right posterolateral disc protrusion which indents the thecal sac.

Answers

1. Myelography is a radiographic spinal examination that involves injection of a contrast agent into the thecal sac prior to the acquisition of radiographs using standard projections. Alternatively, a CT scan may be performed.

2. The technique has been largely superseded by MRI; however, it is still a useful technique whenever MRI is contraindicated or when MR images are limited by artifacts from previous spinal fixation.

3. Two approaches, namely the mid-sagittal and the parasagittal approaches, are commonly used. The advantage of the former is that it is less painful as the ligament is poorly innervated compared to paraspinal muscles. In the parasagittal approach, the needle is advanced into the interlaminar space, and therefore it will not need to be forced through the interspinous ligament (which may be severely calcified) or negotiated through narrowed interspinous spaces.

4. Myelography is generally a safe technique. Some patients develop a headache, vertigo, and vomiting postprocedure secondary to CSF loss. This may be reduced with the use of a smaller needle and by orienting the bevel of the spinal needle parallel to the longitudinal fibers of the thecal sac. The standard spinal needles are 22- and 25-gauge. The latter is enough for intrathecal contrast injection but is insufficient to allow CSF collection.

More serious complications include infection, hematoma, seizures, contrast reactions, and CSF leaks. The latter can be treated by a blood patch. Less commonly the spinal cord may be damaged directly particularly if the conus is low lying or if a cervical approach is being used.

5. The typical postprocedure headache develops within the first few hours and characteristically increases in severity in the upright position and improves in the recumbent position.

Pearls

- Myelography has been largely superseded by MRI but is still useful whenever MRI is contraindicated.
- Complications include infection, hematoma, seizures, contrast reactions, and CSF leaks.
- Two approaches, namely the mid-sagittal and the parasagittal approaches, are commonly used.
- Only nonionic contrast can be injected into the thecal sac.

Suggested Readings

Bischoff RJ, Rodriguez RP, Gupta K, Righi A, Dalton JE, Whitecloud TS. A comparison of computed tomography-myelography, magnetic resonance imaging, and myelography in the diagnosis of herniated nucleus pulposus and spinal stenosis. *J Spinal Disord.* 1993 Aug;6(4):289-295.

http://www.ir.ustl.du/neurorad/internal.sp?NavID=72. Accessed 22nd June 2014.

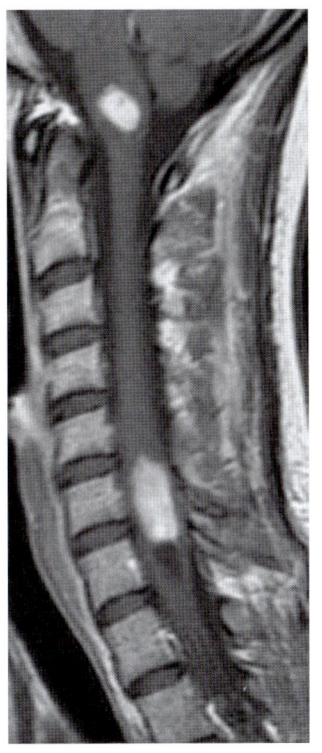 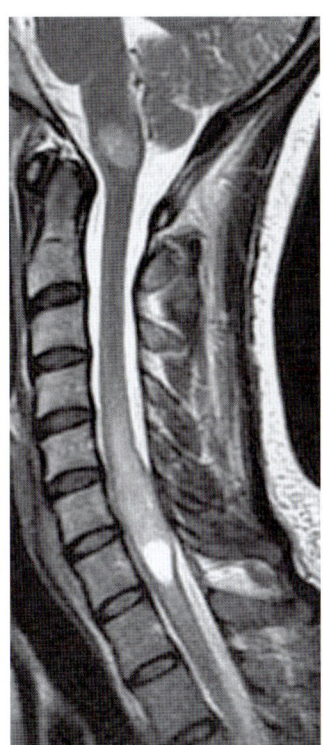

1. What should be included in the differential diagnosis?

2. What are common presenting symptoms?

3. What portion of the cord is most commonly affected?

4. What are the subtypes of this abnormality?

5. What are the treatment options?

Case ranking/difficulty:

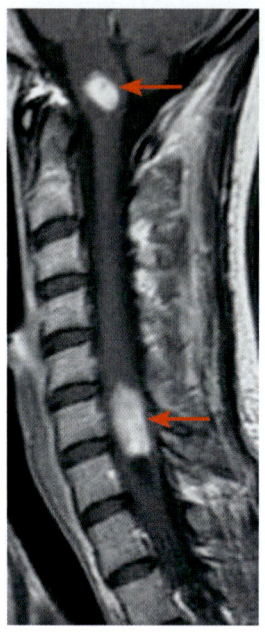

Sagittal T1 image following gadolinium administration demonstrates multiple enhancing foci in the cervical cord; the inferior lesion demonstrates a nonenhancing cystic portion.

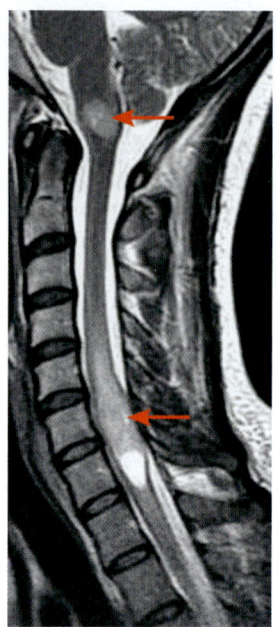

Sagittal T2 image demonstrates multiple T2 hyperintense expansile foci within the cervical cord; the inferior lesion demonstrates a fluid intensity portion.

Answers

1. Any intramedullary lesion should be considered, including ependymoma, astrocytoma, hemangioblastoma, metastasis, and oligodendroglioma; ependymoma is the most common intramedullary tumor in the adult population.

2. Pain is the most common presenting symptoms; others include weakness, radicular symptoms, and sensory deficits.

3. The cervical cord is the most common location of cellular ependymomas, followed by thoracic cord and conus.

4. The subtypes of ependymoma are cellular, myxopapillary, clear cell, and tanycytic; the cellular subtype is the most common intramedullary subtype.

5. Most patients are cured with surgical resection; radiation therapy can be used in patients with recurrent disease or subtotal resection.

Pearls

- Ependymomas are the most common intramedullary spinal cord tumors in adults, accounting for approximately 60% of all intramedullary spinal cord tumors.
- While there is an association with neurofibromatosis type 2 (NF-2), the tumors seen in conjunction with NF-2 are not histologically different from those that occur spontaneously.
- Diagnosis is often delayed secondary to nonspecific presenting symptoms of pain and/or myelopathy.
- These tumors are usually WHO grade II.
- Surgical resection is the treatment of choice with radiation therapy reserved for subtotal resection or recurrent disease.
- There is no role for adjuvant chemotherapy.

Suggested Readings

Bostrom A, von Lehe M, Hartmann W, et al. Surgery for spinal cord ependymomas: outcome and prognostic factors. *Neurosurgery*. 2011;68:302-309.

Whitaker SJ, Bessell EM, Ashley SE, Bloom HJG, Bell BA, Brada M. Postoperative radiotherapy in the management of spinal cord ependymoma. *J Neurosurg*. 1991;74:720-728.

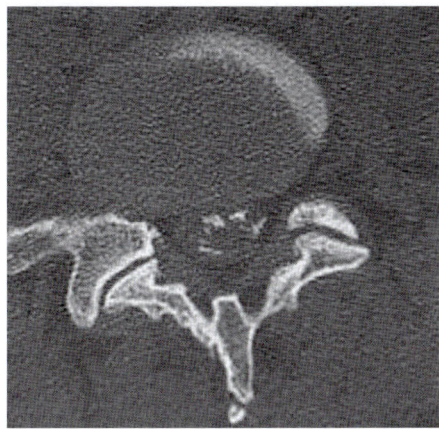 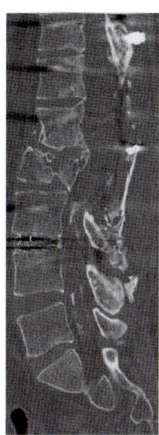

1. What are the most common causes of this abnormality?

2. What are potential etiologies?

3. What is the best modality to evaluate this abnormality?

4. What are the expected MRI findings?

5. What are the treatment options?

Case ranking/difficulty:

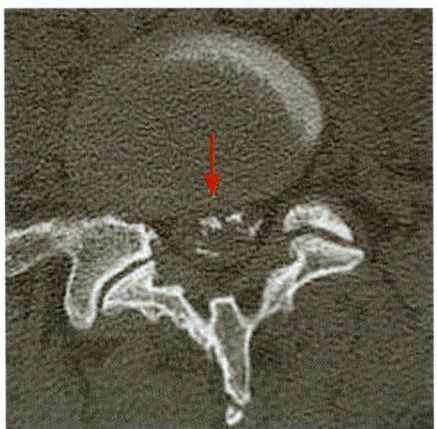

Axial CT image demonstrates calcification of the thecal sac.

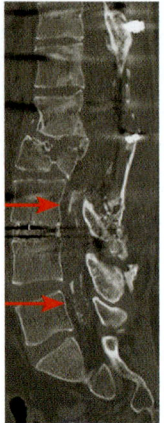

Sagittal CT image demonstrates postoperative changes with calcification of the thecal sac.

Answers

1. Traditionally, spinal meningitis was the most common cause; however, in the modern era, spinal surgery is the most common cause. Other causes include lumbar puncture, subarachnoid hemorrhage, and prior myelogram.

2. The predominant theory is that chronic inflammation leads to osseous metaplasia of the exuberant fibrotic changes. Other theories include organization of intradural blood products with ossification and seeding of bone fragments.

3. Noncontrast CT is the study of choice.

4. Findings are similar to noncalcified arachnoiditis, including clumping of the nerve roots, with superimposed linear or nodular T1 hyperintensity and T2 hypointensity. However, signal abnormality is variable depending on the hydroxylation status of the calcium.

5. Treatment options include analgesia and spinal stimulation, as is performed for noncalcified arachnoiditis. Additionally, some patients benefit from decompressive laminectomy; however, this must encompass the entirety of the abnormality, which is important to document in a radiology report.

Pearls

- Historically arachnoiditis arose secondary to spinal infection; however, it is now more commonly seen in the postoperative patient.
- It manifests with clumping and thickening of the nerve roots.
- It has been classically described as an "empty thecal sac."
- Calcific arachnoiditis has a worse prognosis than the noncalcified variant with a tendency toward progressive neurological decline.

Suggested Readings

Chan CC, Lau PY, Sun LK, Lo SS. Arachnoiditis ossificans. *Hong Kong Med J.* 2009;15:146-148.

Frizzell B, Kaplan P, Dussault R, Sevick R. Arachnoiditis ossificans: MR imaging features in five patients. *AJR.* 2001;177:461-464.

Back pain

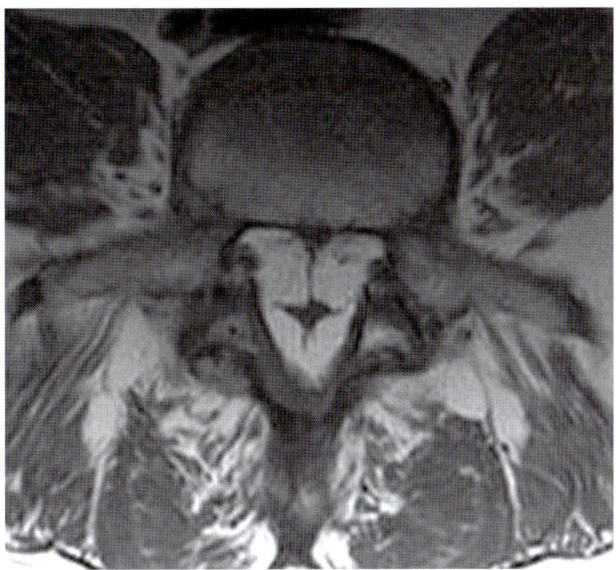 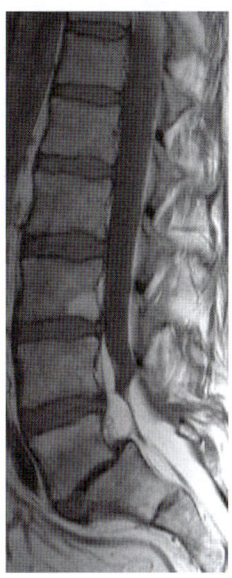

1. What should be included in the differential diagnosis?

2. What are common presenting symptoms?

3. What are potential causative factors?

4. What part of the spine is most commonly involved?

5. What are the treatment options?

Case ranking/difficulty: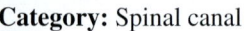

Category: Spinal canal

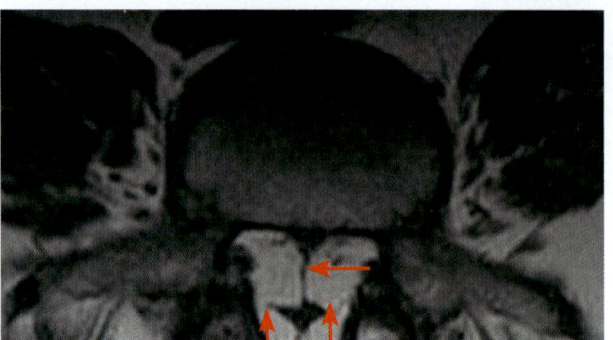

Axial T1 image demonstrates classic Y-shaped configuration of the thecal sac, resulting from limitations of the epidural space by the meningovertebral ligaments.

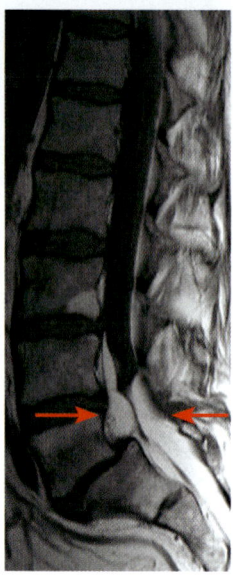

Sagittal T1 image demonstrates focal anterior epidural T1 hyperintensity, consistent with fat, with posterior displacement of the posterior longitudinal ligament. Note also the posterior epidural fat most prevalent below the L4 level.

Answers

1. Processes that involve the epidural space and can have T1 hyperintensity include abscess, hematoma, metastasis, and lipomatosis.

2. Back pain is the most commonly reported symptom; others include myelopathy, radiculopathy, sensory deficit, and incontinence.

3. The most common cause is exogenous steroid use; however, endogenous overproduction is a cause. As the population becomes heavier, obesity is increasing in frequency as a causative factor.

4. The thoracic spine is most commonly involved, followed by the lumbar spine.

5. Weight loss and tapering of exogenous steroids, if possible, are noninvasive treatment options. If symptoms are refractory, surgical decompression should be considered.

Pearls

- Epidural lipomatosis is becoming more common as the population becomes more obese.
- The most common reason to develop epidural lipomatosis is exogenous steroid use.
- This is often an asymptomatic process; however, some patients develop radicular or myelopathic symptoms. In these cases, surgical decompression should be considered and tapering of steroids if possible.
- Epidural lipomatosis is an important entity to recognize and differentiate from other more serious epidural processes, such as abscess, hematoma, or metastatic disease.
- Fat suppressed images can be helpful in the diagnosis.

Suggested Readings

Fassett DR, Schmidt MH. Spinal epidural lipomatosis: a review of its causes and recommendations for treatment. *Neurosurg Focus*. 2004;16:1-3.

Quint DJ, Boulos RS, Sanders WP, Mehta BA, Patel SC, Tiel RL. Epidural lipomatosis. *Radiology*. 1988;169:485-490.

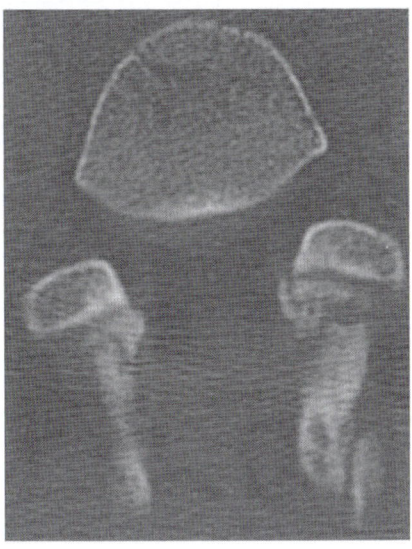 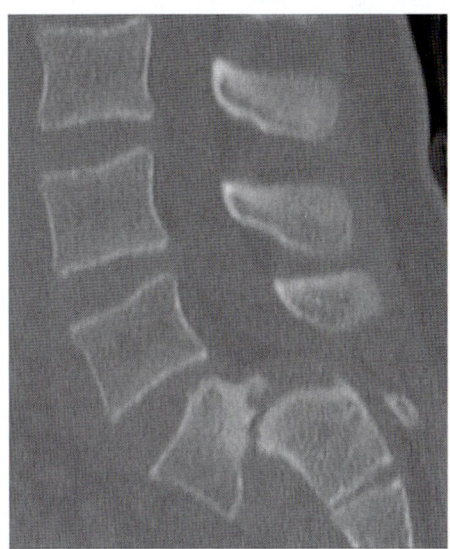

1. What classification scheme is used to grade this abnormality?

2. What are risk factors?

3. What are common presenting symptoms?

4. This abnormality most commonly occurs at what spinal level?

5. What are the treatment options?

Case ranking/difficulty:

Category: Posterior elements

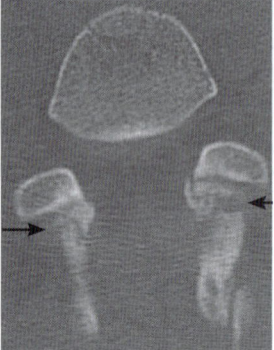

Axial CT image demonstrates bilateral L5 spondylolysis.

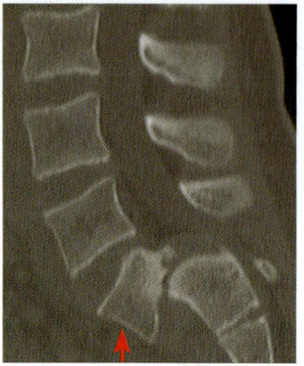

Sagittal CT image demonstrates Grade 4-5 anterolisthesis of L5 on S1.

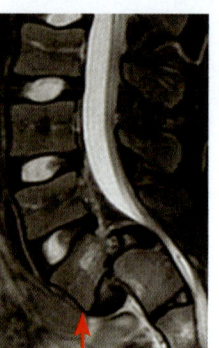

Sagittal T2 image demonstrates Grade 4-5 anterolisthesis of L5 on S1 with uncovering of the disc and severe spinal canal narrowing.

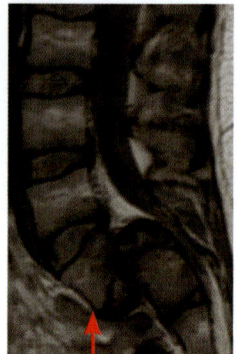

Sagittal PD image demonstrates Grade 4-5 anterolisthesis of L5 on S1 with uncovering of the disc and severe spinal canal narrowing.

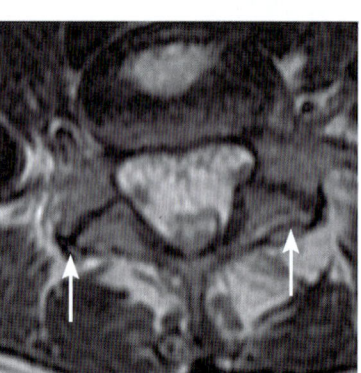

Axial T2 image demonstrates bilateral L5 spondylolyses.

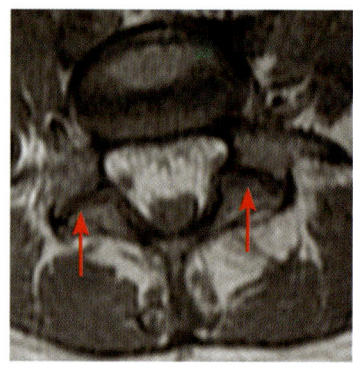

Axial PD image demonstrates bilateral L5 spondylolyses.

Answers

1. Grade I: <25% of vertebral body displacement

    Grade II: 25%-50% of vertebral body displacement

    Grade III: 50%-75% of vertebral body displacement

    Grade IV: 75%-100% of vertebral body displacement

    Grade V: 100% vertebral body displacement

    Grade V spondylolisthesis is also referred to as spondyloptosis.

2. Multiple factors can contribute to spondylolysis, including repetitive microtrauma, spina bifida occulta, abnormal sacral anatomy, and positive family history.

3. Back pain is the most common presenting symptom; others include focal kyphosis, myelopathy, and radiculopathy.

4. Spondyloptosis is most common in the lumbar spine.

5. Depending on patient symptomatology and risk for progression, treatment options can include conservative management, in situ surgical fixation, and surgical reduction and fixation.

Pearls

- Spondyloptosis results when there is complete slippage of one vertebral body relative to the adjacent vertebral body (Grade V spondylolisthesis).
- This is generally due to high-velocity trauma, but can occur from progressive spondylolisthesis secondary to spondylolysis.
- Symptoms usually result from severe spinal canal, lateral recess, and neural foraminal compromise.
- Treatment consists of in situ fixation or reduction and fixation.

Suggested Readings

Curylo LJ, Edwards C, DeWald RW. Radiographic markers in spondyloptosis: implications for spondylolisthesis progression. *Spine*. 2002;27:2021-2025.

Rodriguez DP, Poussaint TY. Imaging of back pain in children. *AJNR*. 2010;31:787-802.

Painful kyphosis

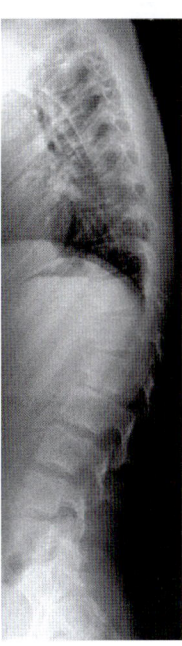

1. What should be included in the differential diagnosis?

2. What are common presenting symptoms?

3. Which location within the spine is most commonly affected?

4. What are the imaging findings?

5. What are the treatment options?

Case ranking/difficulty: **Category:** Vertebral body

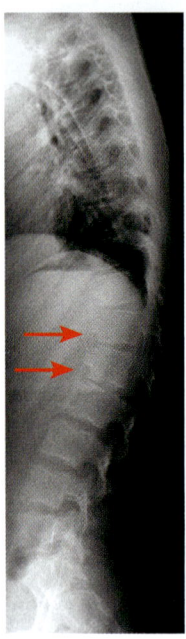

Lateral radiograph demonstrates multiple rounded defects in the anterior vertebral bodies at the thoracolumbar junction.

Answers

1. A combination of kyphosis and endplate irregularity can be seen in compression fracture, infection, osteogenesis imperfecta tarda, and spondyloepiphyseal dysplasia tarda.

2. Pain and kyphosis are the most common presentations; others include scoliosis and myelopathy.

3. Thoracic spine is most commonly affected with the kyphosis apex centered between T7 and T9.

4. Scheuermann disease is related to abnormalities of the epiphyseal growth plates and manifests as anterior wedge compression deformity, apophyseal ring fracture, endplate irregularity, and Schmorl nodes.

5. Treatment options include analgesia, bracing, physical therapy, and surgical fusion. Surgical treatment is indicated in cases of severe kyphosis.

Pearls

- Scheuermann disease is defined as painful kyphosis in association with three or more wedge compression deformities with endplate irregularity.
- It is most common in adolescents, in conjunction with times of rapid growth.
- It is most commonly seen in the thoracic spine.
- Treatment is generally nonoperative bracing; however, surgical fusion may be indicated for patients with severe kyphosis.

Suggested Readings

Jagtap SA, Manuel D, Kesavdas C, et al. Scheuermann disease presenting as compressive myelopathy. *Neurology.* 2012;78:1279.

Rodriguez DP, Poussaint TY. Imaging of back pain in children. *AJNR.* 2010;31:787-802.

Breast cancer

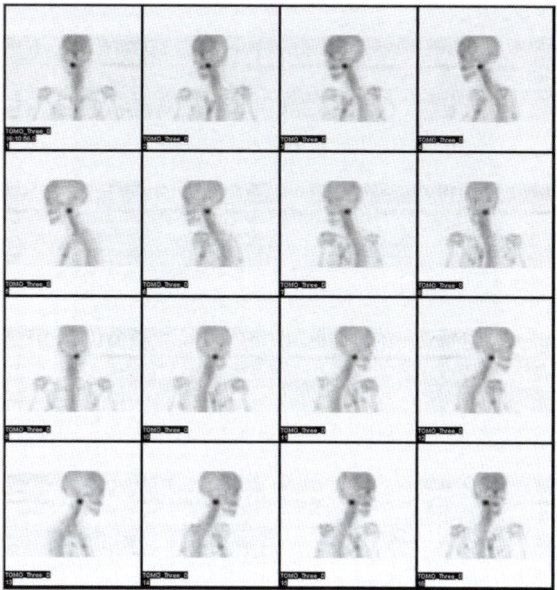

1. What should be included in the differential diagnosis of a vertebral body lesion in an adult?

2. What are common presenting symptoms?

3. What are the most common cancers to metastasize to bone?

4. What portions of the spinal column are most commonly affected?

5. What are the treatment options?

Case ranking/difficulty:

Category: Vertebral body

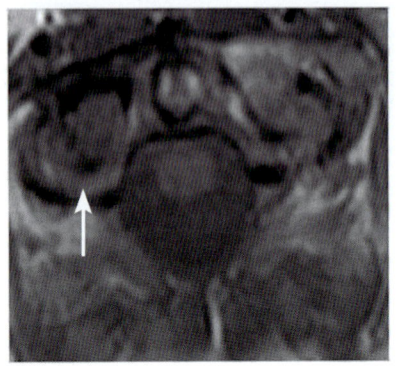

T1 hypointense lesion right lateral mass C1.

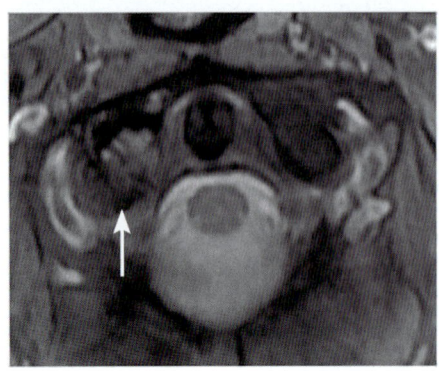

T2 hyperintense mass right lateral mass C1.

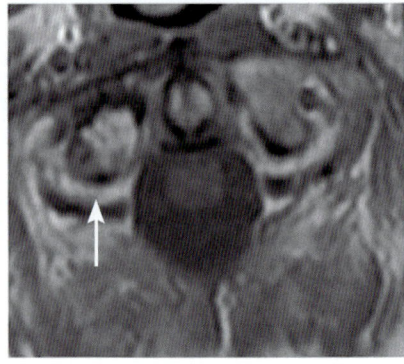

Enhancing mass right lateral mass C1.

Answers

1. Vertebral body lesions include hemangioma, multiple myeloma, metastasis, and infection. The diagnosis may be further complicated by the presence of a superimposed compression fracture.

2. Although nonspecific, one of the most common presentations of osseous metastatic disease is night pain, often severe enough to awaken the patient from sleep.

3. The top five cancers metastatic to bone are prostate, breast, lung, kidney, and thyroid.

4. Osseous metastatic lesions often involve the anterior and middle columns, while sparing the posterior elements.

5. A multimodality treatment approach is usually employed, including analgesia, chemotherapy, radiation/radiosurgery, and resection.

Pearls

- 20% of patients with a primary malignancy will develop symptomatic osseous metastatic lesions.
- Up to half of patients will have skeletal metastases diagnosed at autopsy.
- Treatment options for osseous metastatic lesions (in addition to treating the primary cancer) include radiation, stereotactic radiosurgery, or corpectomy/resection with fusion.
- If osseous metastatic lesions are identified, it is critical to evaluate for extraosseous extension, particularly into the epidural space.

Suggested Reading

Hage WD, Aboulafia AJ, Aboulafia DM. Incidence, location and diagnostic evaluation of metastatic bone disease. *Orthop Clin North Am.* 2000;31:515-528.

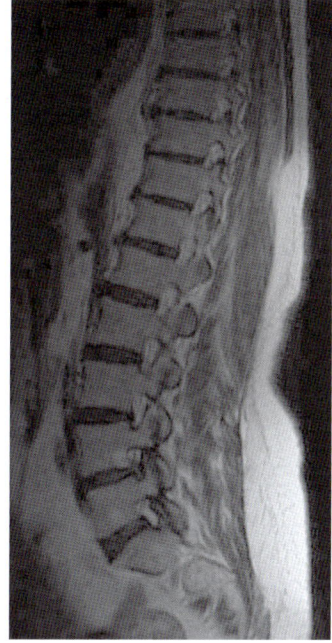 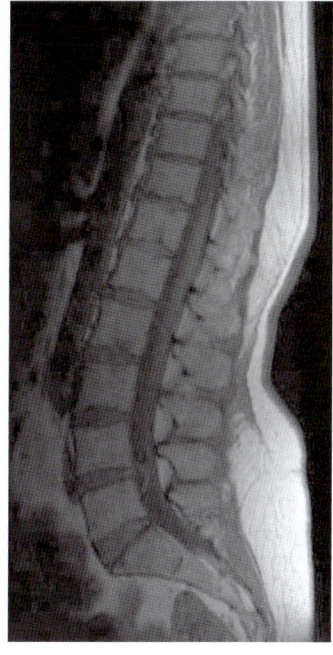 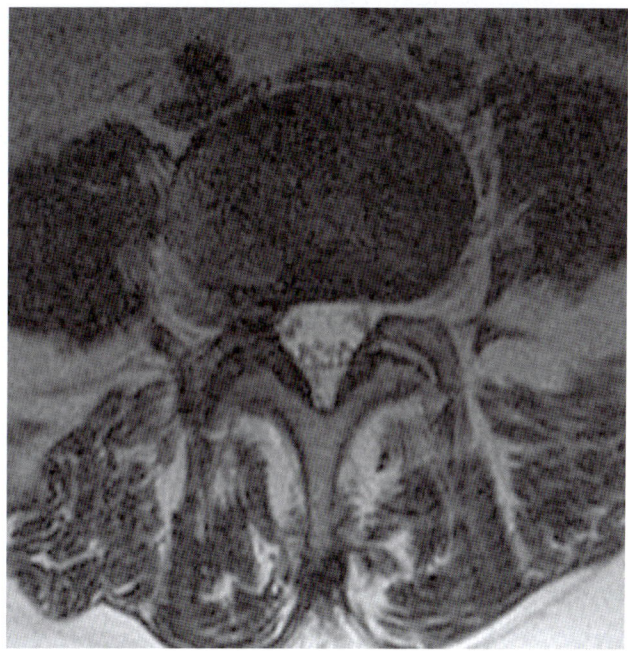

1. What is the most likely diagnosis?

2. What is meant by the term *protrusion*?

3. What is meant by a "focal" herniation?

4. What does the term *herniation* imply?

5. Which is the most common location of disc herniation?

Case ranking/difficulty:

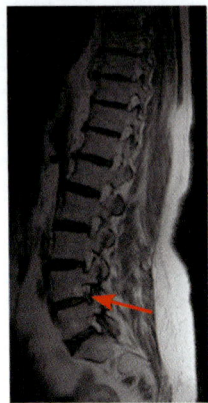

Sagittal T2-weighted sequence of the lumbar spine. There is a right foraminal disc protrusion (*arrow*) at L4-L5. The right L4 exiting nerve root is seen just caudal to the protrusion and the surrounding fat is effaced.

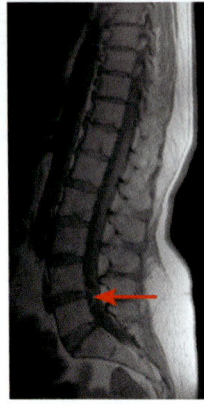

Sagittal T1-weighted sequence of the lumbar spine showing a disc protrusion (*arrow*) at L4-L5. The vertebral body heights and marrow signal are within normal limits.

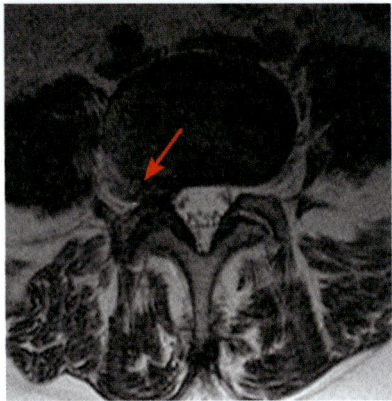

Axial T2-weighted image at the level of L4-L5 intervertebral disc showing a right foraminal disc protrusion (*arrow*). Note that the dome is smaller than the base of the herniation.

Answers

1. Disc "protrusion." In 1995 a multidisciplinary task force from the North American Spine Society recommended the use of a standardized nomenclature.

2. If the distance between the edges of the base of the disc herniation is larger than that between the edges of the herniated material, then it is termed a *protrusion* (ie, the base is wider than its dome). The herniated disc material beyond the disc space remains continuous with disc within the normal disc space.

3. Protrusions are further classified as "focal" or "broad based" depending on whether the base is less than 25% or between 25% and 50% of the circumference of the disc, respectively. Circumferential extension (50%-100%) of disc material beyond the vertebral ring apophysis is not considered a form of herniation and is termed disc bulging.

4. Herniation refers to the localized displacement of disc material (which includes the nucleus pulposus, annular tissue, fragmented apophyseal bone, cartilage, or any combination thereof) beyond the limits of the intervertebral disc space.

5. The axial plane is used to localize herniated discs and the following terminology is used:

    1) Central (Medial): Disc herniations are often slightly eccentric to the left or right as the posterior longitudinal ligament (PLL) is thickest centrally.
    2) Paramedian (Lateral recess): This is the most common location for disc herniations as the PLL is thinner in this region.
    3) Foraminal (Subarticular): Foraminal and extraforaminal herniations account for less than 10% of disc herniations. Herniation of disc material into the intervertebral foramen is often symptomatic due to compression of dorsal root ganglia.
    4) Extraforaminal (Lateral): Disc herniations in this region are uncommon.

Pearls

- Herniation refers to the localized displacement of disc material beyond the limits of the intervertebral disc space.
- If the distance between the edges of the base of the disc herniation is larger than that between the edges of the herniated material, then it is termed a *protrusion* (ie, the base is wider than its dome).
- Protrusions are further classified as "focal" or "broad based."

Suggested Readings

Fardon DF, Milette PC; Combined Task Forces of the North American Spine Society, American Society of Spine Radiology, American Society of Neuroradiology. Nomenclature and classification of lumbar disc pathology. Recommendations of the Combined task Forces of the North American Spine Society, American Society of Spine Radiology, and American Society of Neuroradiology. *Spine (Phila Pa 1976)*. 2001 Mar 1;26(5):E93-E113.

RF Costello, DP Beall. Nomenclature and standard reporting terminology of intervertebral disc herniation. *Magn Reson Imaging Clin N Am.* 2007;15:167-174.

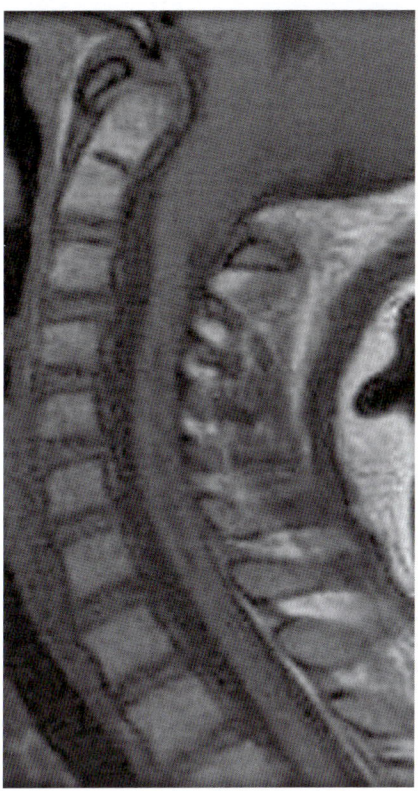 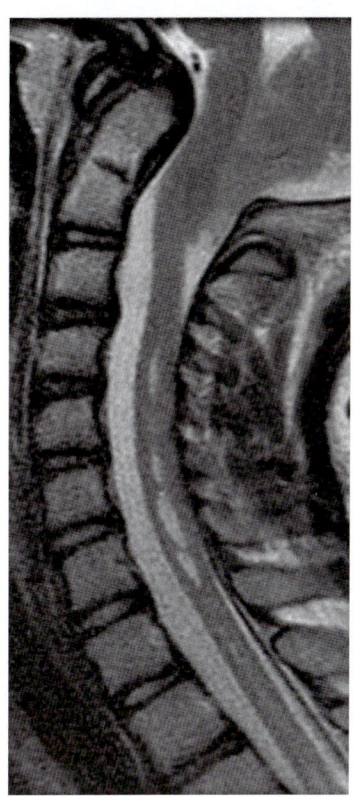

1. What are common presenting symptoms?

2. What are associated findings?

3. Where does syrinx formation most often occur?

4. What are the theoretical causes of this abnormality?

5. What are the treatment options?

Case ranking/difficulty:

Category: Spinal cord

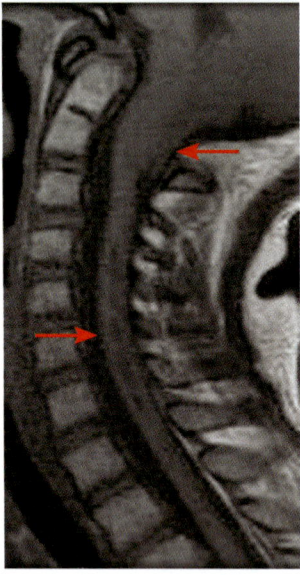

Sagittal T1 image demonstrating inferior displacement and elongation of cerebellar tissue with crowding at the foramen magnum and T1 hypointense fluid collection within the cervical cord.

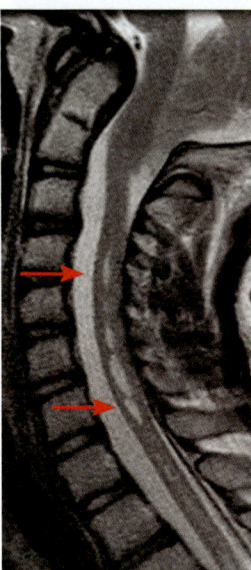

Sagittal T2 image demonstrates multiloculated T2 hyperintense fluid collection within the cervical cord.

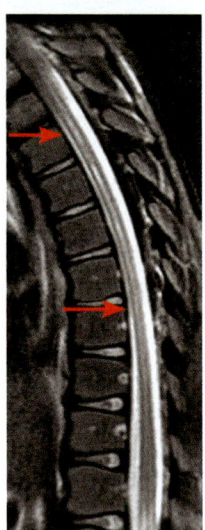

Sagittal T2 image demonstrates caudal extension of syrinx into the thoracic cord.

Answers

1. Symptoms include cough-induced headache, focal sensory loss, lower extremity spasticity, and back pain.

2. Findings in Chiari I malformation include short clivus, hydrocephalus, scoliosis, and platybasia.

3. While syrinx may occur at any level, it is most common at C4-C6.

4. The hydrodynamic/water hammer theory postulates that the low-lying cerebellar tonsils result in pressure forcing cerebrospinal fluid into the central canal. Another leading theory is the *cranial-spinal pressure dissociation* theory, which postulates that sudden changes in venous pressure force cerebrospinal fluid into the central canal.

5. Treatment is primarily directed at relieving the obstruction to flow at the foramen magnum with suboccipital craniectomy and posterior C1 resection; however, shunt placement may be needed in refractory cases, which may be placed within the ventricles or the syrinx itself.

Pearls

- While only 50% of patients with Chiari I malformation have an associated syrinx, up to 90% of symptomatic patients present with syrinx.
- Treatment of Chiari I malformations is primarily directed at relieving obstruction and improving flow dynamics at the foramen magnum.
- This is generally accomplished using a suboccipital craniectomy, and may be augmented by resection of the posterior arch of C1.
- Oftentimes, this will lead to decrease in size of the associated syrinx; however, in cases in which the syrinx is persistent with associated myelopathic symptoms, syringosubarachnoid shunts can be placed.

Suggested Readings

Oldfield EH, Muraszko KM, Shawker TH, Patronas NJ. Pathophysiology of syringomyelia associated with Chiari I malformation of the cerebellar tonsils. *J Neurosurg.* 1994;80:3-15.

Strahle J, Muraszko KM, Kapurch J, Bapuraj JR, Garton HJL, Maher CO. Chiari I malformation Type 1 and syrinx in children undergoing magnetic resonance imaging. *J Neurosurg Pediatrics.* 2011;8:205-213.

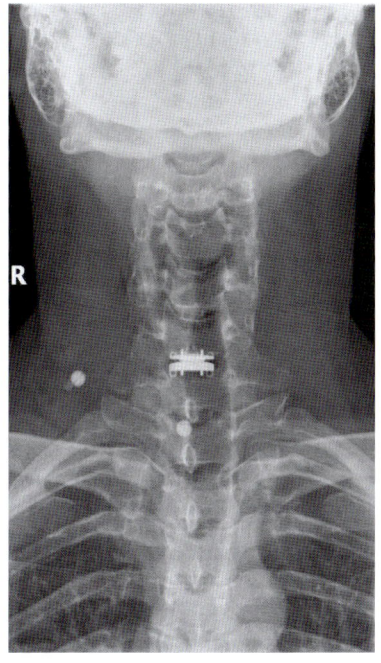 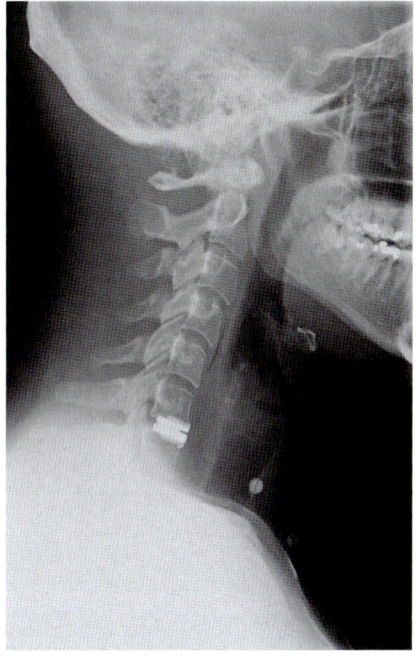 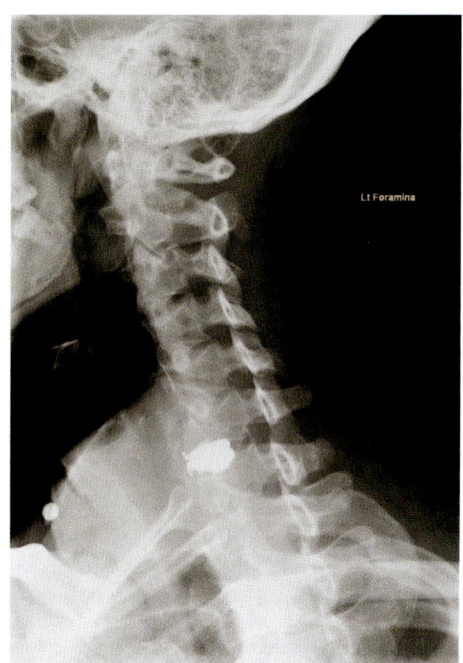

1. What is this procedure called?

2. Name some indications for this procedure.

3. What are the disadvantages of spinal fusion?

4. Name some contraindications to this procedure.

5. Describe ADR device characteristics and surgical implications.

Case ranking/difficulty: **Category:** Disc

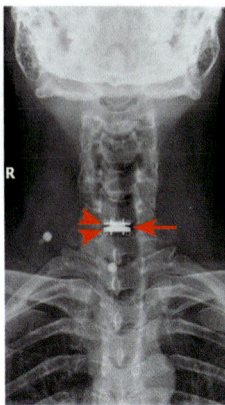

AP radiograph of the cervical spine. There is a prosthetic intervertebral disc between C6 and C7. The artificial disc comprises two metallic endplates (*arrowheads*) that are separated by a more pliable core (*arrow*).

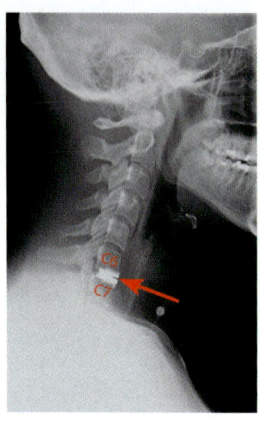

Lateral radiograph of the cervical spine demonstrates an artificial disc replacement (*arrow*) at C6-C7.

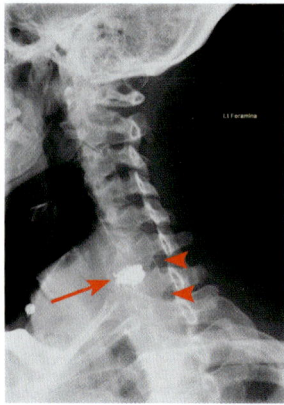

Oblique radiograph of the cervical spine shows a prosthetic disc in situ. The adjacent intervertebral foramina are widely patent.

Answers

1. Artificial disc replacement is a surgical procedure in which artificial mechanical devices are inserted to replace degenerated intervertebral discs in the cervical and lumbar spine.

2. It aims to improve or eliminate chronic, severe neck and back pain secondary to degenerative disc disease. It is an alternative to spinal fusion, which allows continued motion between the affected vertebral bodies and therefore prevents premature breakdown in adjacent spinal levels.

3. Disadvantages of spinal fusion include loss of motion and flexibility, which permanently alter the motion characteristics and biomechanics of the entire spinal column. It has been shown that spinal fusion causes accelerated degeneration of the intervertebral discs above and below the fused level.

4. Relative and absolute contraindications to the procedure include central or lateral recess stenosis, herniated nucleus pulposus with radiculopathy, osteoporosis, scoliosis, facet arthrosis, spondylolysis or spondylolisthesis, and deficiency of the posterior vertebral elements.

5. Depending on the prosthesis used the affected disc is either partially or fully excised. The artificial disc comprises two metallic endplates that are separated by a more pliable core. The latter is usually a plastic spacer made of a polyethylene core and is designed to simulate the biomechanical properties of the nucleus pulposus. The vertebral endplates and paraspinal ligaments are preserved during surgery, which helps maintain the stability of the spinal column. Single discs or several disc levels may be replaced during the same surgery. Artificial disc replacement only gained FDA approval for use in the United States in 2004.

Pearls

- Artificial disc replacement aims to improve or eliminate chronic, severe neck and back pain secondary to degenerative disc disease.
- The artificial disc comprises two metallic endplates that are separated by a more pliable core.
- Contraindications include central or lateral recess stenosis, herniated nucleus pulposus with radiculopathy, osteoporosis, scoliosis, facet arthrosis, spondylolysis or spondylolisthesis, and deficiency of the posterior vertebral elements.
- Single discs or several disc levels may be replaced during the same surgery.

Suggested Readings

Huang RC, Lim MR, Girardi FP, Cammisa FP Jr. The prevalence of contraindications to total disc replacement in a cohort of lumbar surgical patients. *Spine (Phila Pa 1976)*. 2004 Nov 15;29(22):2538-2541.

McDonald CP, Chang V, McDonald M, Ramo N, Bey MJ, Bartol S. Three-dimensional motion analysis of the cervical spine for comparison of anterior cervical decompression and fusion versus artificial disc replacement in 17 patients. *J Neurosurg Spine*. 2013 Dec 20.

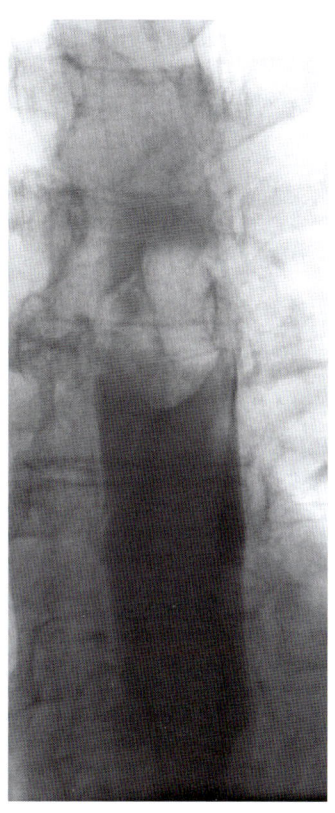 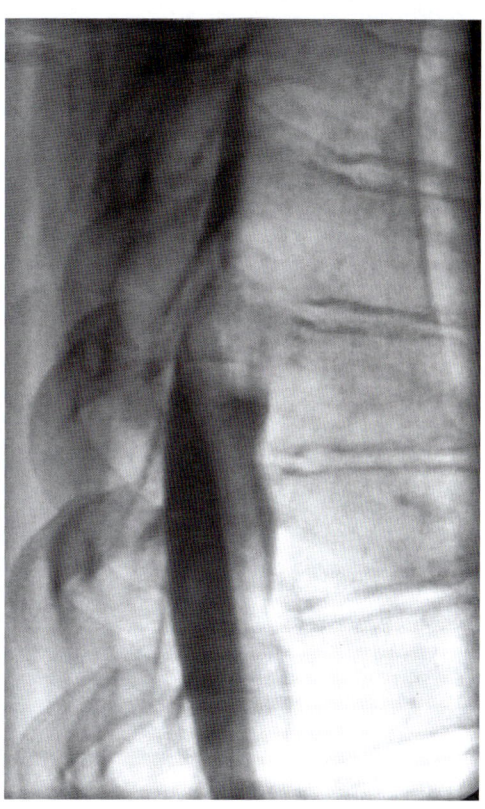

1. What are common imaging findings of this lesion?

2. A posterior position of an intradural extramedullary mass would support the diagnosis of which entity?

3. What is the classic imaging appearance?

4. What portion of the spine is most commonly affected?

5. What are the treatment options?

Case ranking/difficulty:

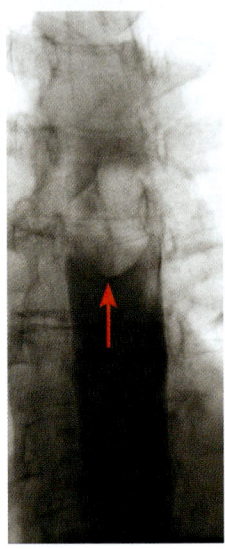

Frontal radiograph demonstrates focal meniscus at the cephalad edge of intrathecal contrast.

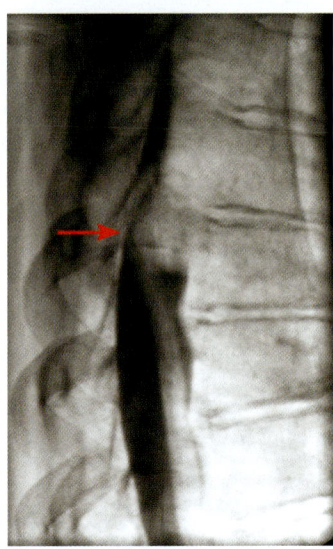

Lateral radiograph demonstrates filling defect in the anterior spinal canal with severe narrowing of the thecal sac.

Answers

1. Meningiomas are more likely to calcify than schwannomas, which are more likely to undergo cystic degeneration. Meningiomas are most common in the thoracic spine, but are overall rarer than intracranial meningiomas.

2. Nerve roots exit the spinal cord in the ventral spinal canal; therefore, a mass in the posterior intradural extramedullary space is unlikely to represent a nerve-based lesion and a meningioma would be favored.

3. Meningiomas are usually isointense to the spinal cord and demonstrate homogeneous enhancement and an enhancing dural tail. Calcification can occur; cystic degeneration is uncommon and favors a diagnosis of schwannoma.

4. Approximately 80% of meningiomas occur in the thoracic spine, followed by the lumbar and cervical spine.

5. Meningiomas are generally amenable to surgical resection with excellent outcomes. However, recurrence can occur if there is subtotal resection, especially in the case of an en plaque or infiltrative lesion and radiotherapy and/or radiosurgery can be considered.

Pearls

- Meningiomas are the second most common tumor of the extramedullary, intradural space.
- They are usually benign and do not present until symptoms of cord or nerve root compression develop.
- The classic imaging appearance is an extramedullary intradural mass with calcifications and an enhancing dural tail.
- Treatment is surgical resection; however, if the mass has been present for a long time, there may be secondary myelomalacia.

Suggested Readings

Beall DP, Googe, DJ, Emery RL, et al. Extramedullary intradural spinal tumors: a pictorial review. *Curr Probl Diagn Radiol*. 2007;36:185-226.

Lee JW, Lee IS, Choi K-U, et al. CT and MRI findings of calcified spinal meningiomas: correlation with pathological findings. *Skeletal Radiol*. 2010;39:345-352.

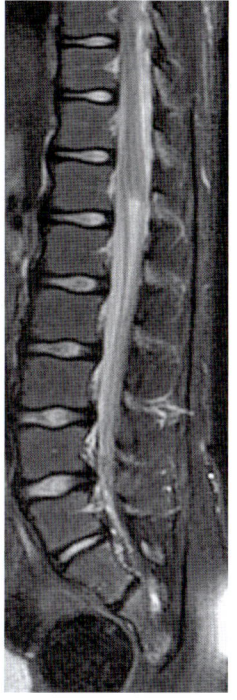 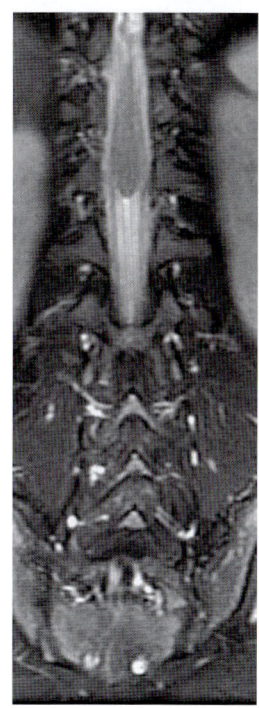

1. What should be included in the differential diagnosis?

2. What are common presenting symptoms?

3. What are potential causative factors?

4. What are differences between Group 1 and Group 2 patients?¡

5. What are the treatment options?

Case ranking/difficulty:

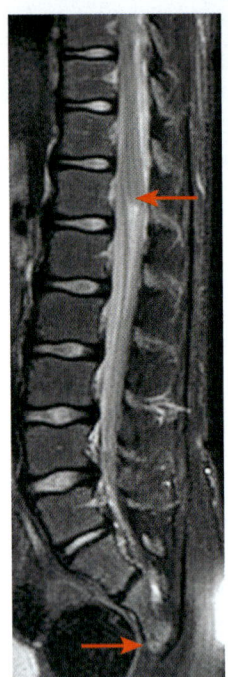

Sagittal T2 image demonstrates agenesis of the coccyx and lower sacrum with a blunted conus, terminating at the L1 level.

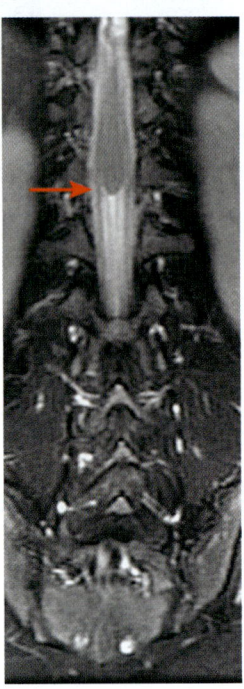

Coronal T2 image demonstrates a blunted conus, terminating at the L1 level.

Answers

1. The differential diagnosis includes tethered cord, myelomeningocele, and terminal lipoma.

2. Presenting symptoms include urinary incontinence, club feet, and lower extremity weakness. In addition, there are associated anomalies of the gastrointestinal and genitourinary tracts, as well as the heart.

3. The exact etiology is uncertain; however, there is a significant increase in incidence in offspring of diabetic mothers, particularly those who are insulin dependent. Other causative factors include vascular insult, toxic exposure, and maternal infection.

4. Group 1 patients are at the more severe end of the spectrum with more severe sacral agenesis. They uniformly have a high location of the conus, which is usually blunted or wedge shaped. Group 2 patients have less severe sacral anomalies and usually have normal to low-lying conus position with occasional tethering lesion.

5. If present, cord tethering should be released. Treatment is then directed at symptomatic lower extremity problems.

Pearls

- Caudal regression syndrome results from an insult prior to the fourth week of gestation.
- There are several etiologies postulated to cause these abnormalities, including hyperglycemia or ischemic insult.
- There is an association with maternal diabetes and VACTERL (Vertebral anomalies, Anorectal malformations, TracheoEsophageal fistulas, Renal, and Limb anomalies).
- While most cases are sporadic, there is an inherited form as well.
- Treatment is geared at untethering the cord (if present) with physical therapy for the lower extremities and treatment for associated incontinence.

Suggested Readings

Gehlot P, Mandliya J. Caudal regression syndrome. *IJBAS*. 2011;1:126-130.

Smith AS, Grable I, Levine D. Caudal regression syndrome in the fetus of a diabetic mother. *Radiology*. 2004;230:229-233.

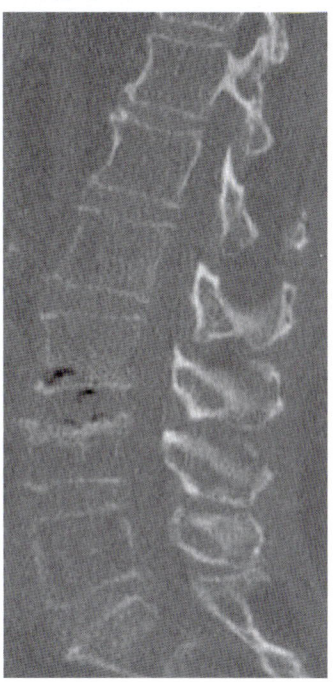 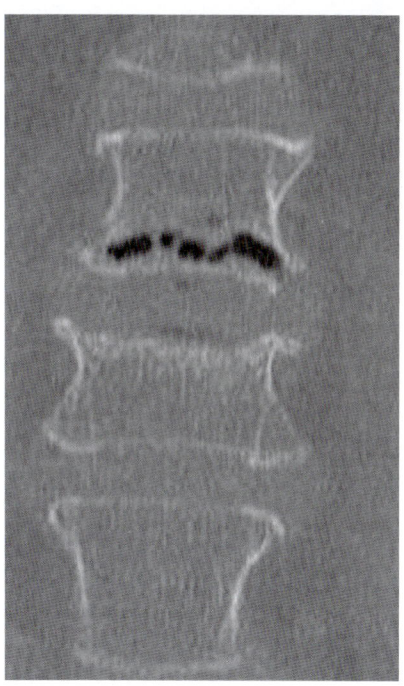

1. What should be included in the differential diagnosis?

2. What are common presenting symptoms?

3. Which location within the spine is most commonly affected?

4. What factors should be considered in selecting treatment options?

5. What are the treatment options?

Case ranking/difficulty:

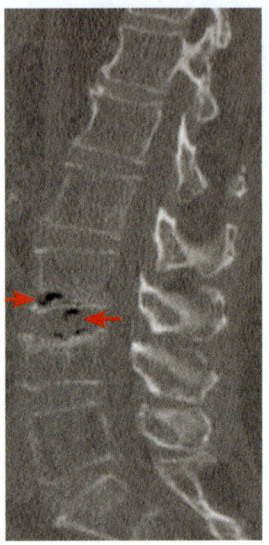

Sagittal CT image demonstrates vacuum disc at L3-L4 with extension into the inferior endplate of L3.

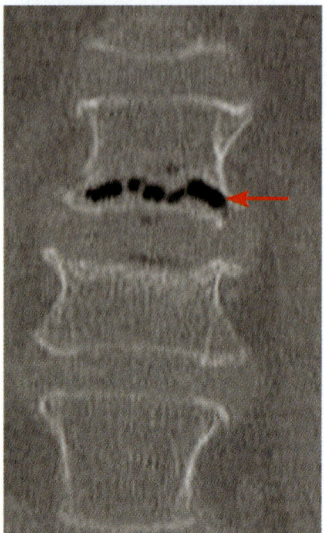

Coronal CT image demonstrates gas within the L3 vertebral body adjacent the inferior endplate.

Answers

1. The differential diagnosis includes infection, Kummell disease, and Schmorl node.

2. The most common presentation is back pain and kyphosis. Presence of bowel and bladder dysfunction, myelopathy, and radiculopathy implies compromise of the spinal canal.

3. The thoracic and lumbar spine are most commonly affected.

4. Patient age, degree of kyphosis, level of disability, pain level, and neurological compromise should all be considered in deciding on treatment options.

5. Potential treatment options include conservative management, analgesia, bracing, and vertebroplasty.

Pearls

- Kummell disease is avascular necrosis of the vertebral body, which often starts in a delayed fashion following trauma.
- The imaging hallmark is the presence of a gas-filled cleft within the vertebral body.

- In this case, there is a compression deformity of the L4 vertebral body; however, the L3 vertebral body height is maintained.
- Given the intrabody air, this vertebra is at high risk for collapse, which can lead to a painful kyphosis.
- Patients tend to be elderly osteopenic women who present with painful focal kyphosis.
- The presence of gas within the vertebral body makes pathologic fracture much less likely.
- Treatment can consist of conservative management and analgesia, to vertebroplasty/kyphoplasty or fusion.

Suggested Readings

Kim SW, Kim H-S. A case of posterior element fracture in Kummell's disease. *Osteoporos Int.* 2012;23:1641-1644.

Ma R, Chow R, Shen FH. Kummell's disease: delayed post-traumatic osteonecrosis of the vertebral body. *Eur Spine J.* 2010;19:1065-1070.

Chronic neck pain with upper extremity weakness

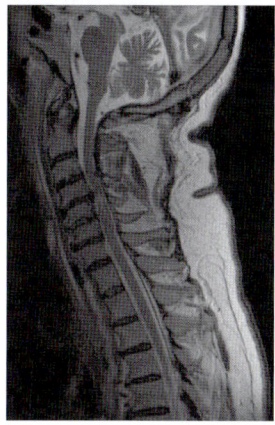 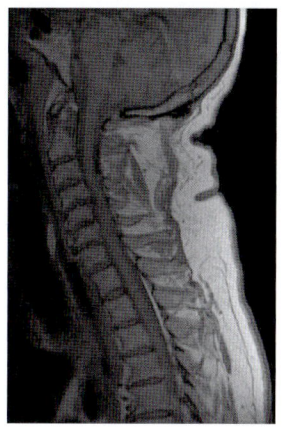 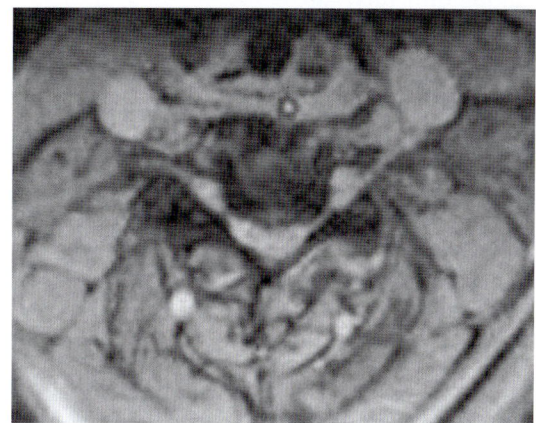

1. What is the most likely diagnosis?

2. How does the condition usually manifest?

3. What should be included in the differential diagnosis?

4. Which imaging modality best images the condition?

5. Which treatments may be beneficial in this condition?

Case ranking/difficulty:

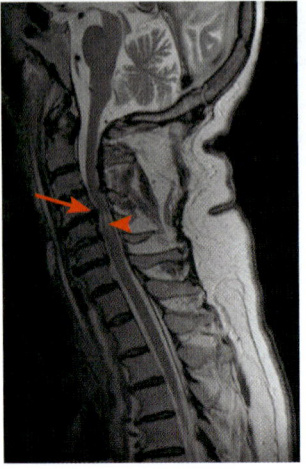

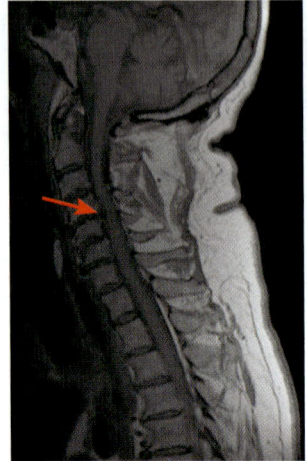

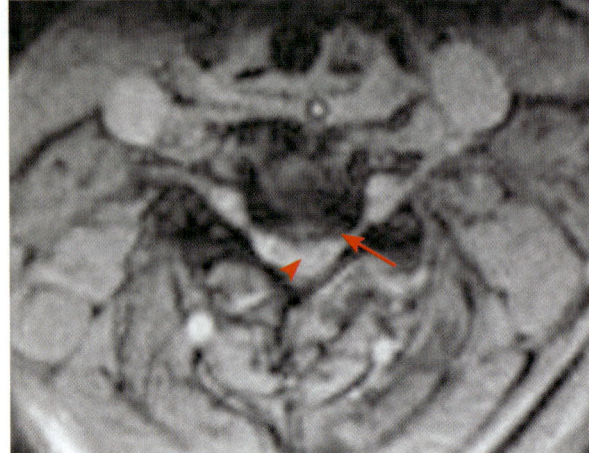

Sagittal T2-weighted sequence of the cervical spine demonstrates degenerative changes in the mid and lower cervical spine. There is a disc/osteophyte protrusion at C4-C5 (*arrow*) that impinges the cervical cord. Intramedullary high signal intensity (*arrowhead*) is noted at C5 level in keeping with cervical spondylotic myelopathy.

Sagittal T1-weighted sequence of the cervical cord. Note a prominent disc/osteophyte bar at C4-C5 (*arrow*) that projects posteriorly into the spinal canal. The associated cord signal abnormality is not appreciated on this sequence.

Axial T2-weighted sequence at the level of C4-C5 intervertebral disc. There is a broad-based disc/osteophyte protrusion (*arrow*) that impinges the cervical cord and results in moderate canal stenosis. Increased intramedullary signal intensity is also noted (*arrowhead*).

altered intramedullary signal intensity particularly on T2-weighted images.

5. Conservative measures aim at providing symptomatic relief and include physical therapy, cervical immobilization, systemic and epidural steroids, and pain relief. Surgery, on the other hand, aims at preventing further neurological deterioration and may achieve some functional recovery.

Answers

1. Cervical spondylotic myelopathy refers to spondylotic changes within the cervical spine that result in neurologic deficits due to cervical cord injury.

2. Affected individuals often present with cervical neck pain, stiffness, and crepitus, which may be associated with or predate brachialgia, upper extremity weakness, and impaired dexterity, and is later followed by neurological dysfunction in the lower limbs. Sensory loss occurs below the affected spinal level and typically results in pain and temperature disturbances with relative sparing of proprioception, vibration, and touch. Gait abnormalities (broad-based, hesitant, shuffling gait) and bowel and bladder instability result from involvement of the long tracts of the cord.

3. Myelopathy could be secondary to causes other than spondylotic including extradural compression of the cord by hemorrhage, abscess formation, and neoplasia. Other causes include inflammatory conditions, vascular disease, drug intoxication, autoimmune conditions, previous trauma, and metabolic abnormalities.

4. Unlike radiography and CT that can only demonstrate cervical spondylotic changes, MRI can evaluate directly the cervical neural structures. It allows for direct visualization of cord impingement and can demonstrate

Pearls

- Cervical spondylotic myelopathy refers to spondylotic changes within the cervical spine, which result in neurologic deficits due to cervical cord injury.
- A clinically symptomatic dysfunction of the cervical cord and radiological demonstration of cord impingement or compression are required to make the diagnosis.
- Several conditions may mimic CSM, and therefore the clinical diagnosis is usually not straightforward.
- Newer techniques like diffusion tensor imaging promise to increase the sensitivity for detecting CSM.

Suggested Readings

König SA, Spetzger U.Surgical management of cervical spondylotic myelopathy—indications for anterior, posterior or combined procedures for decompression and stabilisation. *Acta Neurochir (Wien)*. 2014 Feb;156(2):253-258.

Miyazaki T, Sudo H, Hiratsuka S, Iwasaki N. Cervical spondylotic myelopathy with subacute combined degeneration. *Spine J*. 2014 Feb 1;14(2):381-382.

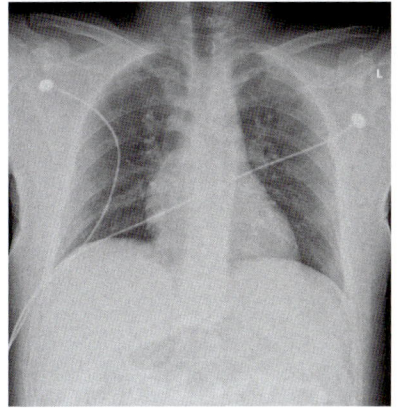 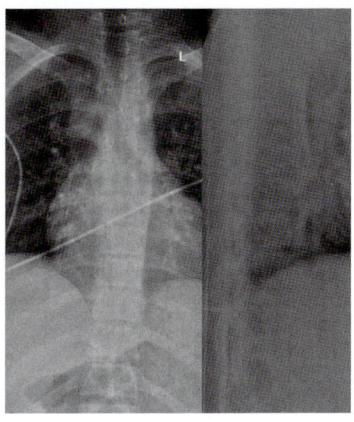 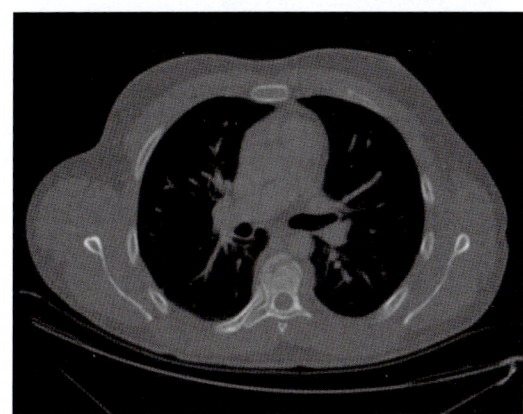

1. What are thoracic paraspinal lines?

2. What is the importance of this soft tissue sign?

3. Describe the radiological appearance of both the right and left paraspinal lines.

4. How often are thoracic paraspinal lines seen?

5. Name some causes of displacement or bulging of thoracic paraspinal lines.

Case ranking/difficulty:

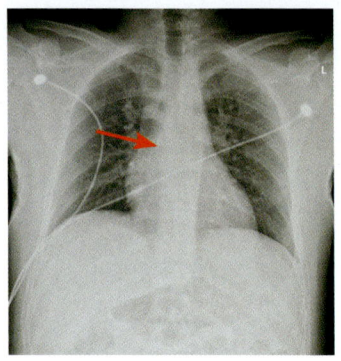

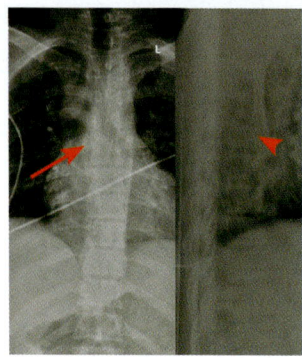

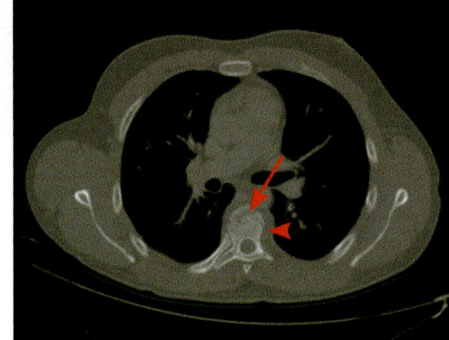

Posteroanterior (PA) chest radiograph in a patient involved in a motor vehicle accident. There is an abnormal focal bulge of the right paraspinal line (*arrow*) at the level of T6 vertebral body. Otherwise the lungs are clear and there are no pleural effusions.

Dedicated thoracic spine radiographs (AP and lateral) were taken, which confirmed the abnormal right paraspinal bulge and a possible upper endplate fracture of T6.

Axial CT scan at the level of T6 shows a wedge fracture of T6 vertebral body (*arrow*) with an associated paraspinal hematoma (*arrowhead*).

Answers

1. Thoracic paraspinal lines (TPL) are a feature of frontal chest radiographs and are formed by the interface between the lungs and posterior mediastinal soft tissues.

2. The ability to recognize soft tissue signs on the chest radiograph can provide valuable clues to spinal and paraspinal pathology. The lines should therefore not be overlooked as they may reveal potentially serious traumatic injuries or posterior mediastinal abnormalities. A localized bulge or diffuse displacement of the thoracic paraspinal lines without an obvious incidental explanation should therefore alert the radiologist of these possibilities and further imaging may be warranted.

3. The left paraspinal line extends from the arch of the aorta to the diaphragm (sometimes extends below it) and lies medial to the lateral aortic wall. Occasionally, it may be seen lateral to the descending thoracic aorta.

    The right paraspinal line is seen as a straight vertical line just lateral to T8 through T12 vertebral levels, and projects below the diaphragm. The lines can be better appreciated on computed tomography.

4. The left paraspinal line is seen in about 35% of chest radiographs and is seen more commonly than its right counterpart, which is only seen in 25% of examinations.

5. Displacement or bulging of paraspinal lines may be due to several etiologies including degenerative change in the thoracic spine, posterior mediastinal lesions (eg, lymphadenopathy, neurogenic tumors, extramedullary hematopoiesis, esophageal pathology, descending thoracic aortic aneurysm, granuloma formation,

and metastatic deposits), abscess formation, and posttraumatic hematoma. The latter three entities are often associated with changes in the adjacent vertebrae, which should therefore be assessed thoroughly. Extensive mediastinal fat in Cushing disease and obese patients may also displace the paraspinal lines.

Pearls

- Thoracic paraspinal lines (TPL) are a feature of frontal chest radiographs and are formed by the interface between the lungs and posterior mediastinal soft tissues.
- Displacement or bulging of paraspinal lines may be due to several etiologies including degenerative changes in the thoracic spine, posterior mediastinal lesions, abscess formation, and posttraumatic hematoma.
- Abnormal thoracic paraspinal lines should not be overlooked as they may reveal potentially serious traumatic injuries or posterior mediastinal abnormalities.

Suggested Readings

Casullo J, Fallone BG. On the perception of the left thoracic paraspinal line. *Acad Radiol.* 1995 Mar;2(3):215-221.

Gupta SK, Mohan V. The thoracic paraspinal line: further signficance. *Clin Radiol.* 1979 May;30(3):329-335.

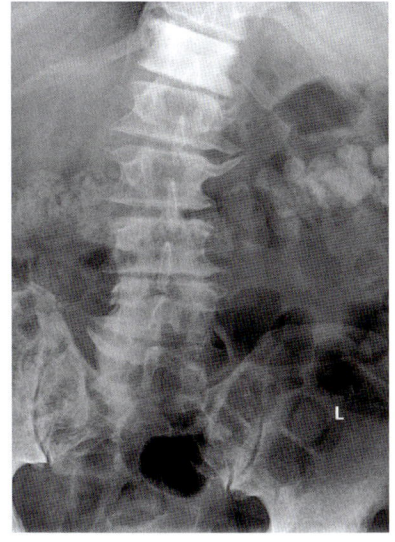 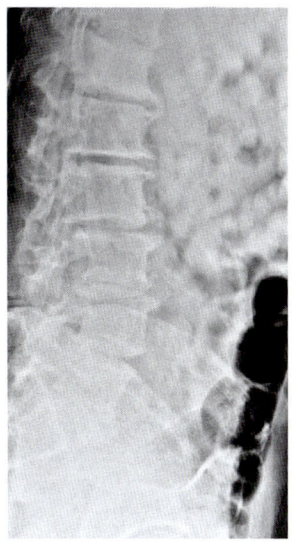 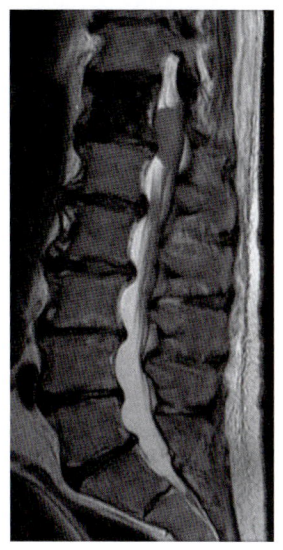 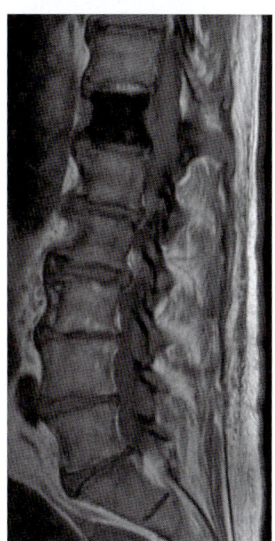

1. What is this radiological finding called?

2. Name some common causes in adults.

3. Name some common causes in children.

4. Describe the typical imaging findings.

5. How can the differential diagnoses be narrowed down?

Case ranking/difficulty:

Category: Vertebral body

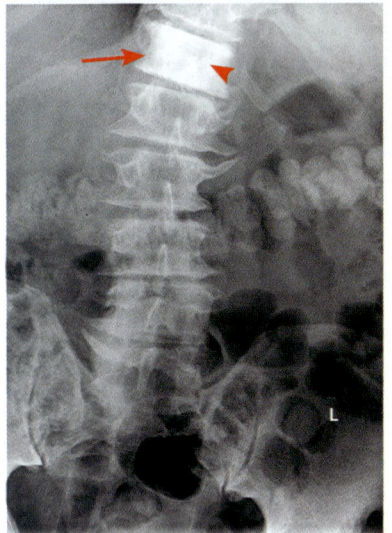 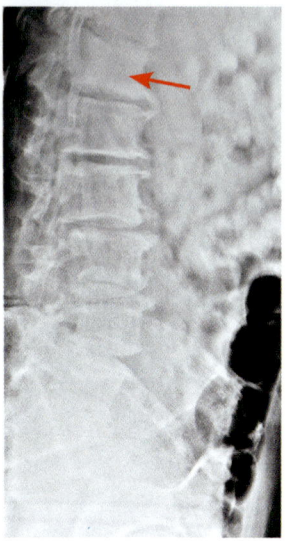 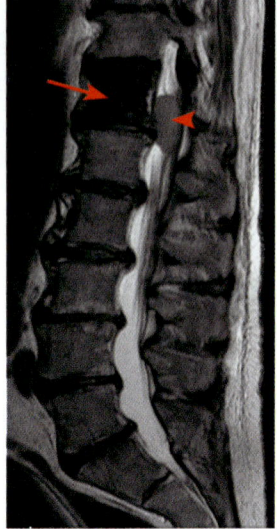 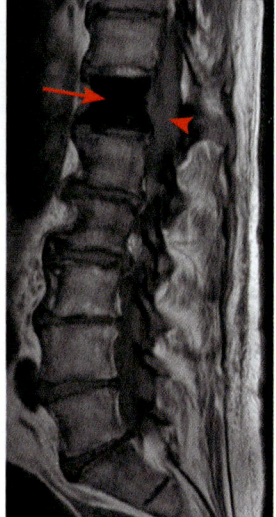

AP radiograph of the lumbar spine. There is a homogenously dense T12 vertebral body (*arrow*) that retains its normal size and contours without change in the adjacent intervertebral discs. The pedicles are not identified in the affected vertebra (*arrowhead*) due to overlapping sclerosis. Appearances are compatible with an "ivory vertebra."

Lateral radiograph of the lumbar spine. Again seen is diffuse sclerosis affecting T12 vertebral body (*arrow*) with no vertebral expansion or cortical destruction. The adjacent discs are not affected.

Sagittal T2-weighted sequence of the lumbar spine. T12 vertebral body (*arrow*) appears very hypointense in keeping with extensive sclerosis. Also note an incidental oval-shaped lesion in the spinal canal (*arrowhead*), which was confirmed to be a meningioma.

Sagittal T1-weighted sequence of the lumbar spine. The normal high signal of the fatty bone marrow is replaced by extensive sclerosis in T12 vertebral body (*arrow*) and appears very hypointense. Again seen in an incidental meningioma (*arrowhead*).

Answers

1. An "ivory vertebra" refers to a solitary homogenously dense vertebral body that otherwise retains its normal size and contours without change in the adjacent intervertebral discs. It was first described by Souques in 1925.

2. In adults, the most common causes are osteoblastic metastases (particularly from breast and prostate carcinoma), lymphoma, infection, post-radiation necrosis, and Paget disease of bone. Less commonly chordoma, SAPHO syndrome, sarcoma, and diffuse condensing osteosis may be responsible.

3. In children, lymphoma, osteosarcoma, osteoblastoma, and metastasis (from neuroblastoma, medulloblastoma and Ewing sarcoma) are often responsible.

4. The affected vertebra appears as a sclerotic dense vertebra with possible involvement of the posterior elements. The vertebral body is not expanded and its contours are preserved. Similar changes are noted on computed tomography where diffuse sclerotic change is seen to involve most of the vertebral body. MRI reveals T1 low signal intensity within the affected vertebral body, which replaces the normal hyperintense fatty bone marrow. The vertebra may demonstrate high signal

intensity on STIR. The affected vertebra may show increased radiotracer uptake on scintigraphy.

5. A thorough clinical history, physical examination, and serological tests may help narrow down the differential diagnoses as some of these are systemic conditions.

Pearls

- An "ivory vertebra" refers to a solitary homogenously dense vertebral body that otherwise retains its normal size and contours without change in the adjacent intervertebral discs.

Suggested Readings

Clifford PD, Jose J. Ivory vertebra sign. *Am J Orthop (Belle Mead NJ)*. 2010 Aug;39(8):400-402.

Graham TS. The ivory vertebra sign. *Radiology*. 2005 May;235(2):614-615.

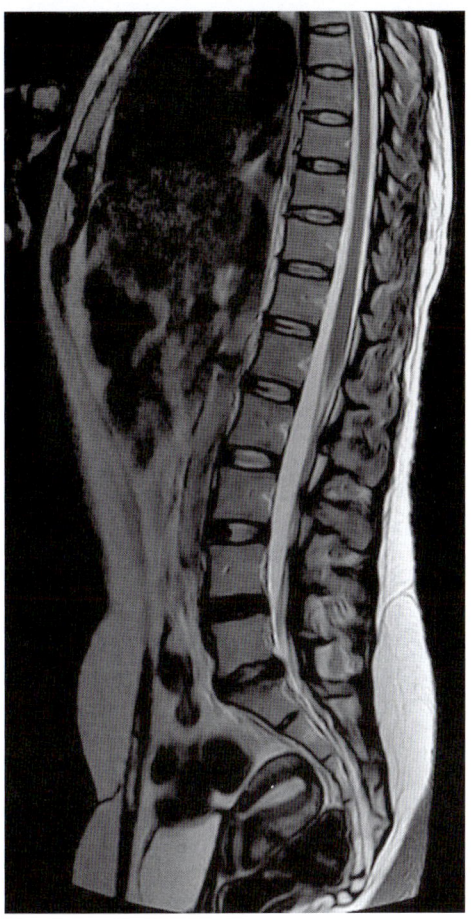 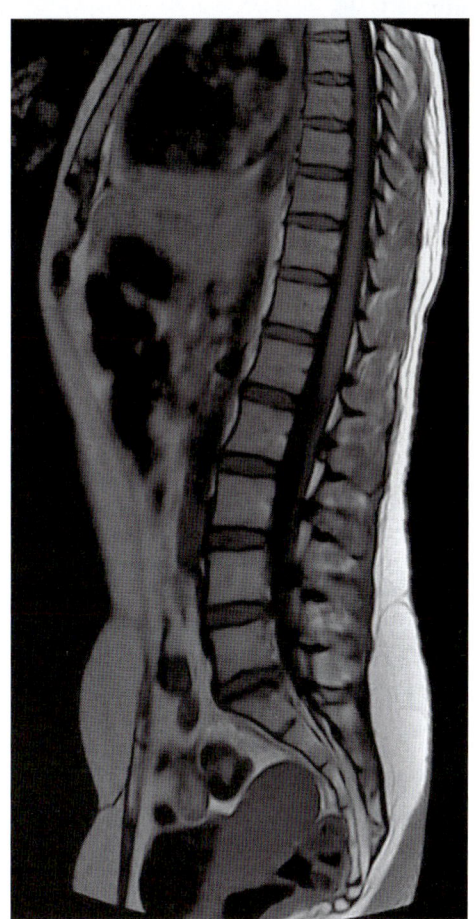

1. What is the most likely diagnosis?

2. What is meant by disc degenerative changes?

3. Describe clinical and genetic implications of this condition.

4. What MRI changes may be seen in this condition?

5. What is the etiology of loss of disc height?

Case ranking/difficulty:

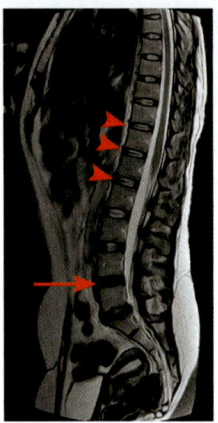

Sagittal T2-weighted sequence of the lumbar spine shows a hypointense intervertebral disc (*arrow*) at L4-L5 with loss of distinction between the inner and outer parts of the disc (Grade 4). A "sandwich-like" configuration of the discs with low signal intensity bands (Grade 2) is also noted (*arrowheads*) at the more cranial levels. Disc degeneration with a small protrusion is also noted at L5/S1.

Answers

1. Disc desiccation is a very common degenerative change of intervertebral discs. It is usually the earliest sign of more severe disc degenerate changes.

2. Intervertebral discs show degenerative changes earlier than other connective tissues in the body. Disc degeneration may manifest as disc space narrowing, altered signal intensity on MRI, annular tears, Schmorl nodes, disc bulging, protrusion, extrusion, and sequestration.

3. The incidence of disc desiccation increases with age and is often considered as a natural process of aging. Pathologically, the hydrophilic glycosaminoglycans within the nucleus pulposus are replaced with fibrocartilage, which reduces the flexibility of the disc. Desiccation affects particularly mobile sections of the spine and is hence most commonly observed in the cervical and lumbar levels.

4. On MRI, the central T2 hyperintensity within the disc is lost and the horizontal midline hypointense cleft can no longer be appreciated.

   Several classifications have been proposed to quantify the extent of disc desiccation. One such classification has five grades as follows:

   I—The nucleus pulposus is homogeneously hyperintense and clearly distinct from the hypointense annular fibers.

   II—The nucleus pulposus is inhomogeneous with horizontal low signal bands in a sandwich-like configuration.

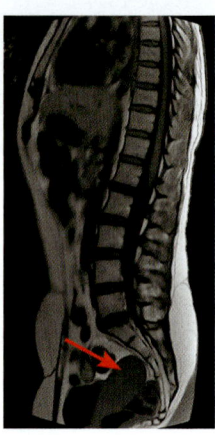

Sagittal T1-weighted sequence of the lumbar spine. The vertebral body heights and marrow signal are within normal limits. Incidental note is made of a retroverted uterus (*arrow*).

   III—The inner parts of the disc are of inhomogeneous intermediate signal intensity.

   IV—The central parts of the disc are of intermediate to low signal intensity with loss of distinction between the inner and outer parts of disc.

   V—Disc collapse.

5. It has been shown that loss of intervertebral disc height is secondary to annular bulging and bowing of the vertebral endplates rather than a reduction in the nucleus pulposus volume.

Pearls

- Pathologically, the hydrophilic glycosaminoglycans within the nucleus pulposus are replaced with fibrocartilage, which reduces the flexibility of the disc.
- Desiccation affects particularly mobile sections of the spine and is hence most commonly observed in the cervical and lumbar levels.
- On MRI, the central T2 hyperintensity within the disc is lost and the horizontal midline hypointense cleft can no longer be appreciated.

Suggested Readings

Alomari RS, Corso JJ, Chaudhary V, Dhillon G. Computer-aided diagnosis of lumbar disc pathology from clinical lower spine MRI. *Int J Comput Assist Radiol Surg*. 2010 May;5(3):287-293.

Dähnert W. *Radiology Review Manual*. Philadelphia, PA: Lippincott Williams Wilkins; 2007.

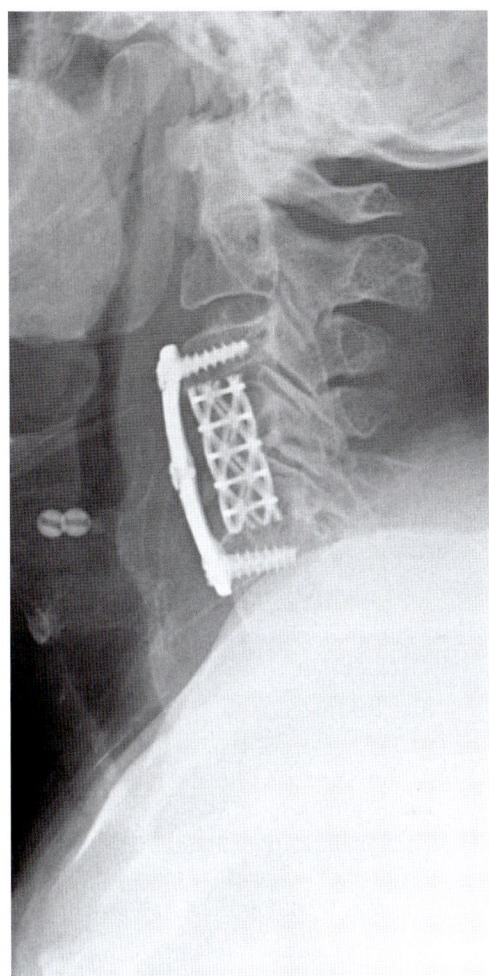
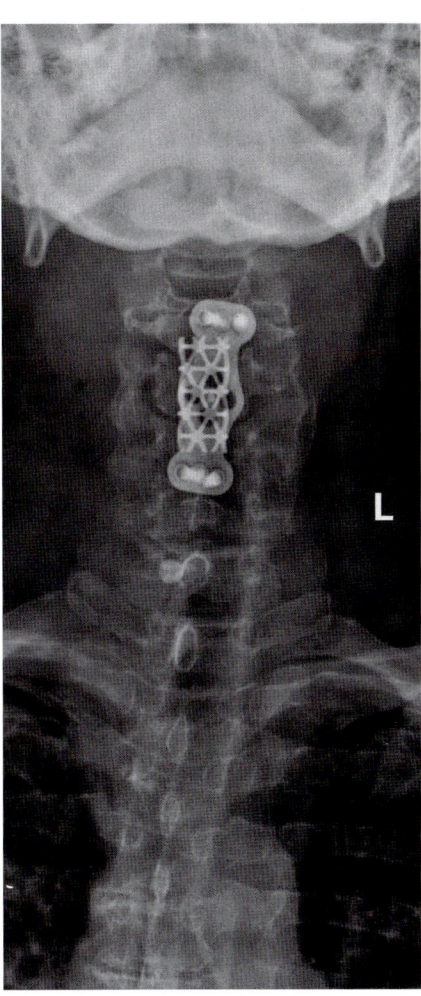

1. What is this procedure called?

2. Describe VBR device characteristics and their surgical implications.

3. Name some disadvantages of carbon fiber devices.

4. What are the objectives of surgical treatment for spinal tumors?

5. Name some recognized complications of this procedure?

Case ranking/difficulty:

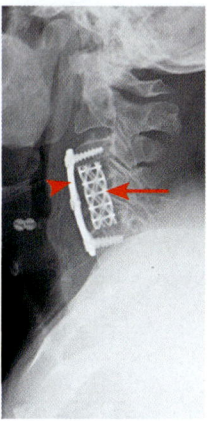

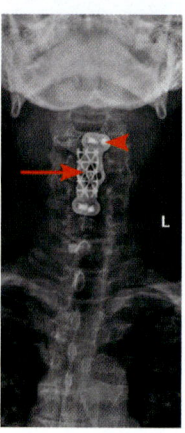

Lateral radiograph of the cervical spine. There is a vertebral body replacement (VBR) device in situ at C4 (*arrow*). The device spans the interbody distance between C3 and C5 and its edges abut the endplates of the respective vertebrae. Anterior fixation of the spine (*arrowhead*) is seen as this device was not designed for use as a standalone device.

Anteroposterior radiograph of the cervical spine. A VBR device (*arrow*) is seen at C4 level. Anterior spinal instrumentation is also noted (*arrowhead*).

Answers

1. Vertebral body replacement refers to the use of prosthetic devices to replace collapsed, damaged, or unstable vertebral bodies due to tumor or trauma.

2. VBR devices come in a variety of lengths, widths, and heights to accommodate most patient anatomies. Others can be set to the required settings during surgery and may have an expansion range enough to replace one or two vertebral bodies.

   Although implant devices may have fixed degrees of lordosis, some have an advanced endplate design, which allows for in situ angulation of up to 10° during surgery in order to precisely match the patient's anatomic need.

   A variety of materials have been used in the construction of vertebral body implants, which include titanium cages and meshes, ceramic, ceramic/glass, and carbon fiber.

   Some titanium mesh cages have spikes at their end tips and sharp edges that allow them to be anchored into the adjacent vertebral bodies. This provides extra torsional stability. Most expandable cages are not designed for use as a standalone device, and therefore anterior (with or without additional posterior) instrumentation is required.

3. Carbon fiber has the advantage of being radiolucent and therefore allows better postoperative fusion assessment. However, carbon fiber implants have several disadvantages including inflammatory responses with possible foreign body reactions, material brittleness that can result in breakage, as well as composite material failure.

4. The objectives of surgical treatment for spine tumors include pain amelioration, decompression of the neural elements, spinal stabilization, and wide resection of the primary or metastatic tumors.

5. Complications of vertebral body replacement may result from either the surgical approach or the placement of spinal instrumentation. These include hemorrhage secondary to vascular injury, infection, injury to internal organs, the lumbosacral plexus, and the sympathetic chain.

   Most manufacturers recommend annual radiographic assessment and pain assessment scores in order to detect loss of device height and implant failure.

Pearls

- Vertebral body replacement refers to the use of prosthetic devices to replace collapsed, damaged, or unstable vertebral bodies due to tumor or trauma.
- Several implants with different specifications and characteristics have been devised and are available on the market.

Suggested Readings

Daentzer D, Bianchi N, Böker DK, Deinsberger W. Multilevel segmental interbody fusion versus vertebral body replacement: comparison of two operative methods. *Orthopade*. 2013 Dec 19.

Rohlmann A, Dreischarf M, Zander T, Graichen F, Bergmann G. Loads on a vertebral body replacement during locomotion measured in vivo. *Gait Posture*. 2013 Oct 19.

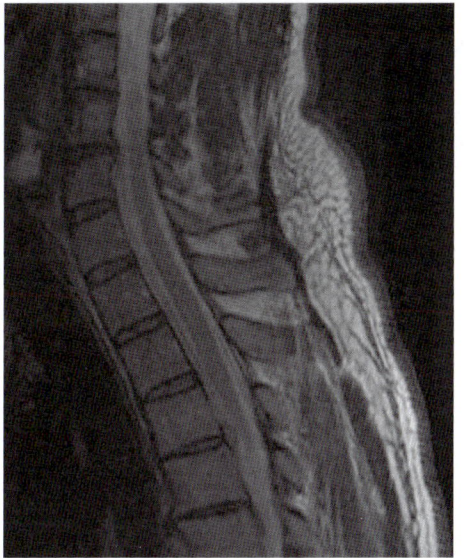
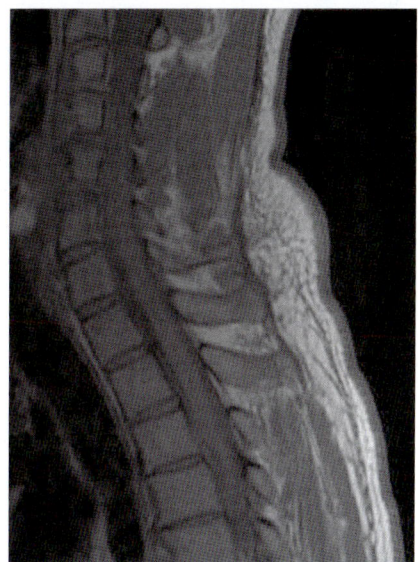

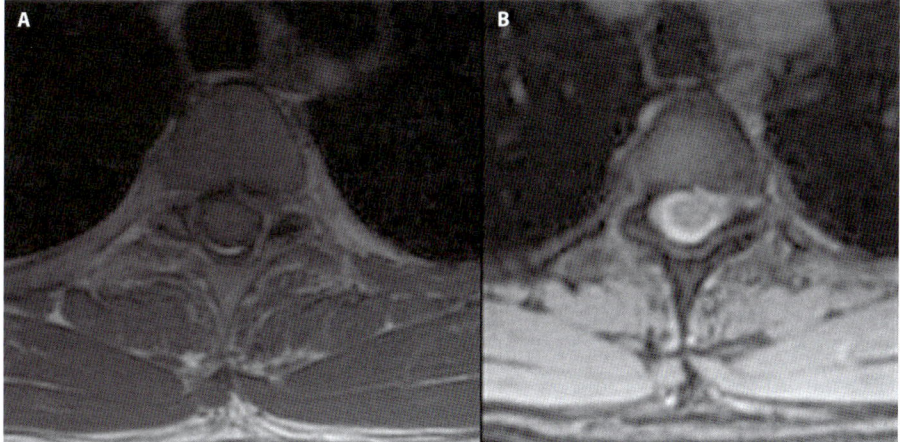

1. What is the most likely diagnosis?

2. Where do most disc herniations occur?

3. Name subdivisions of this condition.

4. What is the etiology of this condition?

5. Integrity of which anatomical structure is used
   to differentiate "contained" from "uncontained"
   disc herniations?

Case ranking/difficulty:

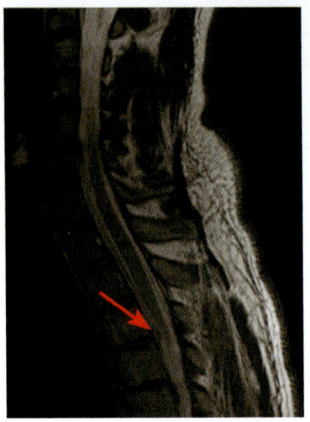

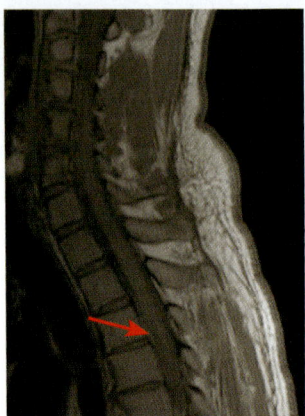

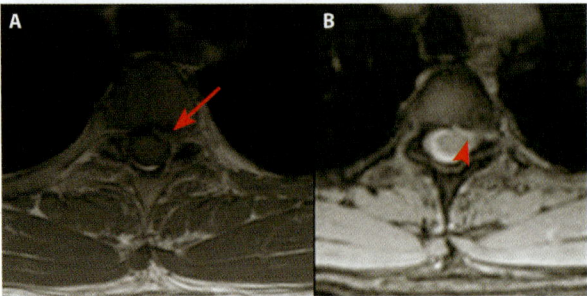

Axial images at the level of T3-T4. There is a paracentral disc herniation (*arrow*, panel A) filling the left lateral recess and displacing the dural sac (*arrowhead*, panel B) medially.

Sagittal T2-weighted sequence of the cervical and upper thoracic spine. There is disc herniation (*arrow*) at T3-T4 intervertebral disc space that is of the same signal intensity as the nucleus pulposus. The herniated material is contained posteriorly by the posterior longitudinal ligament (PLL). Note is also made of mild degenerative changes in the lower cervical spine.

Sagittal T1-weighted sequence of the cervical and upper thoracic spine. Note that the herniated material (*arrow*) follows the same signal intensity as the central part of the intervertebral disc and represents herniated nucleus pulposus. There is mild loss of the affected intervertebral disc height.

The term is not synonymous with ruptured disc, which is equivalent to disc herniation.

5. Intervertebral disc herniations are also characterized as "contained" when the displaced disc material is covered by the intact outer annulus and "uncontained" when such covering is absent. Although the disc material may still be covered by the posterior longitudinal ligament (PLL) and the peridural membranes, the term *uncontained* is still recommended if the outer annulus is breeched.

Answers

1. The annulus fibrosus is composed of 15-20 consecutive rings called laminae composed of type 1 collagen, which run obliquely to span the distance between adjacent vertebrae. The direction of such fibers alternates between one lamina and another with their orientation with respect to the vertical being approximately 65°-70°. The inner portion of the annulus fibrosus is composed of weaker fibrocartilage that blends gradually with the central nucleus pulposus.

2. The annulus is thinner and the collagen fibers are more disorganized posterolaterally, rendering this part of the disc weaker. The latter accounts for the increased risk of disc herniation posterolaterally.

3. Annulus fibrosus ruptures may be further subdivided into circumferential or radial ruptures.

4. In 1995, a multidisciplinary task force from the North American Spine Society addressed the lack of standardization in the terminology of intervertebral disc disorders and recommended a nomenclature for use in clinical practice.

   Rupture of the annulus refers to disruption of the annulus fibrosus and the term implies a posttraumatic etiology.

Pearls

- Rupture of the annulus refers to disruption of the annulus fibrosus and the term implies a posttraumatic etiology.
- Annulus fibrosus ruptures may be further subdivided into circumferential or radial ruptures.

Suggested Readings

Fardon DF, Milette PC; Combined Task Forces of the North American Spine Society, American Society of Spine Radiology, American Society of Neuroradiology. Nomenclature and classification of lumbar disc pathology. Recommendations of the Combined task Forces of the North American Spine Society, American Society of Spine Radiology, and American Society of Neuroradiology. *Spine (Phila Pa 1976)*. 2001 Mar 1;26(5):E93-E113.

Standring S (Ed.). *Gray's Anatomy*. 39th ed. London: Elsevier. Churchill Livingstone; 2011.

Incidental finding on a chest radiograph

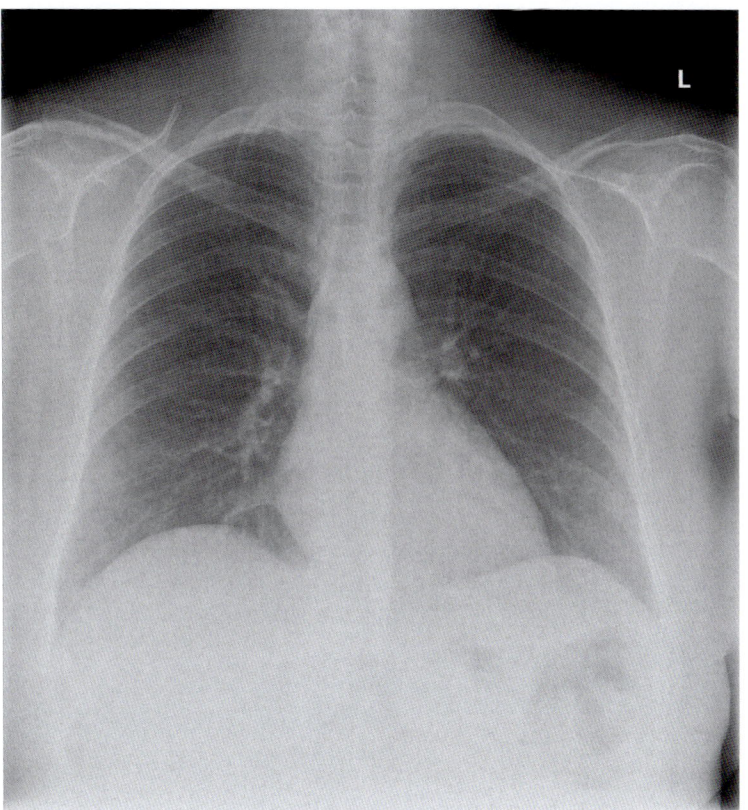

1. What is the most likely diagnosis?

2. How does the condition usually manifest?

3. Describe the imaging findings in this condition.

4. Describe clinical and pathological characteristics of this condition.

5. What is meant by a *false cervical rib*?

Case ranking/difficulty:

Category: Miscellanous

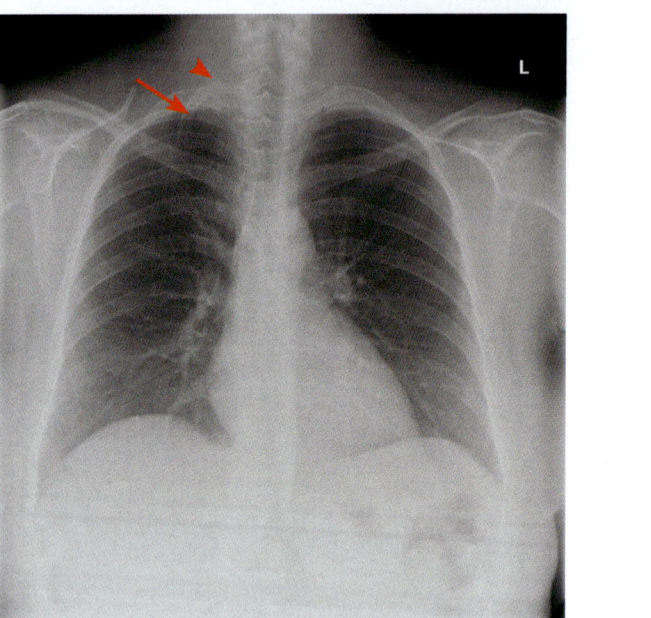

Frontal chest radiograph. There is a right cervical rib (*arrow*) that articulates via a costotransverse joint (*arrowhead*) with C7 vertebra.

Answers

1. Cervical ribs are supernumerary ribs that form true articulations with the transverse process of the seventh cervical vertebra.

2. When symptomatic, cervical ribs often present around the fourth or fifth decade and the dominant arm is more frequently affected. Neurological symptoms (97%) predominate (pain, wasting of hand muscles, paresthesiae) with venous (2%) and arterial manifestations (1%) being much rarer. Venous occlusion by either mechanical compression or venous thrombosis results in ipsilateral upper limb swelling whereas arterial compromise often results in Raynauds-like presentation. Dynamic tests including Wright test and Adson test may confirm the presence of thoracic outlet syndrome.

3. The diagnosis can be made on plain films of the cervical spine. A costotransverse joint needs to be present to make the diagnosis. The length of cervical ribs varies from a rudimentary stump to a fully formed rib that articulates anteriorly with the sternoclavicular junction. Fusion with the first rib is common as is pseudoarthrosis of the cervical rib. Coronal oblique MR sequences will also depict the relation between the cervical rib and the thoracic outlet, neural and vascular structures. Deviation of brachial plexus roots, focal vessel dilatations, vascular deviations or kinks, and collateral circulation may be seen.

4. They may be uni- (33%) or bilateral (66%) and occur in 0.5% of the general population. They are more commonly found in females. Up to 15% of patients with Klippel-Feil syndrome have a cervical rib. Although they arise most commonly at the level of C7 (95%), they have been described as high as C4 level. The condition is sometimes called dorsalization of the cervical spine. Cervical ribs vary significantly in their shape, size, and anatomical course, and it is impossible to determine radiographically whether cervical ribs will be symptomatic or not. This is because short cervical ribs may be associated with long fibrous bands that cause compression of neural or vascular structures.

5. Elongation of the transverse process of C7 that curves and tapers distally but lacks a costotransverse and costovertebral joints is called a *false cervical rib* or apophysomegaly. The latter is rarely symptomatic but may still have associated fibrous bands that may impinge into the scalene triangle.

Pearls

- Cervical ribs are supernumerary ribs that form true articulations with the transverse process of the seventh cervical vertebra.
- They are often asymptomatic but may result in thoracic outlet syndrome due to compression of the ipsilateral brachial plexus or subclavian vessels.
- They may be uni- (33%) or bilateral (66%) and occur in 0.5% of the general population.
- A costotransverse joint needs to be present to make the diagnosis.
- The length of cervical ribs varies from a rudimentary stump to a fully formed rib that articulates anteriorly with the sternoclavicular junction.
- Coronal oblique MR sequences will also depict the relation between the cervical rib and the thoracic outlet, neural and vascular structures.

Suggested Readings

Millan G, Casal D, Sagaribay A, Marques V, Martins JE. Neurogenic thoracic outlet syndrome associated with cervical rib. *Acta Reumatol Port.* 2013 Apr-Jun;38(2):98-103.

Weber AE, Criado E. Relevance of bone anomalies in patients with thoracic outlet syndrome. *Ann Vasc Surg.* 2013 Dec 5.

Chronic low back pain

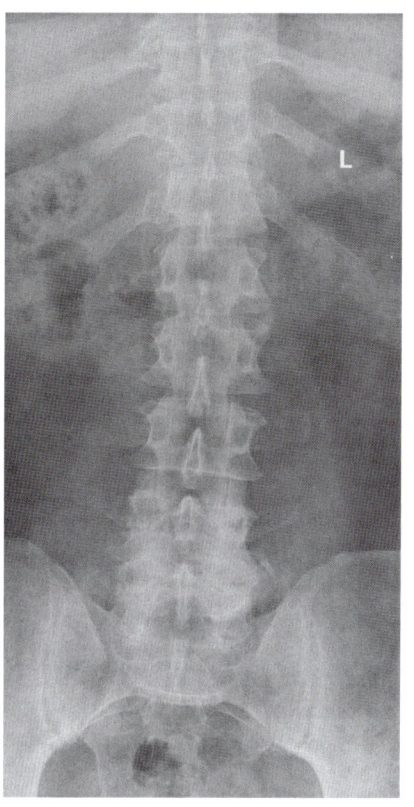 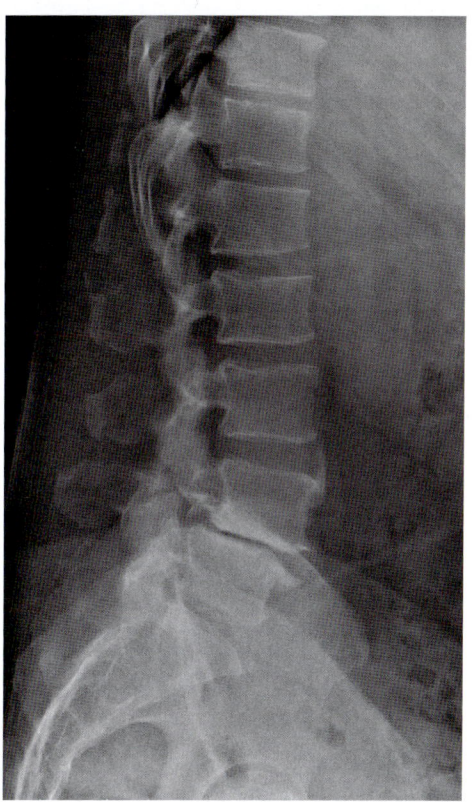

1. What is the most likely diagnosis?

2. Describe clinical and pathological characteristics of this condition.

3. How does the condition manifest clinically?

4. Describe the typical imaging findings.

5. Which treatments may be beneficial in this condition?

Case ranking/difficulty:

Category: Posterior elements

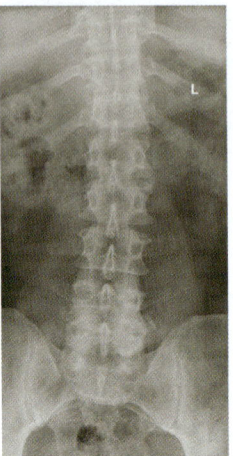

AP radiograph of the lumbar spine. The vertebral endplates and pedicles are intact. Note that the pars interarticularis defect is not seen on this projection.

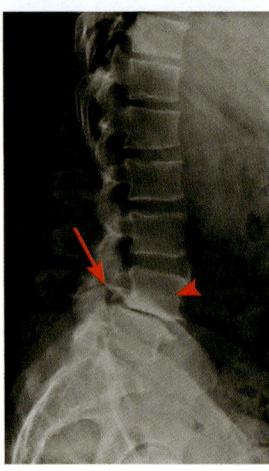

Lateral radiograph of the lumbar spine demonstrates a defect in the pars interarticularis (*arrow*) of L4 vertebra that has resulted in grade 1 anterolisthesis of L4 vertebra (*arrowhead*).

Answers

1. Spondylolysis refers to a defect in the neural arch, specifically in the pars interarticularis.

2. Spondylolysis is a stress fracture of the pars interarticularis secondary to repeated microtrauma particularly in individuals involved in strenuous sports including football and gymnastics. Heredity is also believed to play an important role. The condition has a male predominance and is more common in patients with spina bifida occulta. The pars interarticularis is very vulnerable when the spine is subjected to an axial force in the extended position such as when landing on one's feet. Such pressure can cause a fracture in susceptible individuals. Bilateral spondylolysis can progress to spondylolisthesis.

3. Pars defects are commonly asymptomatic but some patients may experience pain with extension or rotation of the lumbar spine.

4. The diagnosis can be made on radiography. Lateral projections are the most sensitive whereas oblique views are the most specific for detection of pars fractures. Oblique radiographs characteristically demonstrate a collar around the neck of the "Scottie dog." Radiography may, however, be limited by its inability to demonstrate stress reactions in the affected pars interarticularis before progression to a complete fracture. MRI, CT, and scintigraphic studies are much more sensitive to detect these early changes.

5. Treatment involves physiotherapy and rest from strenuous activities. A Boston overlap brace (antilordotic brace) is also effective. Nonsteroidal anti-inflammatory drugs (NSAIDs) are used to relieve the pain and reduce inflammation. Surgical options include laminectomy and posterior lumbar fusion and may be offered to symptomatic patients who do not respond to conservative measures.

Pearls

- Spondylolysis refers to a defect in the neural arch, specifically in the pars interarticularis.
- Most cases (95%) occur at L5 level but spondylolysis may affect any lumbar vertebra and less commonly the thoracic vertebrae.
- Pars defects are commonly asymptomatic but some patients may experience pain with extension or rotation of the lumbar spine.

Suggested Readings

Standaert CJ, Herring SA. Spondylolysis: a critical review. *Br J Sports Med*. 2000 Dec;34(6):415-422.

Syrmou E, Tsitsopoulos PP, Marinopoulos D, Tsonidis C, Anagnostopoulos I, Tsitsopoulos PD. Spondylolysis: a review and reappraisal. *Hippokratia*. 2010 Jan;14(1):17-21.

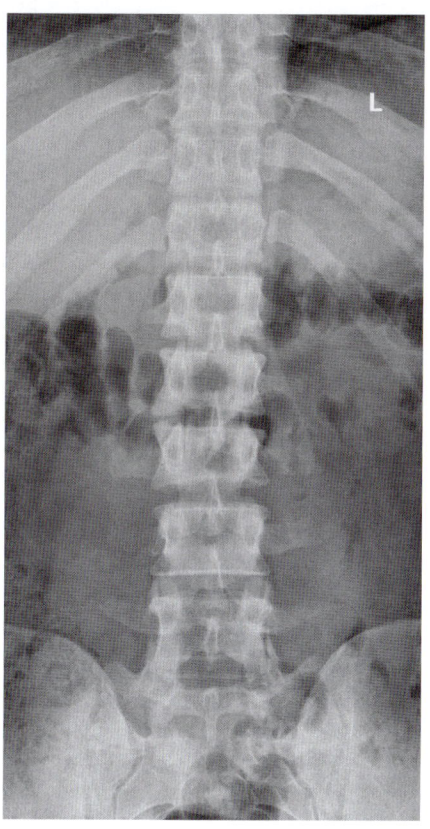 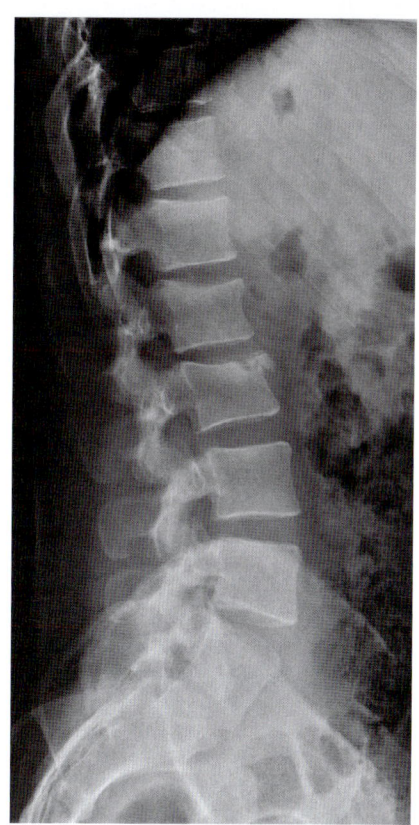

1. What is the most likely diagnosis?

2. Why shouldn't this finding be overlooked?

3. Which are the four subtypes described by Castellvi et al?

4. Describe the typical imaging findings.

5. Which landmarks are used to characterize lumbosacral transitional vertebrae?

Case ranking/difficulty: **Category:** Vertebral body

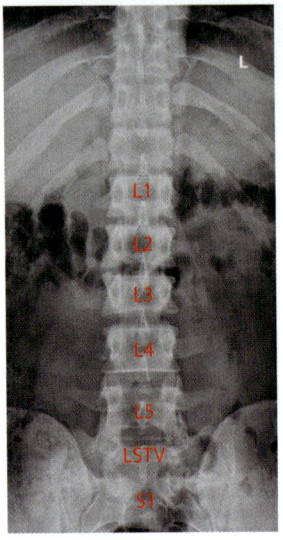

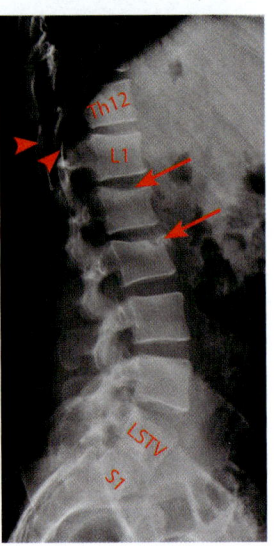

AP radiograph of the lumbar spine. There are six rib-free lumbar-type vertebrae (labelled L1—LSTV) in keeping with a lumbosacral transitional vertebra. Posttraumatic upper end plate fractures of L2 and L3 are seen, which are better appreciated on the lateral film.

Lateral radiograph of the lumbar spine. There are upper end plate fractures of L2 and L3 vertebrae (*arrows*). The vertebral alignment is preserved. The most caudal ribs (*arrowheads*) articulate with Th12 vertebra. Note that there are six lumbar vertebrae in keeping with an LSTV. Squaring of the lumbarized upper sacral segment is noted. The intervertebral disc above the LSTV shows some loss of disc height.

Answers

1. Lumbosacral transitional vertebrae (LSTV) are common congenital spinal anomalies seen in 4%-30% of the general population.

2. They have been implicated as a cause of chronic back pain. Lumbosacral transitional vertebrae should not be overlooked as failure to recognize the anomaly or a poor description in the radiological report may lead to spinal interventions or surgery being performed at an incorrect level.

3. Castellvi et al proposed a classification of lumbosacral transitional vertebrae:

   Type 1—a dysplastic transverse process with a height of >90 mm

   Type 2—incomplete lumbarization or sacralization

   Type 3—complete lumbarization or sacralization with complete fusion with the neighboring sacral basis

   Type 4—mixed type

4. Lumbarization of S1 is less common than sacralization and is encountered in about 2% of the population. Six rib-free lumbar-type vertebrae are seen on radiography. Anomalous (often rudimentary) facet joints and intervertebral disc between S1 and S2 are seen. Other radiographic findings include squaring of the lumbarized upper sacral segment or wedging of the sacralized lowest lumbar segment. The intervertebral disc above the LSTV often shows increased degenerative changes.

5. A sagittal cervicothoracic MR localizer may be used to accurately characterize transitional vertebrae. Another technique to correctly number LSTV is to identify the iliolumbar ligament, which usually arises from the transverse process of L5 and is a relatively constant landmark. The use of other anatomical markers including the aortic bifurcation, right renal artery, and conus medullaris has been described, but these are less reliable.

Pearls

- Lumbosacral transitional vertebrae (LSTV) are common congenital spinal anomalies seen in 4%-30% of the general population.
- Failure to recognize LSTV may lead to spinal interventions or surgery being performed at an incorrect level.

Suggested Readings

Castellvi AE, Goldstein LA, Chan DPK. Lumbosacral transitional vertebra and their relationship with lumbar extadural defects. *Spine*. 1983;9:493-495.

Konin GP, Walz DM. Lumbosacral transitional vertebrae: classification, imaging findings, and clinical relevance. *AJNR Am J Neuroradiol*. 2010 Nov;31(10):1778-1786.

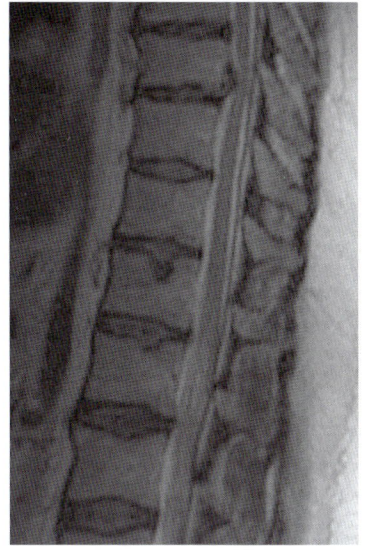 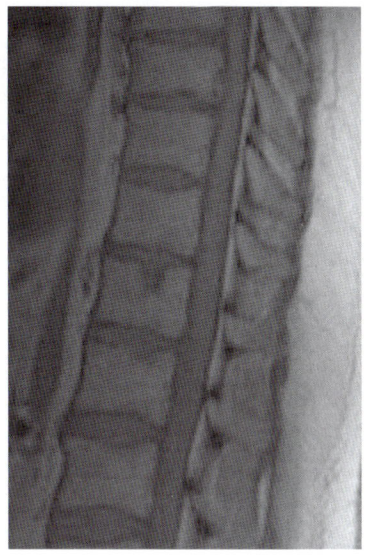 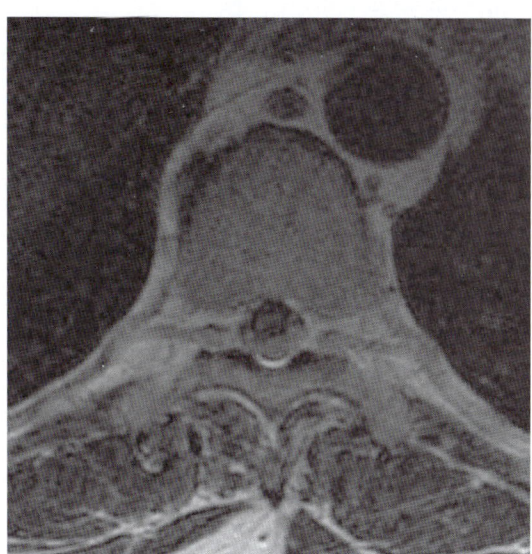

1. What is the most likely diagnosis?

2. What is meant by the term *extrusion*?

3. What might herniated disc material consist of?

4. What does the term *herniation* imply?

5. Name some forms of disc "herniation."

Case ranking/difficulty:

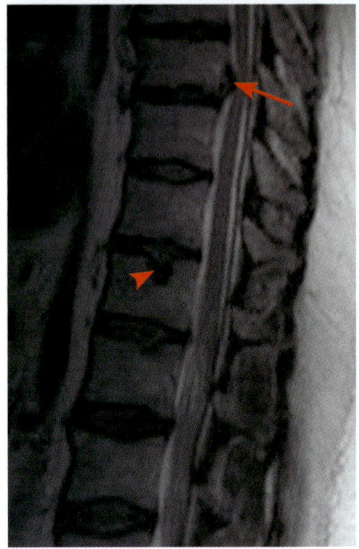

Sagittal T2-weighted sequence of the lumbar spine. There is a disc extrusion (*arrow*) at T9-T10 with cranial migration. The herniated disc material is in continuity with the parent disc. A Schmorl node (*arrowhead*) is noted in the superior endplate of T12.

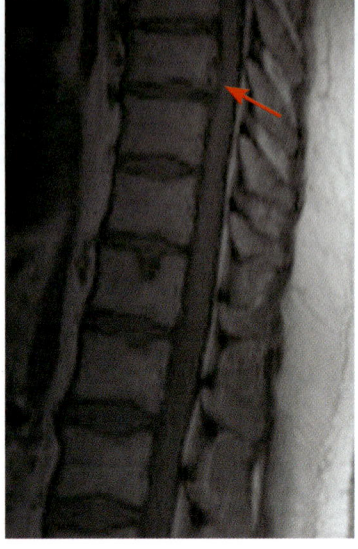

Sagittal T1-weighted sequence of the lumbar spine showing a disc extrusion at T9-T10 (*arrow*).

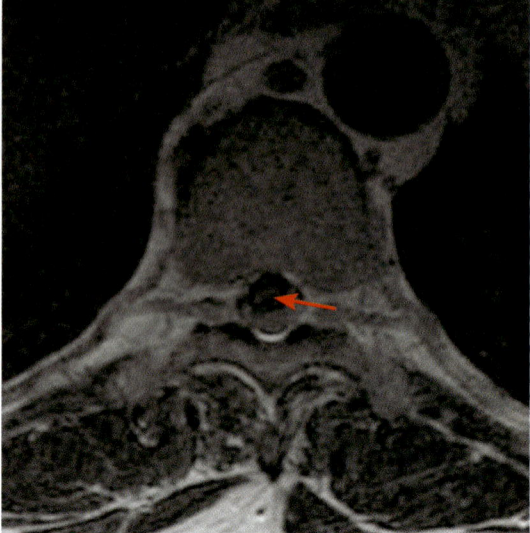

Axial T2-weighted image at the level of T9 vertebral body. There is an extradural lesion (*arrow*) within the spinal canal, which represents extruded disc material.

Answers

1. Disc extrusion.

2. Herniated discs may be further subclassified as *protrusion* or *extrusion* according to the shape of herniated material.

   Extrusion occurs when the distance between edges of herniated disc material is greater than the edges of the base of the herniation in any particular plane (ie, it has a broader dome than neck).

3. The herniated material may consist of nucleus pulposus, annular tissue, fibrocartilage, and fragmented apophyseal bone.

4. Disc herniation is defined as displacement of disc material beyond the normal limits of the intervertebral disc space. The latter is defined craniocaudally by the adjacent vertebral endplates and peripherally by the vertebral ring apophysis excluding any osteophytic formations.

   Displacement of disc material may only occur when there is a disruption in the annulus fibrosus or a break in the vertebral endplate resulting in intravertebral herniation, which is also known as a Schmorl node.

5. When disc material extends circumferentially beyond the vertebral ring apophysis, the term *bulging* is used, which is not considered a form of disc herniation.

Sequestration is a subtype of extrusion in which herniated disc material has lost continuity with the disc of origin. *Migration* implies that the herniated disc material is displaced away from the site of extrusion both if continuation with the parent disc is maintained or whether there is sequestered fragment. Hence, the term migration refers only to the position and not to continuity of the extruded material.

Pearls

- Disc herniation is defined as displacement of disc material beyond the normal limits of the intervertebral disc space.
- *Extrusion* occurs when the distance between edges of herniated disc material is greater than the edges of the base of the herniation in any particular plane (ie, it has a broader dome than neck).

Suggested Reading

Fardon DF, Milette PC; Combined Task Forces of the North American Spine Society, American Society of Spine Radiology, American Society of Neuroradiology. Nomenclature and classification of lumbar disc pathology. Recommendations of the Combined task Forces of the North American Spine Society, American Society of Spine Radiology, and American Society of Neuroradiology. *Spine (Phila Pa 1976)*. 2001 Mar 1;26(5):E93-E113.

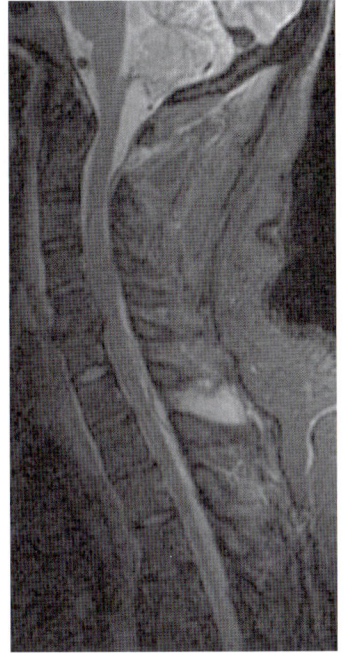 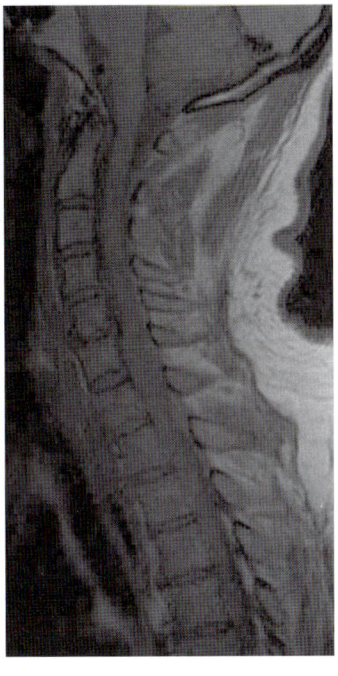 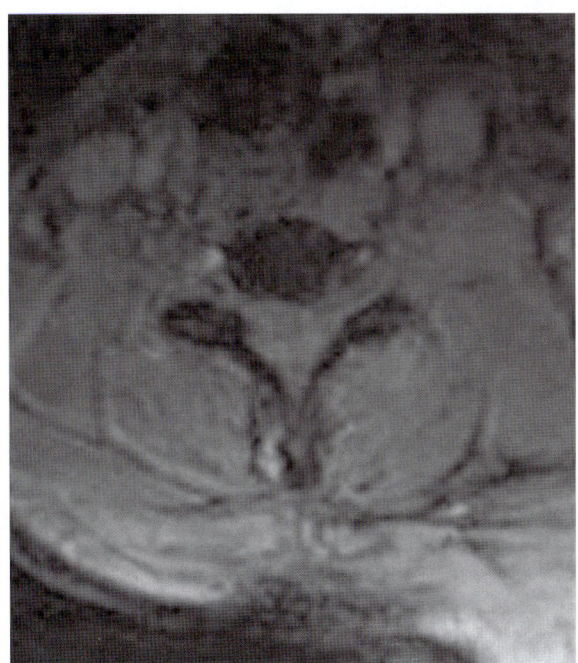

1. What is the most likely diagnosis?

2. How does this condition present clinically?

3. Name some predisposing conditions.

4. Which imaging modality best images this condition?

5. Which is the most common pathogen cultivated in this condition?

Case ranking/difficulty:

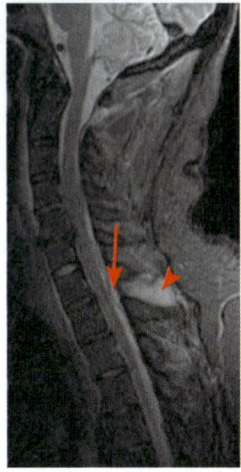

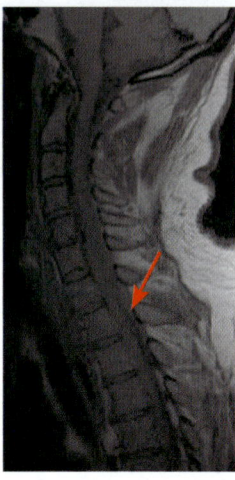

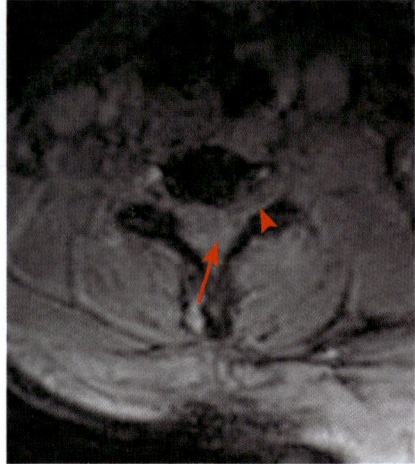

Sagittal T2-weighted sequence (with fat suppression) of the cervical and upper thoracic spine. There is a T2 hyperintense dorsal epidural collection that lifts the dura into the spinal canal (*arrow*). Note the hyperintensity in the paraspinal muscles (*arrowhead*) posterior to the collection in keeping with adjacent myositis.

Sagittal T1-weighted sequence of the cervical and upper thoracic spine. Note that the hypointense epidural collection (*arrow*) is difficult to distinguish from the adjacent CSF signal.

Axial T2-weighted sequence confirms the epidural location of the abscess (*arrow*). The collection extends along the extradural space into the left exiting foramen (*arrowhead*). Note the high signal intensity along the right side of the spinous process.

Answers

1. The anatomy of the spinal epidural space is crucial to understand the development and progression of epidural abscesses. Anteriorly the dura is tightly adherent to ligaments and vertebral bodies whereas posteriorly the dura is more lax allowing infections to spread over several levels. Abscess formation is therefore more frequent in the posterior epidural space, particularly in the thoracic region.

   Spread of infection to the posterior space is often hematogenic from a distant source of infection.

2. The initial presentation is often nonspecific and includes back pain and malaise. Additional symptoms may include fever, radiculopathy, and sphincter dysfunction. Headache and neck pain may occur with cervical epidural abscesses. Some studies have found that posterior spinal epidural abscesses are more likely to present with severe neurologic deficits compared to ventral epidural abscesses. It is estimated that up to 50% of cases are initially misdiagnosed or have a delayed diagnosis.

3. Hematogenic spread of infection to the epidural spread may occur from bacterial endocarditis, urinary tract infections, peritoneal and retroperitoneal infections, and infected indwelling catheters. The anterior epidural space is, on the other hand, prone to direct extension from vertebral osteomyelitis, particularly in adults. Iatrogenic causes include epidural injections or catheter placement, which may lead to direct inoculation of the epidural space. The source of infection remains unidentified in many cases.

4. MRI is the imaging modality of choice. It will not only confirm the presence of an epidural abscess but also determine the extent of involvement and the presence of canal or cord compromise. It may also help in planning surgical treatment.

5. *Staphylococcus aureus* is commonly cultivated and accounts for up to 65% of cases.

Pearls

- *Staphylococcus aureus* is commonly cultivated and accounts for up to 65% of cases.
- Early diagnosis and treatment are associated with improved outcomes.

Suggested Readings

Huang PY, Chen SF, Chang WN, et al. Spinal epidural abscess in adults caused by *Staphylococcus aureus*: clinical characteristics and prognostic factors. *Clin Neurol Neurosurg*. 2012 Jul;114(6):572-576.

Lang IM, Hughes DG, Jenkins JP, St Clair Forbes W, McKenna F. MR imaging appearances of cervical epidural abscess. *Clin Radiol*. 1995 Jul;50(7):466-471.

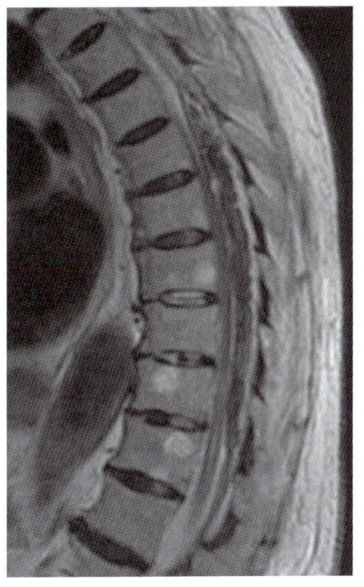 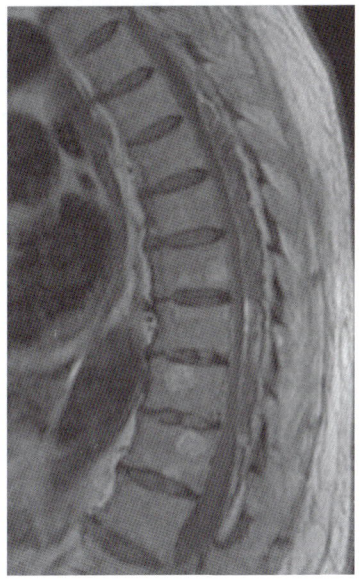 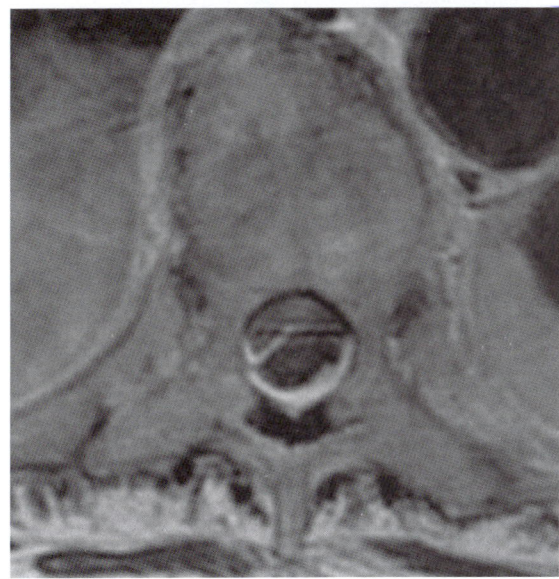

1. What is the most likely diagnosis?

2. What should be included in the differential diagnosis?

3. How does the condition manifest clinically?

4. Which imaging modality best images this condition?

5. Name some predisposing factors.

Case ranking/difficulty:

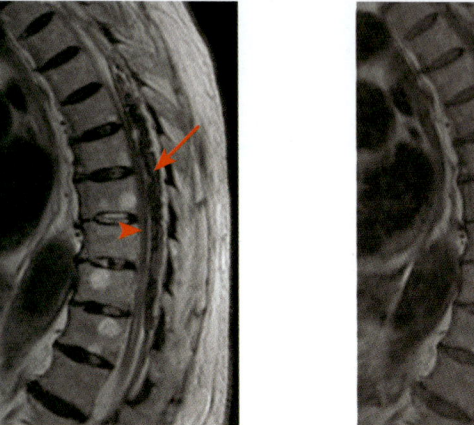

Sagittal T2-weighted sequence of the thoracic spine showing an extensive extradural collection (*arrow*) dorsal to the thoracic cord (*arrow*). The collection is heterogenous and mostly of low signal intensity. Incidental note is made of multiple scattered vertebral hemangiomas.

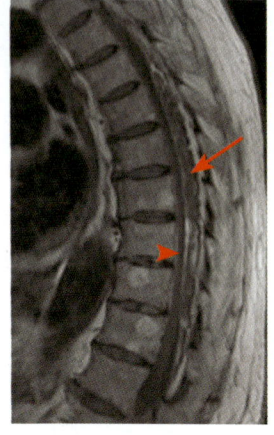

Sagittal T1-weighted sequence of the thoracic spine again shows a heterogenous epidural collection (*arrow*) posterior to the cord (*arrowhead*). Incidental note is made of multiple scattered vertebral hemangiomas.

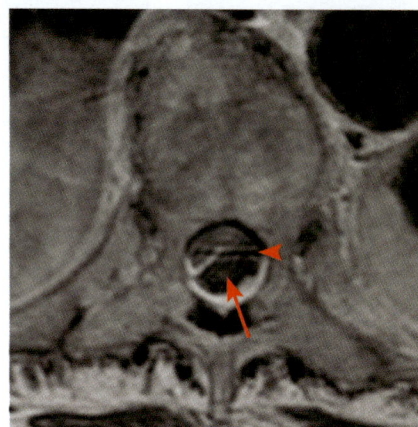

Axial T2-weighted sequence at the level of the lower thoracic spine. Note that the thecal sac (*arrowhead*) is displaced ventrally by a low signal intensity collection (*arrow*), which causes severe canal narrowing.

Answers

1. Spontaneous spinal epidural hematoma (EDH) is a rare condition requiring urgent management. It has been reported to occur in all age groups but it is extremely rare in the pediatric population.

2. Differential diagnoses include acute intervertebral disc herniation, spinal cord infarction, epidural tumor or abscess, spondylitis, transverse myelitis, dissecting aortic aneurysm, and acute myocardial infarction.

3. Patients typically present with an acute onset of severe stabbing back pain with rapidly developing signs of spinal cord or cauda equina compression (including paraparesis and quadriparesis).

4. MRI is the gold standard imaging modality and is useful in establishing the diagnosis. It demonstrates biconvex epidural hematomas in the epidural space with well-defined borders tapering superiorly and inferiorly. Subacute hematomas show characteristic T1 hyperintensity. T2 heterogeneous hyperintensity with focal hypointensity should suggest the diagnosis of acute spinal EDH. Central or peripheral contrast enhancement may be seen. Hyperemia of the adjacent dura mater has been postulated as a cause of peripheral enhancement of spinal EDH. Central enhancement may either be secondary to an underlying lesion or contrast extravasation from leaking vessels. A CT scan should be obtained if MRI is contraindicated or unavailable.

5. A venous source is thought to be responsible in spontaneous spinal EDH or that following minimal trauma. Predisposing factors that have been implicated include coagulopathy, anticoagulant and thrombolytic drugs, spinal vascular anomalies, intervertebral disc herniation, Paget disease of bone, Valsalva maneuver, and hypertension. Rupture of valveless veins in Batson plexus even by the slightest change of posture may cause epidural bleeding. Less commonly the source of bleeding is arterial from spinal epidural arteries and paraspinal muscular branches. The latter is more common in postoperative EDH.

Pearls

- Spontaneous spinal epidural hematoma (EDH) is a rare condition requiring urgent management.
- MRI is the gold standard imaging modality and is useful in establishing the diagnosis.

Suggested Readings

Baek BS, Hur JW, Kwon KY, Lee HK. Spontaneous spinal epidural hematoma. *J Korean Neurosurg Soc.* 2008;44(1):40-42.

Fukui MB, Swarnkar AS, Williams RL. Acute spontaneous spinal epidural hematomas. *AJNR Am J Neuroradiol.*1999 Aug;20(7):1365-1372.

Chronic low back pain

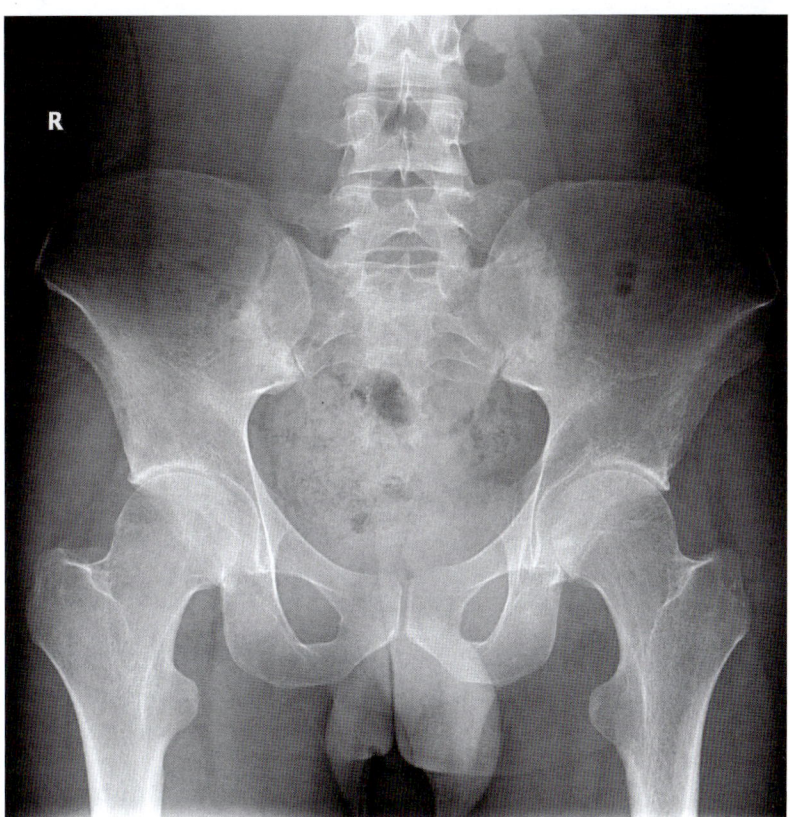

1. What is the most likely diagnosis?

2. Which radiological findings are typical of this condition?

3. Which spinal levels are particularly affected?

4. Which imaging modality best images this condition?

5. Which treatments may be beneficial?

Case ranking/difficulty:

Category: Posterior elements

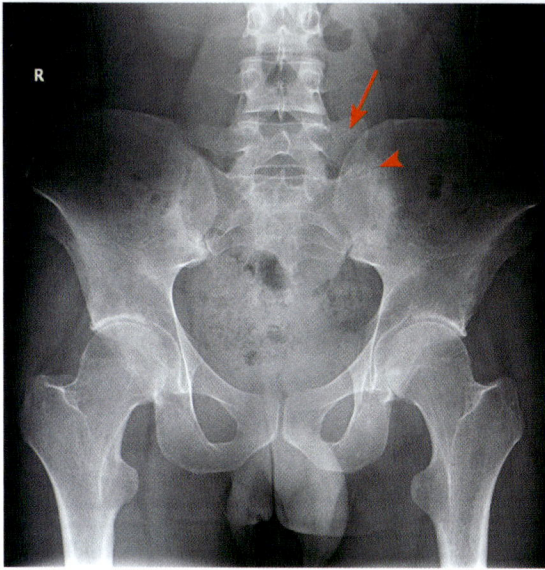

Frontal radiograph of the pelvis shows anomalous enlargement of the left L5 transverse process. The patulous transverse process (*arrow*) forms a pseudoarticulation with the left sacral ala (*arrowhead*).

Answers

1. Bertolotti syndrome refers to lower back pain secondary to lumbosacral transitional vertebrae.

2. The transitional L5 vertebra will have unilateral patulous enlargement of its transverse process, which may articulate or fuse with the sacrum. Less commonly it may articulate with the ilium.

3. The anomalous articulation results in limited motion at the lumbosacral articulation. To compensate for this, increased movement occurs at a more cranial lumbar segment, resulting in increased strain on the L4-L5 disc. Presentation is often with a sciatic or radicular type of pain, which corresponds to the fifth lumbar nerve root.

   Various studies have shown that the intervertebral discs immediately above the transitional vertebra were much more degenerate than the disc between the transitional vertebra and the sacrum. The articulation was also associated with increased strain and degenerative changes in the opposite facet joint.

   Aihara et al found that the iliolumbar ligaments cranial to the transitional vertebrae were much thinner and weaker than in unaffected individuals. The same authors postulated that this finding may explain the accelerated degeneration of the lumbar discs due to hypermobility and abnormal torque of the intervertebral spaces above the transitional vertebra.

4. Radiographs may be diagnostic and demonstrate anomalous enlargement of the transverse process of a transitional vertebra.

   MRI is the gold standard examination. It will not only characterize the articulation or fusion but also demonstrate preferential disc degeneration at the L4/5 level. Disc herniation and exiting nerve impingement may also be evaluated. Coronal images are particularly helpful to demonstrate the abnormal articulation.

5. Posterolateral fusion or resection of the anomalous articulation may be offered. Nonsurgical treatments include guided steroid injections within the cavity of the pseudarthrosis or radiofrequency sensory ablation.

   Bertolotti syndrome should be included in the list of differential diagnoses in young people presenting with lower back pain.

Pearls

- Bertolotti syndrome refers to lower back pain secondary to lumbosacral transitional vertebrae.
- The transitional L5 vertebra will have unilateral spatulas enlargement of its transverse process, which may articulate or fuse with the sacrum or ilium.
- Presentation is with sciatica or radiculopathy, which corresponds to the fifth lumbar nerve root.
- MRI is the gold standard examination and both surgical and conservative approaches are used.
- Bertolotti syndrome should be included in the list of differential diagnoses in young people presenting with lower back pain.

Suggested Readings

Aihara T, Takahashi K, Ogasawara A, Itadera E, Ono Y, Moriya H. Intervertebral disc degeneration associated with lumbosacral transitional vertebrae: a clinical and anatomical study. *J Bone Joint Surg Br*. 2005;87:687-691.

Castellvi AE, Goldstein LA, Chan DPK. Lumbosacral transitional vertebra and their relationship with lumbar extadural defects. *Spine*. 1983;9:493-495.

Quinlan JF, Duke D, Eustace S. Bertolotti's syndrome. A cause of back pain in young people. *J Bone Joint Surg Br*. 2006 Sep;88(9):1183-1186.

Chronic low back pain

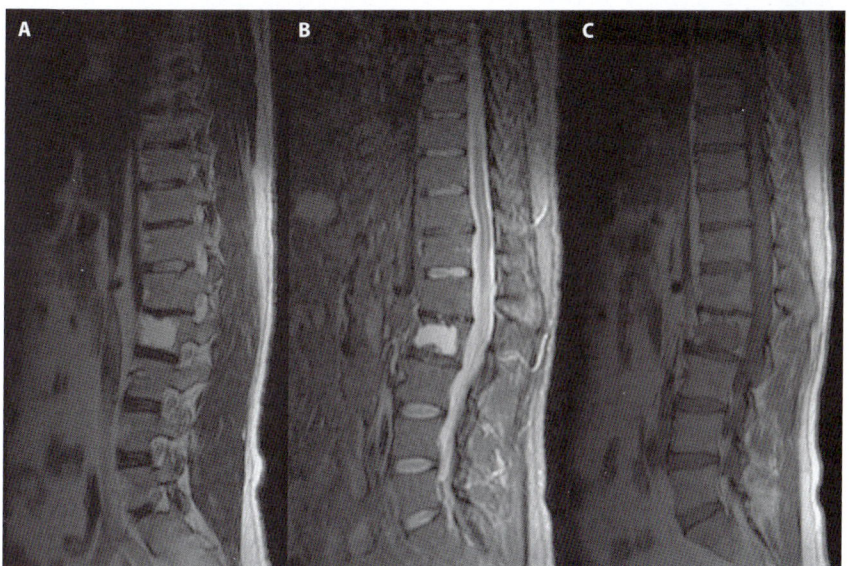

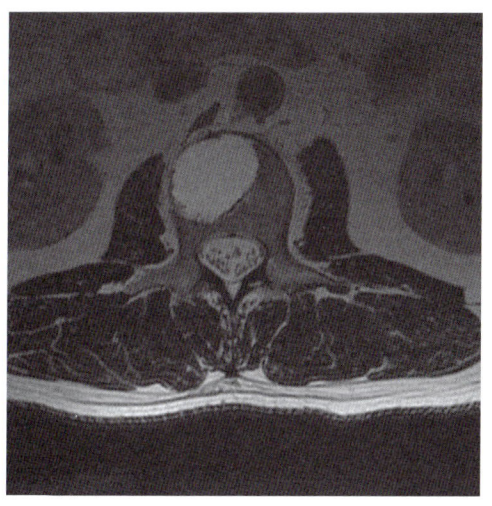
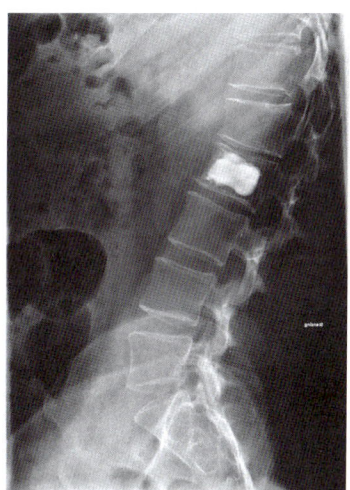
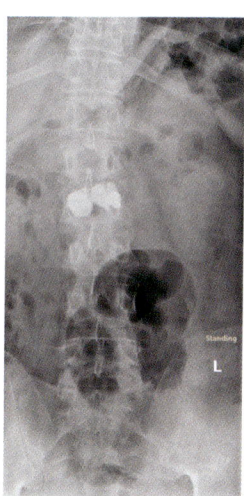

1. What is this procedure called?

2. Name some indications for this procedure.

3. Name some contraindications to the procedure.

4. Are there any recognized complications?

5. What is the purpose of this procedure?

Case ranking/difficulty:

Category: Vertebral body

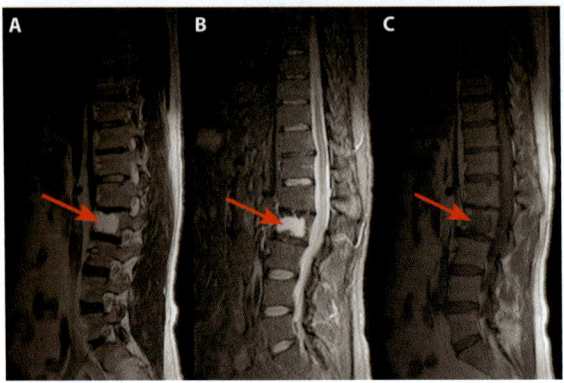

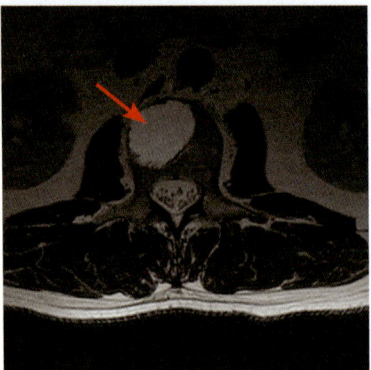

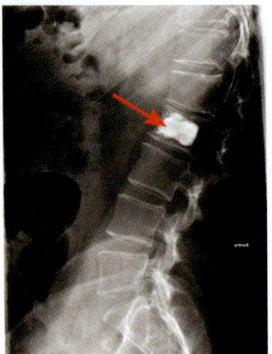

Sagittal sequences of the lumbar spine (Panel A = T2 weighted, Panel B = STIR, and Panel C = T1 weighted). There is a well-defined cystic lesion (*arrow*) occupying most of L2 vertebral body, which was histologically confirmed to be a solitary bone cyst.

Axial T2-weighted sequence at the level of L2. Again seen is a cystic lesion (*arrow*) occupying most of the cross-sectional area of the vertebral body.

Lateral radiograph of the lumbar spine. There is radiopaque material (*arrow*) filling the previously demonstrated cystic lesion in L2 vertebral body.

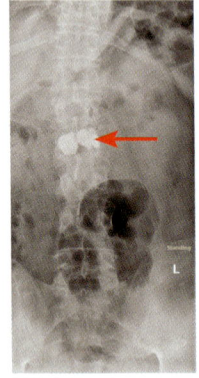

Frontal radiograph of the lumbar spine. Note that the polymethylmethacrylate (*arrow*) fills both sides of the vertebral body.

4. Complications of percutaneous vertebroplasty include neurologic deficits, fractures, hemorrhage, infection, allergic reactions, pulmonary embolism, and pneumothorax.

5. Percutaneous vertebroplasty not only provides pain relief but may also improve functional outcomes.

Pearls

- Percutaneous vertebroplasty is a minimally invasive treatment used in painful osteoporotic and malignant fractures refractory to medical therapy.
- Complications include neurologic deficits, fractures, hemorrhage, infection, allergic reactions, pulmonary embolus, and pneumothorax.

Answers

1. Percutaneous vertebroplasty involves image-guided percutaneous injection of cement (polymethylmethacrylate—PMMA) into the affected vertebral bodies.

2. Percutaneous vertebroplasty is used in painful osteoporotic and malignant fractures refractory to medical therapy. The procedure has also been used in vertebral angioma and as a prophylactic procedure in pathologically weakened vertebrae.

3. The procedure is contraindicated in active osteomyelitis, allergy to PMMA, and patients with uncorrectable coagulopathy.

   Major complications occur in <1% of patients treated for osteoporotic fractures and in <5% of neoplastic vertebral fractures.

Suggested Readings

Buchbinder R, Osborne RH, Ebeling PR, et al. A randomized trial of vertebroplasty for painful osteoporotic vertebral fractures. *N Engl J Med.* 2009 Aug 6;361(6):557-568.

Deramond H, Depriester C, Galibert P, Le Gars D. Percutaneous vertebroplasty with polymethylmethacrylate. Technique, indications, and results. *Radiol Clin North Am.* 1998 May;36(3):533-546.

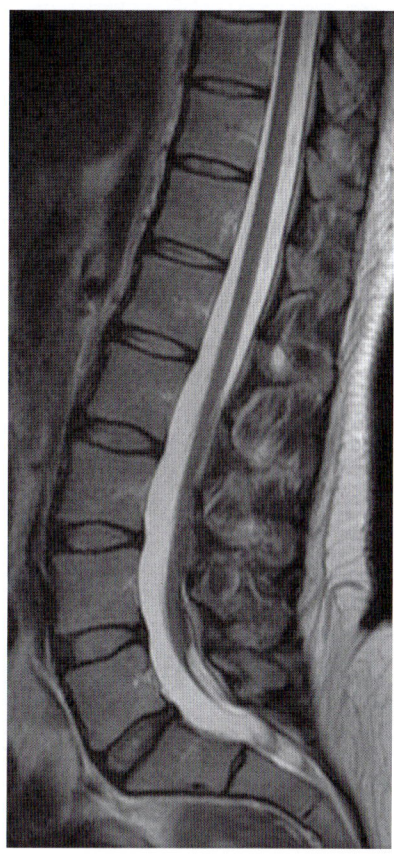 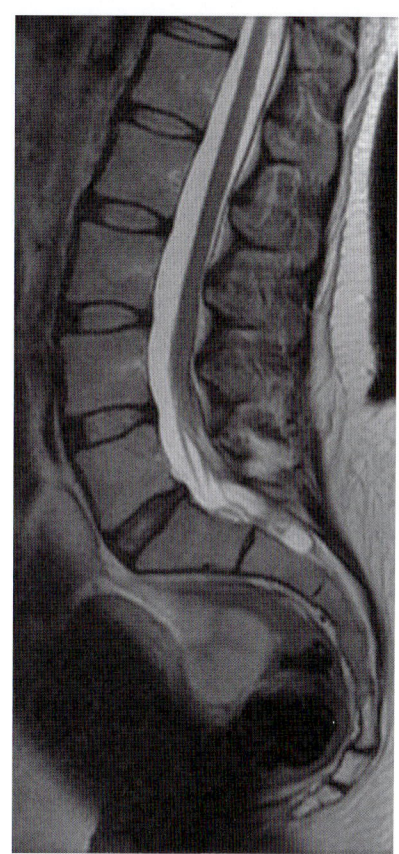

1. What is the most likely diagnosis?

2. Describe clinical and pathological characteristics of this condition.

3. Which other spinal findings are associated with this condition?

4. Which imaging modality best images this condition?

5. Which imaging findings are typical of this condition?

Case ranking/difficulty:

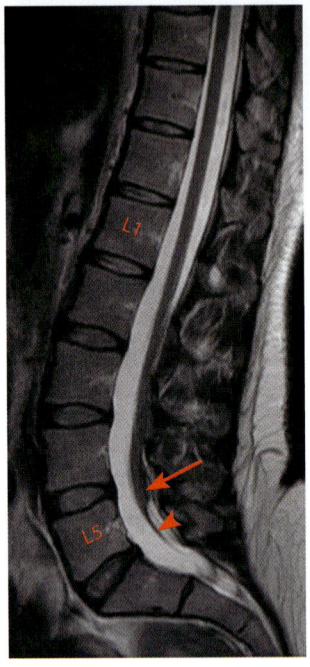

Sagittal T2-weighted sequence of the lumbar spine showing a low-lying spinal cord. Note that the conus medullaris (*arrow*) is abnormally low and lies at the level of L5 vertebral body. The filum terminale (*arrowhead*) is thickened, and there is no evidence of associated spinal dysraphism.

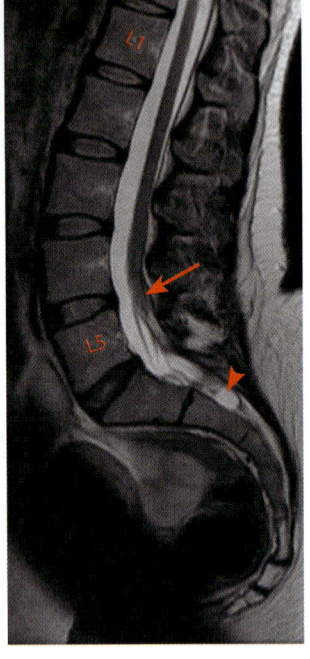

Sagittal T2-weighted sequence of the sacrum. A slightly more caudal sequence was acquired to exclude associated lesions such as myelomeningocele and cord lipoma. Note an incidental Tarlov cyst (*arrowhead*) within the sacral canal. The conus medullaris lies at the level of the superior endplate of L5.

Answers

1. Tethered spinal cord refers to incomplete involution of the distal spinal cord with failure of ascent of the conus medullaris. Abnormal tissue attachments within the spinal canal limit the developmental ascent of the spinal cord. Tethered cord syndrome describes the constellation of symptoms secondary to tethering of the cord. The condition may be further subdivided into primary when it is seen as an isolated anomaly or secondary when it occurs in the setting of other abnormalities such as myelomeningocele and lipoma of the filum terminale.

2. Presentation in childhood is with the cutaneous stigmata of associated spinal dysraphism. The condition more commonly presents between 5 and 15 years, particularly during periods of growth spurts. The condition may, however, go undiagnosed until adulthood and present with sensory, motor, or autonomic dysfunction. Neurological dysfunction is secondary to chronic

stretching of the spinal cord, which leads to vascular insufficiency at the level of the conus medullaris. If left untreated, tethered cord syndrome will have a progressive course. Surgical release may improve neurological function dramatically.

3. Cord tethering may be associated with filar lipoma and cyst, diastematomyelia, and imperforate anus. Scoliosis is seen in up to 20% of affected individuals.

4. MRI is diagnostic of the condition and is regarded as the gold standard imaging modality.

5. MR will confirm a low-lying conus medullaris (ie, caudal to L2), define the thickness of the filum terminale (>2mm), and evaluate for associated spinal dysraphism. An abnormal course of the nerve roots relative to the spinal cord (>15°) may also be appreciated.

In the pediatric population, ultrasonography is also an important screening tool. The lack of ossified posterior elements in normal infants provides an excellent acoustic window. Reduced or absent pulsatile movement of the cord and nerve roots is observed on M-mode scanning.

Pearls

- Tethered cord syndrome describes the constellation of symptoms secondary to tethering of the spinal cord.
- The condition may be further subdivided into primary when it is seen as an isolated anomaly or secondary when it occurs in the setting of other abnormalities.
- The condition commonly presents between 5 and 15 years, particularly during periods of growth spurts.
- It may, however, go undiagnosed until adulthood and present with sensory, motor, or autonomic dysfunction.
- Cord tethering may be associated with filar lipoma and cyst, diastematomyelia, and imperforate anus.
- MRI is diagnostic of the condition and is regarded as the gold standard imaging modality.
- In the pediatric population, ultrasonography is also an important screening tool.
- Surgical release may improve neurological function dramatically.

Suggested Readings

Ng WH, Seow WT. Tethered cord syndrome preceding syrinx formation—serial radiological documentation. *Childs Nerv Syst.* 2001;17(8):494-496.

Raghavan N, Barkovich AJ, Edwards M et al. MR imaging in the tethered spinal cord syndrome. *AJR Am J Roentgenol.* 1989;152(4):843-852.

Unremitting back pain

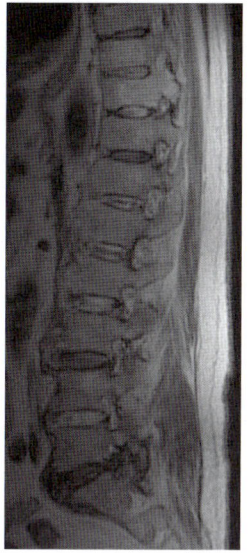 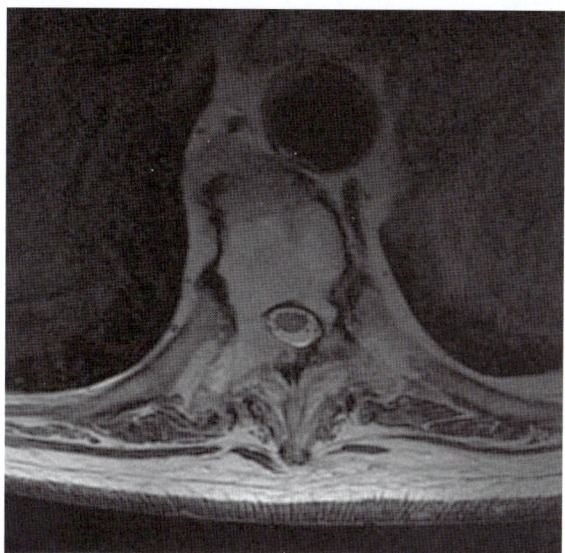

1. What is the most likely diagnosis?

2. Which bones are often affected in this condition?

3. Which symptoms does this condition present with?

4. What are the characteristic imaging findings?

5. Which treatments may be beneficial in this condition?

Case ranking/difficulty: **Category:** Vertebral body

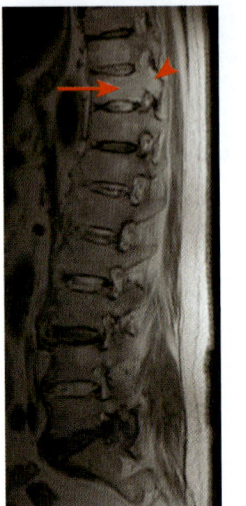

T2-weighted sequence of the lumbar spine shows a hyperintense lesion in T10 (*arrow*) that extends to involve the posterior elements (*arrowhead*).

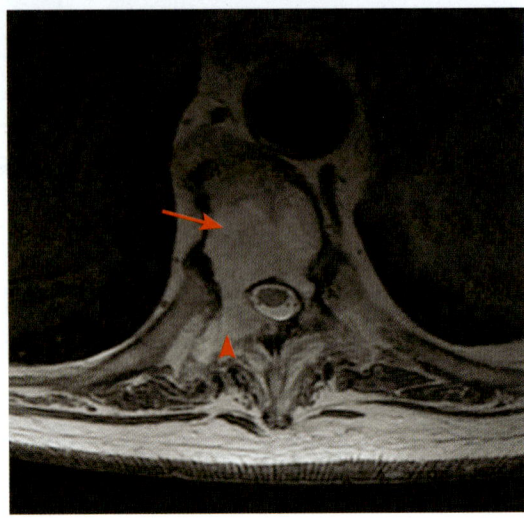

Axial T2-weighted sequence again demonstrates the hyperintense lesion (*arrow*) centered within the vertebral body with direct extension into the right pedicle and transverse process.

Answers

1. Solitary plasmacytoma of bone (SPB) is a rare hematologic malignancy. It represents the solitary form of the spectrum of plasma cell neoplasms that are characterized by neoplastic proliferation of a monoclonal plasma cell infiltrate.

2. The lesion has a predilection for the axial skeleton, particularly the thoracic spine. The ribs, sternum, clavicle, and scapula are also commonly affected.

3. Compression of the cord may also occur and the neurological deficits are sometimes the presenting symptoms. More commonly presentation is with unremitting back pain or pathological fractures. Up to 50% of solitary plasmacytomas have been shown to evolve into multiple myeloma within 10 years (average 3.5 years) from the initial diagnosis.

4. The lesion appears as a purely lytic lesion with a narrow zone of transition on plain films. MRI is the imaging modality of choice and demonstrates a focal area of bone marrow replacement. Signal characteristics are not specific since the lesion appears hypointense on T1-weighted and hyperintense on T2-weighted and STIR sequences. An extraosseous soft-tissue component may be demonstrated and possible impingement on the cord or spinal nerves should be evaluated.

5. Targeted radiotherapy is the treatment of choice in solitary plasmacytoma of bone and often relieves the associated symptoms.

Pearls

- Solitary plasmacytoma of bone (SPB) is characterized by neoplastic proliferation of a monoclonal plasma cell infiltrate.
- It has a predilection for the axial skeleton, particularly the thoracic spine.
- Targeted radiotherapy is the treatment of choice.

Suggested Readings

Afonso PD, Almeida A. Solitary plasmacytoma of the spine: an unusual presentation. *AJNR Am J Neuroradiol*. 2010 Jan;31(1):E5.

Dimopoulos MA, Moulopoulos LA, Maniatis A, Alexanian R. Solitary plasmacytoma of bone and asymptomatic multiple myeloma. *Blood*. 2000 Sep 15;96(6):2037-2044.

Worsening back pain

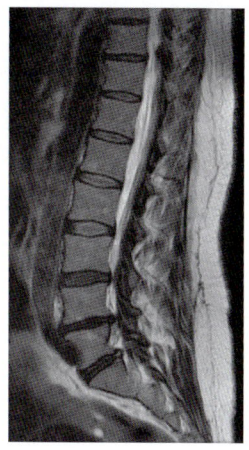 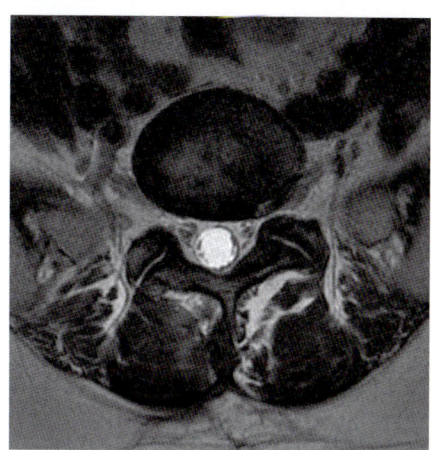

1. What is the most likely diagnosis?

2. How does the condition usually present?

3. What may give rise to this condition?

4. Which imaging modality best images this condition?

5. How many subtypes of this condition are described?

Case ranking/difficulty:

Category: Disc

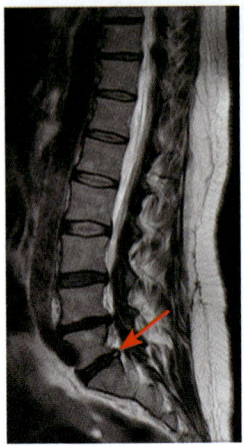

Sagittal T2-weighted sequence of the lumbar spine showing a hyperintense linear focus (*arrow*) within the otherwise hypointense annulus fibrosus. Multilevel disc desiccation is noted between L3 through to S1.

Answers

1. Annular fissure refers to the deficiency in the fibers of the annulus fibrosus. The term fissure is preferred over tear as the latter may erroneously imply acute disc injury.

2. Annular fissures are very common and most are asymptomatic. However, ingrowth of nerve endings and formation of granulation tissue within the defect may result in pain. This occurs particularly when fissures occur close to dorsal root ganglia.

3. Disruptions may be due to separation between the annular fibers, avulsion of the annular fibers from their vertebral insertions, and breaks that involve one or more layers of the annular lamellae. The breaks may extend in a radial, transverse, or concentric fashion.

4. They are seen as T2 hyperintense regions in the otherwise low signal annulus on MRI. Contrast enhancement is seen in up to 96% of cases. Discography can further characterize annular fissures and may distinguish a partial-from a full-thickness tear. The clinical relevance of the latter is, however, disputed.

5. Yu et al described three types of annular fissures as follows:

   Type 1 (concentric tears)—rupture of the transverse fibers connecting adjacent annular lamellae. The longitudinal fibers are intact and these tears are not visualized on MR.

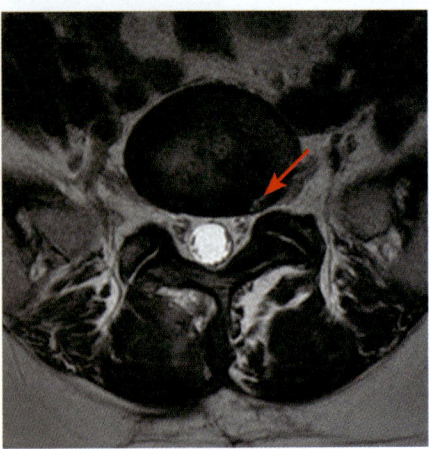

Axial T2-weighted image at the level of L5-S1 intervertebral disc. There is a linear hyperintensity (*arrow*) in the posterolateral aspect of the annulus fibrosus, which is compatible with an annular fissure.

Type 2 (radial tears)—fissures that extend from the periphery of the annulus fibrosus to the nucleus pulposus, which disrupt the longitudinal fibers. The abnormality is seen as a hyperintense focus on T2-weighted sequence.

Type 3 tears (transverse tears)—disruption of Sharpey fibers adjacent to their vertebral insertion. They are also seen as focal T2 high signal intensity zones.

Pearls

- Annular fissure refers to deficiency in the fibers of the annulus fibrosus.
- The breaks may extend in a radial, transverse, or concentric fashion.
- Ingrowth of nerve endings and formation of granulation tissue within the defect may result in pain.

Suggested Readings

RF Costello, DP Beall. Nomenclature and standard reporting terminology of intervertebral disc herniation. *Magn Reson Imaging Clin N Am.* 2007;15:167-174.

Yu S, Sether LA, Ho PS, Wagner M, Haughton VM. Tears of the anulus fibrosus: correlation between MR and pathologic findings in cadavers. *AJNR Am J Neuroradiol.* 1988;9:367-370.

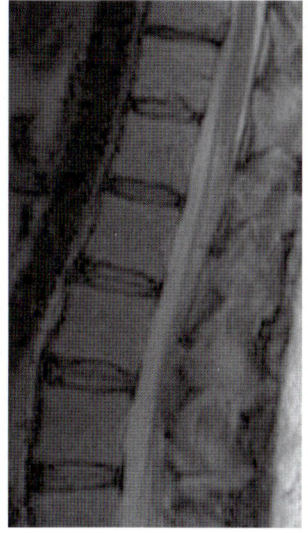 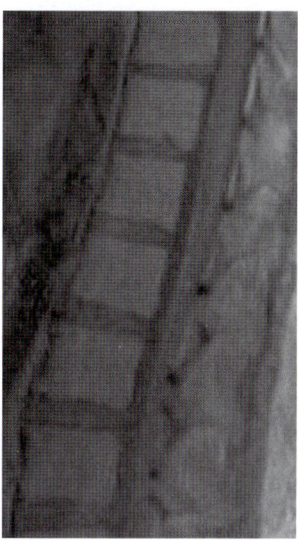 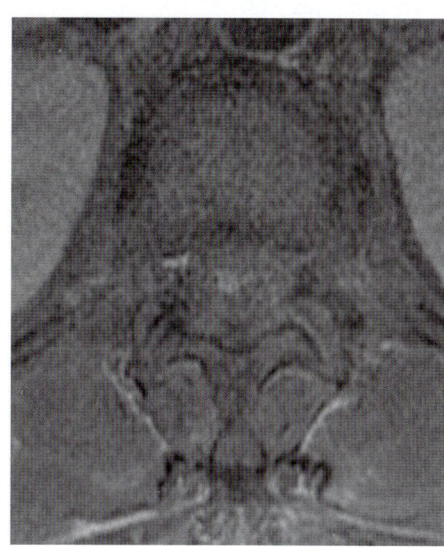

1. What is the most likely diagnosis?

2. What should be included in the differential diagnosis?

3. Which primary tumors are often implicated?

4. Which imaging modality best images this condition?

5. Which treatments may be beneficial in this condition?

Case ranking/difficulty:

Category: Nerve roots/Nerve plexus/Peripheral nerves

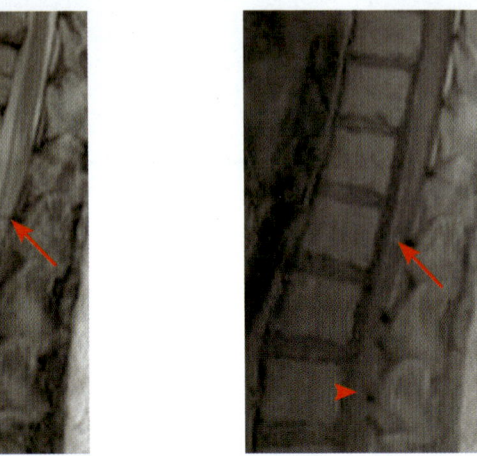

Sagittal T2-weighted sequence of the lumbar spine. Note subtle nodularity (*arrow*) along the cauda equina roots. The cord terminates at T12 and the lumbar vertebrae have preserved body heights and marrow signal.

Contrast-enhanced T1-weighted sequence of the lumbar spine. There are enhancing nodules (*arrow*) and diffuse leptomeningeal enhancement (*arrowhead*) along the cauda equina roots.

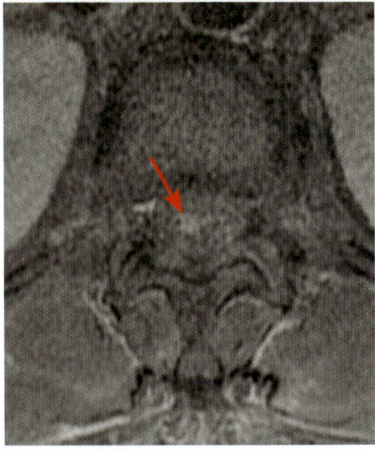

Contrast-enhanced axial T1-weighted image at the level of L2. Note pathological nodular enhancement (*arrow*) along the cauda equina roots in this fat saturated sequence.

Answers

1. Leptomeningeal metastasis rarely complicates cancer and refers to the invasion and proliferation of neoplastic cells within the subarachnoid space.

2. Differential diagnoses of leptomeningeal enhancement include infectious, granulomatous, neoplastic, and connective tissue disorders.

3. The most common cancers to metastasize to the leptomeninges are breast cancer, lung cancer, and malignant melanoma. Leptomeningeal metastasis occurs both with solid tumors when it is called leptomeningeal carcinomatosis and with nonsolid tumors when the condition is referred to as tumor or lymphomatous/leukemic meningitis.

4. Contrast-enhanced MRI is the imaging investigation of choice and demonstrates pathological leptomeningeal enhancement, which extends into the cerebral sulci and cerebellar folia or presents as enhancing subarachnoid tumor nodules. Multifocal or diffuse infiltration in a sheet-like fashion can be seen along the spinal cord and cauda equina roots. Associated findings in the spine include cord enlargement, intraparenchymal nodules, and epidural compression. Lumbar puncture is the standard diagnostic procedure. Multiple punctures may be required as positive cytology is only demonstrated in 50%-70% on initial sampling. The CSF opening pressure and CSF protein may also be increased.

5. Treatment often involves focal radiotherapy to symptomatic sites in combination with systemic chemotherapy. Intrathecal chemotherapy requires normal CSF flow dynamics. It is rarely efficacious except for treatment of hematopoietic neoplasms. Some studies have also demonstrated the beneficial use of intrathecal therapy in leptomeningeal spread complicating breast cancer.

Pearls

- Leptomeningeal metastasis refers to the invasion and proliferation of neoplastic cells within the subarachnoid space.
- The most common cancers to metastasize to the leptomeninges are breast cancer, lung cancer, and malignant melanoma.
- Contrast-enhanced MRI is the imaging investigation of choice and demonstrates pathological leptomeningeal enhancement.

Suggested Readings

Bruna J, Simó M, Velasco R. Leptomeningeal metastases. *Curr Treat Options Neurol*. 2012 Aug;14(4):402-415.

Chamberlain MC. Leptomeningeal metastasis. *Curr Opin Neurol*. 2009 Dec;22(6):665-674.

Worsening back pain

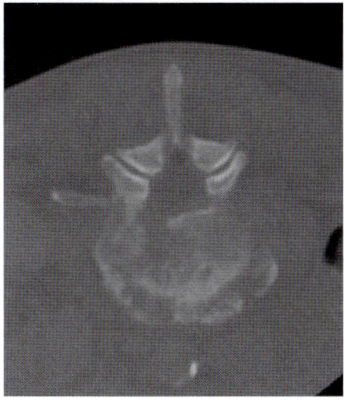
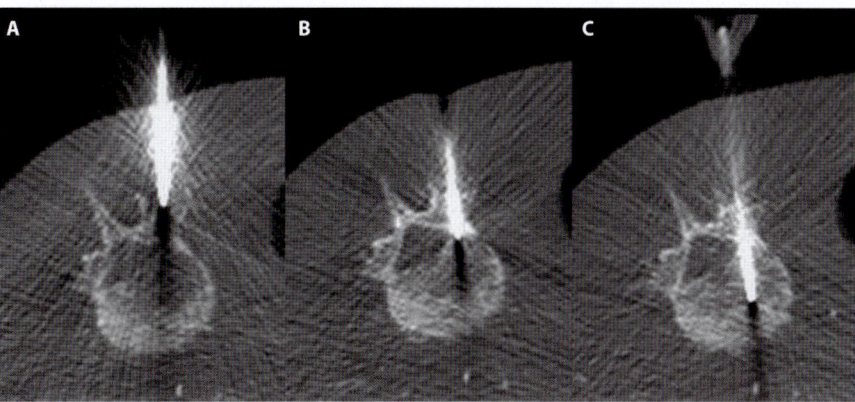

1. What is this procedure called?

2. Which approaches are commonly used?

3. What are the potential benefits of the coaxial technique?

4. Name some recognized complications of this procedure.

5. Name some contraindications to this procedure.

Case ranking/difficulty:

Category: Vertebral body

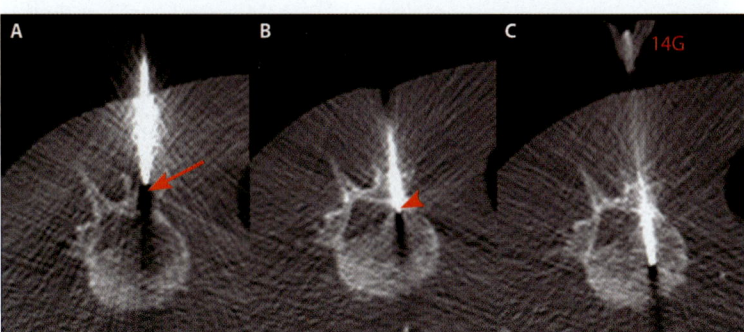

Axial CT image with the patient in the prone position showing a destructive lesion centered in the body of L3 vertebra and extending into the right pedicle.

Percutaneous biopsy of L3 vertebral body via a transpedicular approach. A 14G biopsy needle was advanced until it reached the periosteum (*arrow*, panel A). It was then advanced along the pedicle (*arrow*, panel B) into the central part of the vertebral body.

Answers

1. Vertebral biopsy is indicated when a definite diagnosis cannot be made on neuroimaging and when histological evaluation of a vertebral lesion is required. Open biopsy is associated with significant morbidity and complications. On the other hand, percutaneous vertebral biopsy has been shown to be a safe and highly accurate procedure. It can be performed under intravenous sedation and local anesthesia. General anesthetic may be used in patients with severe back pain.

2. Three approaches are commonly used—the posterolateral, transpedicular, and transcostotransversal— the latter being used in the thoracic region. The choice of the approach often depends on the location of the lesion. The posterolateral approach is often used if the lesion is located in the lower part of the vertebra or if it is predominantly located in the disc space. The transpedicular approach was shown to be more effective if the pedicle and the posterior half of the vertebral body were involved. The accuracy of vertebral biopsies using the transpedicular approach was shown to be higher compared to that of the posterolateral approach.

3. The coaxial technique is preferred as it often allows intact specimens of adequate size to be obtained. It also enables multiple biopsies to be obtained through a single tract, increasing the diagnostic accuracy. Bleeding at the biopsy site may also be controlled by the insertion of Gelfoam through the cannula.

4. CT-guided vertebral biopsy has a reported accuracy of 67%-97% with a complication rate of 0%-26%. Fluoroscopic guidance may also be used where rapid CT scanning is not available. Complications of percutaneous vertebral biopsy include infections, pulmonary and neurologic complications.

5. Vertebral biopsy is contraindicated in patients with uncorrected bleeding diathesis.

Pearls

- Percutaneous vertebral biopsy has been shown to be a safe and highly accurate procedure.
- It can be performed under intravenous sedation and local anesthesia. CT-guided vertebral biopsy has a reported accuracy of 67%-97% with a complication rate of 0%-26%.
- Fluoroscopic guidance may also be used where rapid CT scanning is not available.
- Complications of percutaneous vertebral biopsy include infections, pulmonary and neurologic complications.
- Three approaches are commonly used— the posterolateral, transpedicular, and transcostotransversal—the latter being used in the thoracic region.
- The coaxial technique is preferred as it often allows intact specimens of adequate size to be obtained.
- Vertebral biopsy is contraindicated in patients with uncorrected bleeding diathesis.

Suggested Readings

Pierot L, Boulin A. Percutaneous biopsy of the thoracic and lumbar spine: transpedicular approach under fluoroscopic guidance. *AJNR Am J Neuroradiol*. 1999 Jan;20(1):23-25.

Yaffe D, Greenberg G, Leitner J, Gipstein R, Shapiro M, Bachar GN. CT-guided percutaneous biopsy of thoracic and lumbar spine: a new coaxial technique. *AJNR Am J Neuroradiol*. 2003 Nov-Dec;24(10):2111-2113.

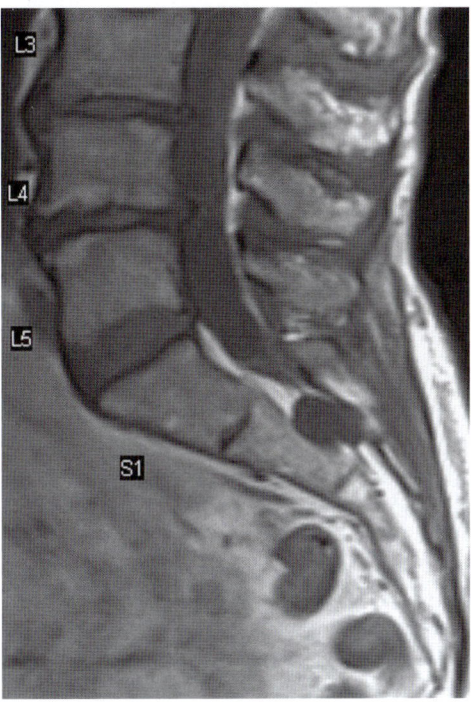 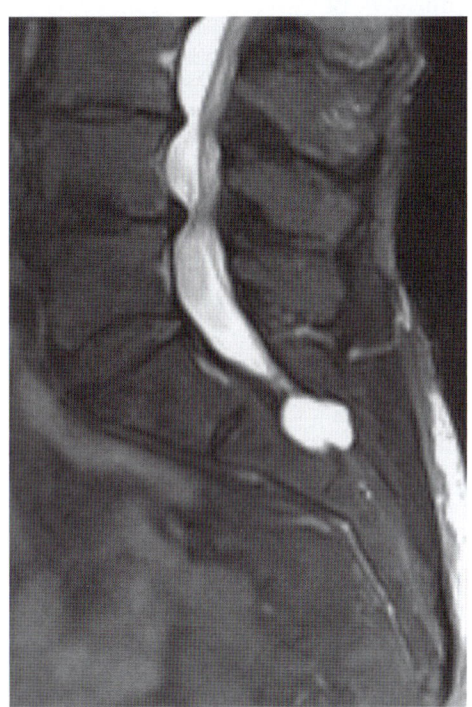

1. What is the likely diagnosis?

2. The lesion most commonly occurs at what level?

3. The lesion is typically located proximal to the dorsal root ganglion. True or False?

4. What is the typical appearance on conventional or CT myelography?

5. Nerve fibers are usually within the walls of these lesions. True or False?

Case ranking/difficulty: **Category:** Thecal sac

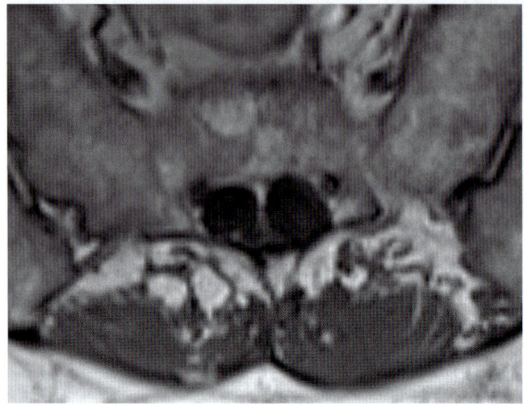

Osseous remodeling.

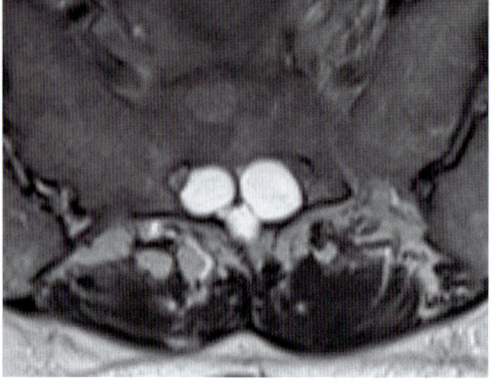

Similar findings. Nerve fibers are within the walls, but difficult to appreciate.

Answers

1. The presence of a cerebrospinal fluid (CSF) filled lesion in the sacral canal with remodeling of bone is diagnostic for a Tarlov cyst.

2. The vast majority of Tarlov cysts occur at the S1-4 level, although they uncommonly occur elsewhere in the spine. This helps differentiate from meningeal diverticulae, which usually occur in the thoracic spine.

3. False. Tarlov cysts occur at or distal to the junction of the posterior nerve root and dorsal root ganglia unlike meningeal diverticulae, which occur proximally.

4. Most Tarlov cysts have a potential or limited communication with the subarachnoid space. Therefore, with oil-based contrast myelographic contrast material that has been used in the past, there may be no filling or delayed filling of the cyst. The delayed filling is due to exudation though the cyst wall, or via CSF hydrostatic pressure. This finding is less pronounced when using water-soluble contrast media.

   Meningeal diverticulae, with their larger communication, usually fill immediately.

5. True. Nerve fibers are usually within the walls of Tarlov cysts, and sometimes within the cyst cavity itself, helping to differentiate them from meningeal diverticulae, which have no neural elements.

Pearls

- Tarlov cysts are very common, affecting 5%-10% of the general population.
- Most are asymptomatic, but a large size (greater than 1.5 cm) may result in symptoms.
- Symptoms include loss of bladder, bowel and sexual function, chronic back pain, and sensory deficit.
- Lesions are most commonly at the S1-4 level, and are frequently multiple.
- CT and MRI will show a fluid-filled structure with bone remodeling in some cases. The nerve roots are in the cyst wall and sometimes within the cyst cavity. These cysts can extend into the foramina and cause expansion.
- Cysts occur distal to the dorsal root ganglia, unlike arachnoid diverticulae

Suggested Readings

Paulsen RD, Call GA, Murtagh FR. Prevalence and percutaneous drainage of cysts of the sacral nerve root sheath (Tarlov cysts). *AJNR Am J Neuroradiol.* 1994 Feb;15(2):293-297; discussion 298-299.

Sen RK, Goyal T, Tripathy SK, Chakraborty S. Tarlov cysts: a report of two cases. *J Orthop Surg (Hong Kong).* 2012 Apr;20(1):87-89.

Xu J, Sun Y, Huang X, Luan W. Management of symptomatic sacral perineural cysts. *PLoS One.* 2012 Jul;7(6):e39958.

Generalized bone pain

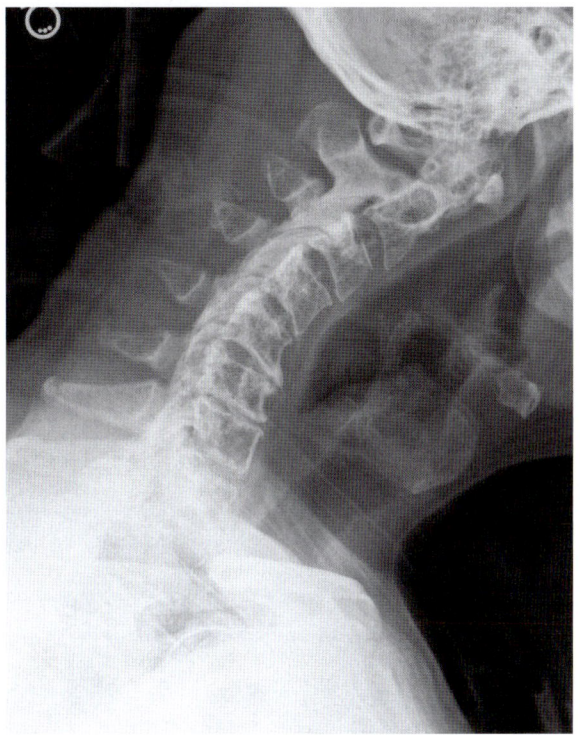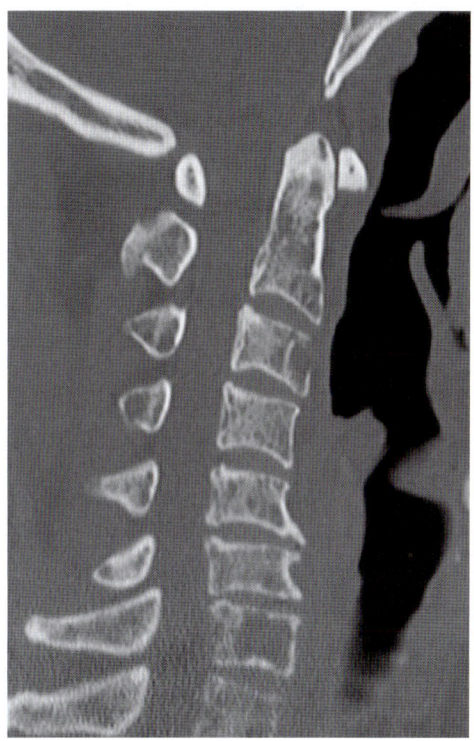

1. What are the imaging features of this entity?

2. What are the complications of this disease?

3. This disease is caused by clonal proliferation of which type of cell?

4. What are risk factors for this condition?

5. What are the possible treatments?

Case ranking/difficulty: **Category:** More than one category

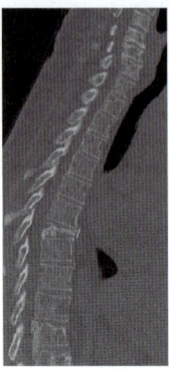

Diffuse osteopenia, with multiple focal areas of osteolysis. Collapse of a thoracic vertebra, with mild wedging of several others.

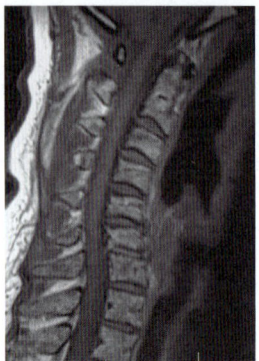

Heterogenous T1 signal.

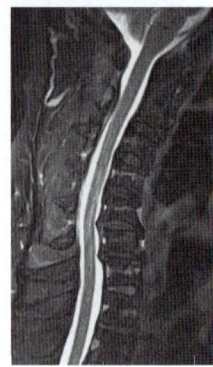

Signal is not significantly increased on T2-weighted images.

Answers

1. MRI is the most sensitive test for myeloma. Marrow infiltration by myeloma results in low T1 marrow signal, although the STIR signal can be variable.

   Pathological fractures result from the weakening of bone due to lytic lesions.

   Myeloma has typically low uptake on radionuclide scans; however, a lesion may show increased uptake in the presence of a pathological fracture.

2. Myeloma does not cause thrombocytosis. As a consequence of marrow infiltration by plasma cells, thrombocyte production is reduced, leading to thrombocytopenia.

   Secondary amyloidosis can cause effects in multiple organs including liver, kidneys, and lungs.

   Cord compression can result from spinal deposits with epidural soft tissue masses. Pathological fractures are relatively common.

3. Monoclonal proliferation of plasma cells results in multiple myeloma. The immunoglobulin light chains are detected in the serum and urine (Bence-Jones protein), which forms the basis of laboratory diagnosis.

4. There are no definite risk factors for multiple myeloma, although there is a very slightly higher incidence in first-degree relatives, and the disease is more common in blacks. There is no known genetic predisposition, with mutations acquired, rather than hereditary. Hence, it is extremely rare below 40 years of age.

5. Stem cell transplant offers the best chance of disease remission, although it can often not be tolerated in the elderly population that tend to have the disease. There is no possibility of cure with surgery, as the disease by definition is a systemic disorder of plasma cell monoclonal proliferation. The complications of bone pain, hypercalcemia, and pathological fracture can be treated.

Pearls

- Multiple myeloma is the most common primary bone tumor. It must always be considered in the differential diagnosis of multiple lytic lesions, especially in the appropriate age group (over 50 years).
- A plasmacytoma is a focal collection of myelomatous cells and may represent early stage disease, with a high incidence of conversion to diffuse multiple myeloma. It has a better prognosis than multiple myeloma.
- A skeletal survey is often performed to stage the extent of the disease.
- MRI is, however, the gold standard where resources permit, as the full extent of marrow replacement can be appreciated, as well as any associated soft tissue components.
- Imaging features consist of diffuse lytic lesions on plain films and diffuse marrow infiltration with low T1 signal lesions on MRI.
- The MRI signal on T2-weighted images is variable and should not be relied upon exclusively for diagnosis.
- Similarly lesions can be "warm" or "hot" on a bone scan in the presence of a fracture.
- Complications of myeloma include pathological fracture; hence, it is as important to highlight to the clinician sites prone to fracture, as it is to comment on the presence of established fractures.

Suggested Readings

Li SD, Wang YF, Qi JY, Qiu LG. Clinical features of bone complications and prognostic value of bone lesions detected by X-ray skeletal survey in previously untreated patients with multiple myeloma. *Indian J Hematol Blood Transfus.* 2010 Sep;26(3):83-88.

Sedlic A, Chingkoe C, Lee KW, Duddalwar VA, Chang SD. Abdominal extraosseous lesions of multiple myeloma: imaging findings. *Can Assoc Radiol J.* 2012 Mar;65(1):2-8.

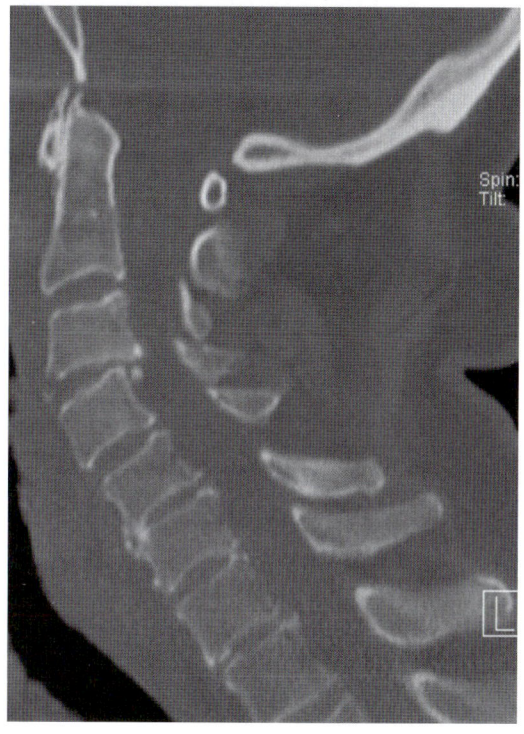 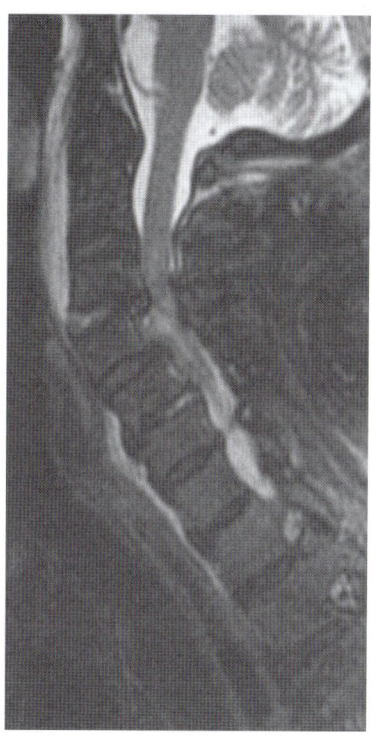

1. What are the major radiologic findings?

2. What is the likely mechanism of injury?

3. Which part of the spine is most commonly affected?

4. With regard to hyperextension and hyperflexion injuries, which are more stable?

5. When neurologic compromise occurs, what are the usual symptoms?

Case ranking/difficulty:

Category: Vertebral body

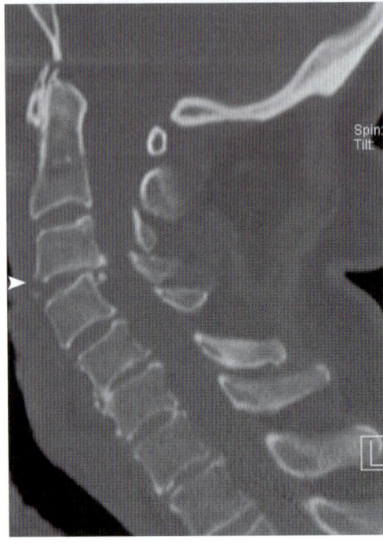

Extension teardrop fracture at C3, with mild retrolisthesis.

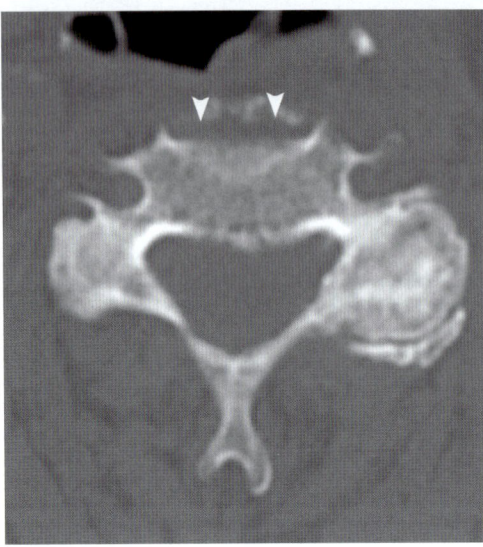

Fracture can be difficult to appreciate on axial images, especially if the orientation of the axial slices is suboptimal.

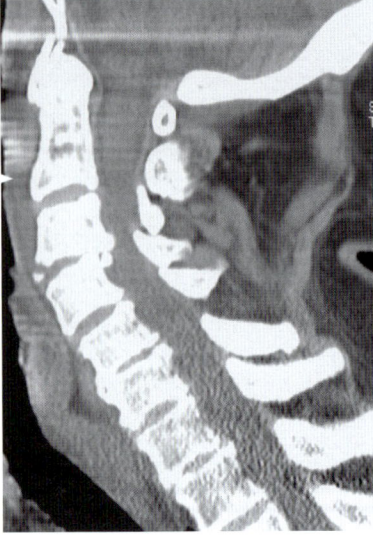

Prevertebral soft tissue swelling.

Answers

1. There is an extension teardrop fracture at the anterior inferior C3 body, with prevertebral soft tissue swelling and mild retrolisthesis of C3 resulting in cord compression.

2. The most likely mechanism, in an upper vertebral body corner fracture in an older patient, is hyperextension.

3. The upper cervical spine, especially C2, is most commonly affected in hyperextension injuries. Hyperflexion injuries predominate in the lower cervical spine.

4. Hyperextension injuries are more stable. Hyperflexion injuries, which predominate in the lower cervical spine, are more unstable and often result in cord compression.

5. The cord compression and edema classically results in an anterior cord syndrome, with quadriplegia and loss of pain, touch and temperature but with preservation of posterior column function such as proprioception and vibration.

- Fractures are more stable than their hyperflexion counterparts in the lower cervical spine.
- Cord compression, when it occurs, is due to retrolisthesis or compression from the hyperkyphotic vertebral segment. The anterior longitudinal ligament (ALL) avulses a triangular fragment of bone from the anterior inferior vertebral body. The fragment height is equal to or greater than its transverse dimension.
- The facet and interspinous distances may be widened.
- Prevertebral soft tissue swelling is usually present, but may be minimal or absent in older patients.
- Treatment is usually with cervical orthosis, but cervical fusion is indicated in some cases.

Suggested Readings

Rao SK, Wasyliw C, Nunez DB. Spectrum of imaging findings in hyperextension injuries of the neck. *Radiographics.* 2005;25(5):1239-1254.

Torretti JA, Sengupta DK. Cervical spine trauma. *Indian J Orthop.* 2007 Oct;41(4):255-267.

Pearls

- Extension teardrop fractures usually occurs in older patients with osteoporotic bone.
- C2 and C3 are most often affected. Hyperflexion injuries predominate in the lower cervical spine.

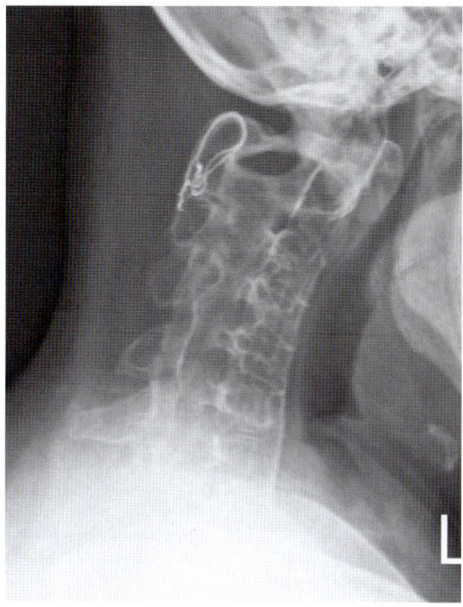 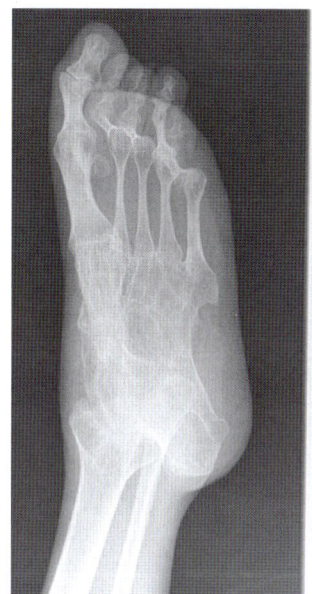 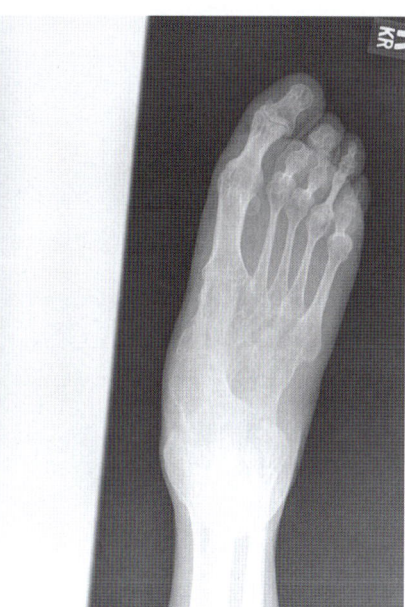

1. What are the radiographic findings?

2. What is the differential diagnosis, and what is the most likely diagnosis?

3. What are the major forms of this condition, using the American College of Rheumatology (ACR) criteria?

4. The pauciarticular type of this condition typically affects which joints?

5. In this case, what is the typical range of HLA-B27 positivity?

Case ranking/difficulty:

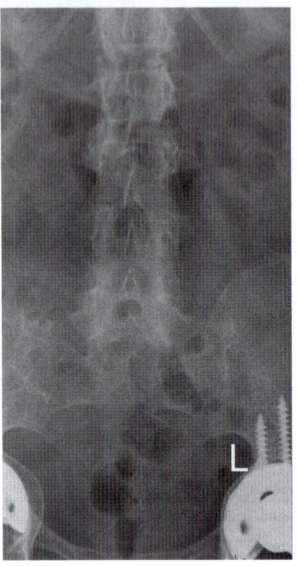

Sacroiliac joint, vertebral and posterior element fusion.

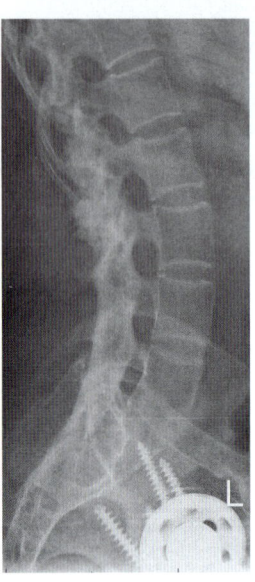

Posterior element fusion.

Answers

1. There is ankylosis of the cervical spine with tarsal ankylosis. Although the predental space can be widened and the dens eroded, these features are not present in this case.

2. Extensive bony ankylosis can be seen in juvenile idiopathic arthritis (JIA) and ankylosing spondylitis. This case demonstrates extensive spinal involvement that can be seen in both entities, and along with SI joint fusion, can make the diagnosis difficult. The presence of extensive tarsal ankylosis, however, suggests JIA as the diagnosis.

3. The three major types of JIA recognized by the ACR are the polyarticular, pauciarticular, and systemic types.

4. The pauciarticular type typically affects the large joints such as the knees and ankles. The polyarticular type affects the small joints of the hands and feet.

5. HLA-B27 is frequently positive in patients with late onset pauciarticular JIA, with the development of enthesitis and sacroiliitis. HLA-B27 is positive in approximately 80% of these cases.

- The systemic form is characterized by mainly systemic symptoms, with arthralgia, pleuritis, and pericarditis among a range of other symptoms.
- Soft tissue swelling, effusions, and periosteal reaction are typical. Hyperemia may result in overgrowth of the epiphyses.
- Bony ankylosis is characteristic and may affect the small and large joints. Ankylosis is not typically a feature of adult rheumatoid arthritis, except in the cervical spine.
- Cervical spine involvement in JIA is more common than lumbar and thoracic spine. In these patients, HLA-B27 is positive in up to 80% of cases, and SI joint fusion is also common. There is often a family history of spondyloarthropathy.
- Cervical spine features include facet erosions and ankylosis, predental space widening, dens erosion, and atlantoaxial subluxation.
- Ultrasound and MRI are useful in evaluating early peripheral changes, and monitoring the response to therapy.

Pearls

- Juvenile idiopathic arthritis has three main forms: polyarticular, pauciarticular, and systemic.
- Polyarticular form affects the small joints of the hands and feet.
- Pauciarticular form affects larger joints such as knees and ankles.

Suggested Readings

Johnson K. Imaging of juvenile idiopathic arthritis. *Pediatr Radiol.* 2006 Aug;36(8):743-758.

Johnson K, Wittkop B, Haigh F, Ryder C, Gardner-Medwin JM. The early magnetic resonance imaging features of the knee in juvenile idiopathic arthritis. *Clin Radiol.* 2002 Jun;57(6):466-471.

Short stature

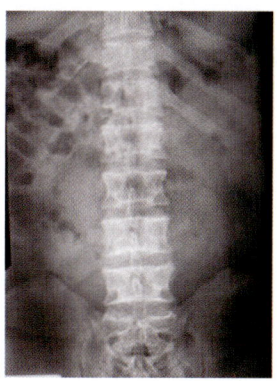 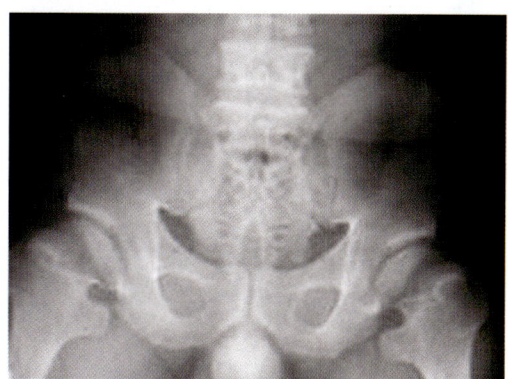

1. What are the findings on the radiographs?

2. What is the most likely diagnosis?

3. What form of dwarfism is demonstrated in this condition?

4. What is the inheritance pattern?

5. What are the main causes of mortality in these patients?

Case ranking/difficulty:

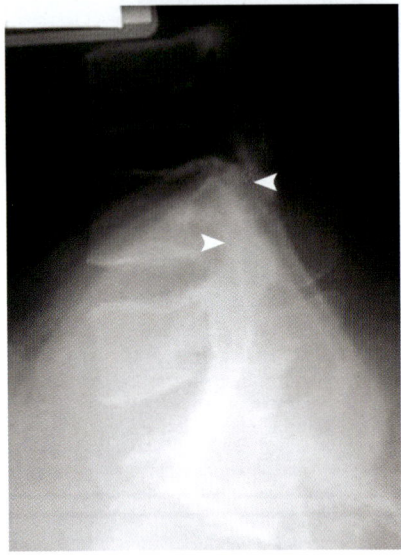

The pedicles are short and broad.

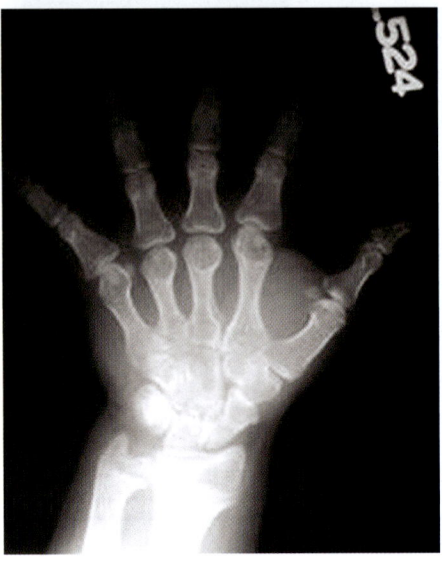

Short broad metacarpals and phalanges, with a trident hand.

Answers

1. Narrowed interpedicular distance, "Champagne" glass pelvis, horizontal sacrum, and acetabulae with short, broad femoral heads and necks.

2. The findings are consistent with achondroplasia.

3. Achondroplasia is a disproportionate rhizomelic (proximal) dwarfism.

4. 85% of cases are a result of a spontaneous genetic mutation, and 15% are due to an autosomal dominant inheritance.

5. In patients under 4 years, brainstem compression is the leading cause of death. Between 5 and 24 years central nervous system and respiratory causes predominate, and between 25 and 54 years cardiovascular complications are the leading cause of death.

Pearls

- Achondroplasia is a proximal (rhizomelic) dwarfism.
- Endochondral ossification is affected, with normal periosteal and membranous bone growth.
- Affected bones are short with normal thickness.
- There is metaphyseal flaring with a ball in socket epiphysis.
- There are also trident hands, which are fingers of equal length that are widely opposed
- The vertebrae are bullet shaped with posterior scalloping and spinal stenosis. Brainstem compression may occur.
- A "champagne" glass pelvis is seen.
- The foramen magnum is narrowed, which can lead to brainstem compression.
- Mortality is increased, usually due to brainstem compression in young patients, and respiratory and cardiovascular complications in older patients.

Suggested Readings

Kao SC, Waziri MH, Smith WL, Sato Y, Yuh WT, Franken EA. MR imaging of the craniovertebral junction, cranium, and brain in children with achondroplasia. *AJR Am J Roentgenol.* 1989 Sep;153(3):565-569.

Song HR, Choonia AT, Hong SJ, Lee SH, Suh SW, Cha IH, Park JT. Rotational profile of the lower extremity in achondroplasia: computed tomographic examination of 25 patients. *Skeletal Radiol.* 2006 Dec;35(12):929-934.

Chronic back pain

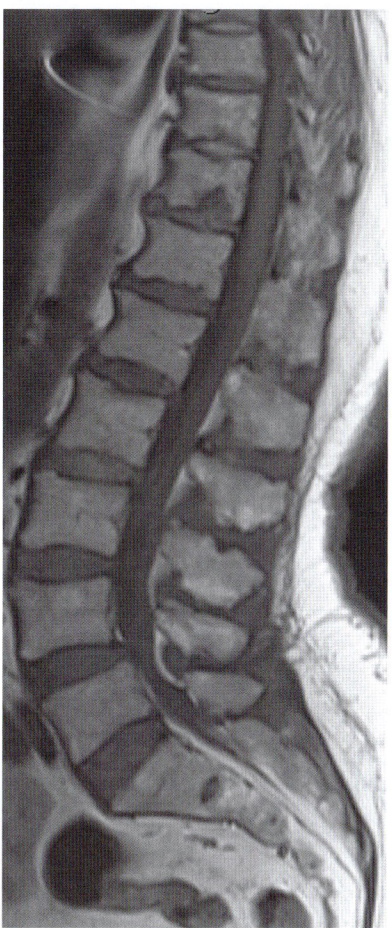 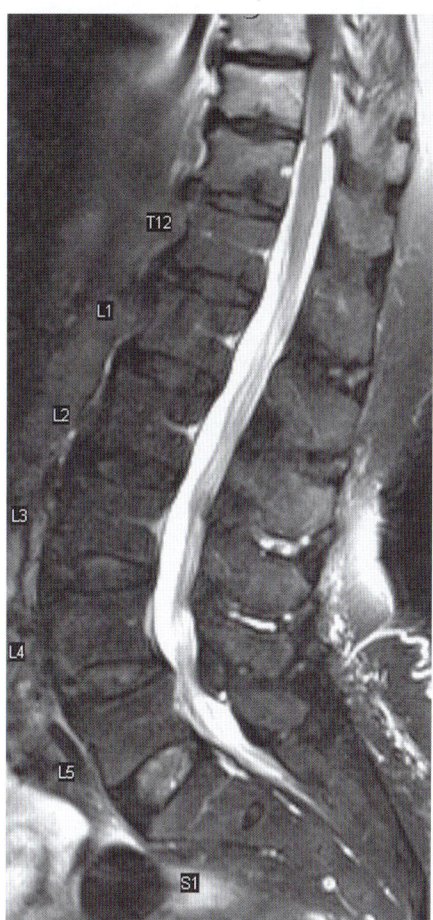

1. What are the salient MRI findings?

2. What is the diagnosis?

3. What are contributory factors to this entity?

4. The condition is most commonly seen in the lumbar spine. True or False?

5. Surgical excision of the spinous processes is curative. True or False?

Case ranking/difficulty:

Category: Posterior elements

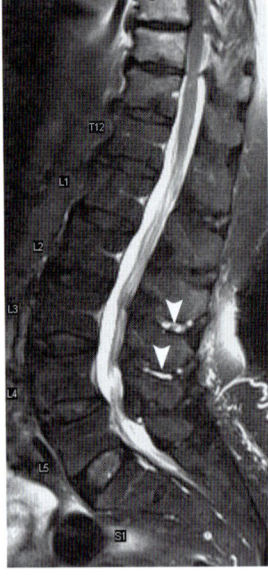

Note interspinous bursitis (*arrowheads*).

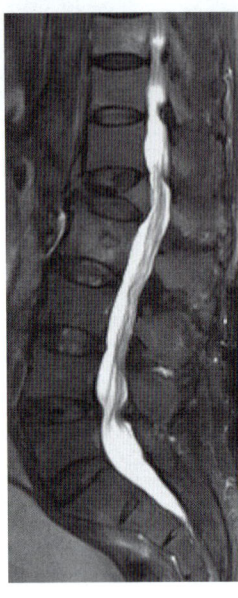

Another patient with a compression fracture and loss of vertebral height. The extent to which associated vertebral and disc disease is contributory is uncertain.

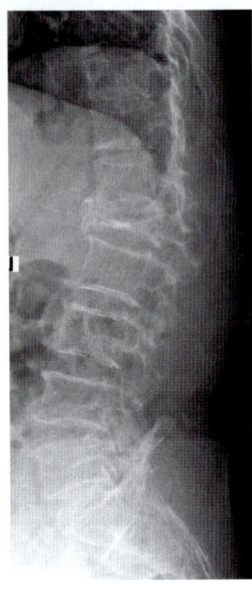

Note the enlarged spinous processes.

Answers

1. The spinous processes are enlarged with interspinous bursitis. Although degenerative disc disease with height loss is a frequent association, it is not present in this case.

2. The findings are compatible with a diagnosis of Baastrup phenomenon.

3. Baastrup phenomenon is associated with advancing age, with a prevalence of more than 80% above age 80. Degenerative disc disease or vertebral height loss are frequent associations; however, the condition may be seen when the rest of the spine is entirely normal. The contact between the spinous processes is accentuated in extension.

4. True. Baastrup phenomena is almost always seen in the lumbar spine, although the thoracic spine may be affected very infrequently.

5. False. Although there are undoubtedly nociceptors formed at the spinous processes of these patients, the result of surgical excision of the spinous processes has been disappointing. Therefore, failure to address other causes of back pain in these individuals may result in ongoing pain.

Pearls

- Baastrup phenomenon is a condition where the spinous processes of the spine (usually the lumbar) become enlarged, flat, and sclerotic and are in contact with each other.
- The contact between the spinous processes is accentuated in extension.
- Adventitial bursae form between the spinous processes, and are readily detected on MRI.
- Associated degenerative disc disease with loss of disc height is frequent. The degree to which Baastrup is contributory to back pain is therefore uncertain.
- The incidence increases with advancing age, with a prevalence of more than 80% over age 80.
- Treatment is typically conservative.

Suggested Readings

Kwong Y, Rao N, Latief K. MDCT findings in Baastrup disease: disease or normal feature of the aging spine? *AJR Am J Roentgenol*. 2011 May;196(5):1156-1159.

Maes R, Morrison WB, Parker L, Schweitzer ME, Carrino JA. Lumbar interspinous bursitis (Baastrup disease) in a symptomatic population: prevalence on magnetic resonance imaging. *Spine (Phila Pa 1976)*. 2008 Apr;33(7):E211-E215.

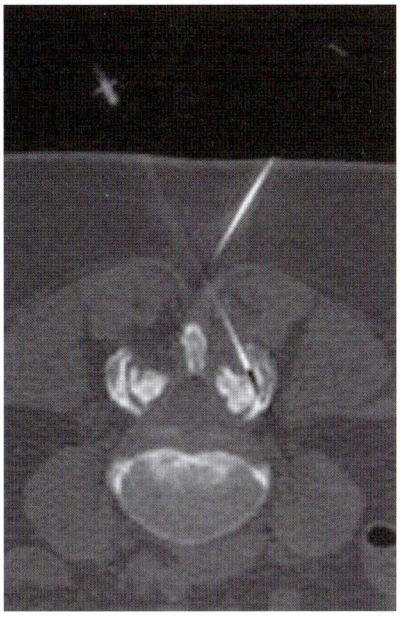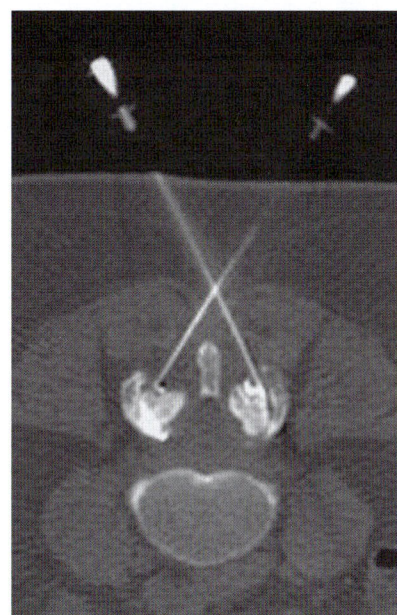

1. What is this procedure called?

2. Name some indications for this procedure.

3. Name some contraindications to the procedure.

4. Which drugs are used for infiltration?

5. Are there any recognized complications of this procedure?

Case ranking/difficulty:

Category: Posterior elements

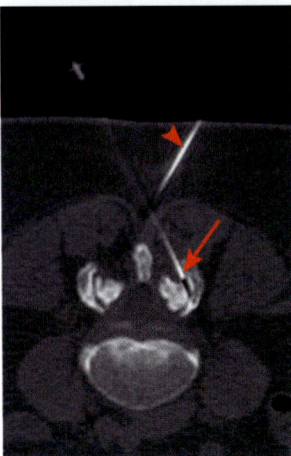

Axial CT image with the patient in the prone position. Bilateral percutaneous needle placement into L4-5 facet joints. The tip of the first needle is already placed within the capsule (*arrow*) and the second needle (*arrowhead*) is being advanced to reach the left sided L4-5 facet joint.

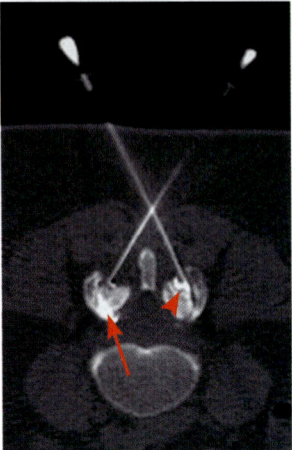

A small amount of contrast injection confirmed the intracapsular position of the needle tips (*arrow* and *arrowhead*). The joints were then infiltrated using 20 mg of Depo-Medrol and 0.5 mL of 0.5% Bupivacaine under strict aseptic technique.

The procedure is performed under imaging guidance using fluoroscopy, computed tomography, ultrasound, or MR guidance, which confirms the needle placement and increases the precision of the procedure.

4. The procedure is performed under local anesthetic using strict aseptic precautions. The joint is infiltrated with a long-acting steroid depot preparation and a long-acting local anesthetic agent via a 23G spinal needle inserted percutaneously. The injected anesthetic agent acts on the nociceptive fibers within the synovium, whereas the corticosteroids reduce synovial inflammation.

The position of the needle tip may be confirmed by injecting contrast within the capsule prior to injection of the mixture, although studies have shown that precise intra-articular injection is not required.

5. Complications are very rare and include septic arthritis, spondylodiscitis, and allergy to the injectates. The outcome of facet joint injection is variable and some patients may not achieve the desired benefit. In patients who experience symptom relief, the therapeutic benefit may be short lived and may necessitate repeated injections.

The capacity of the normal facet joint is about 2 mL, and care must be taken when injecting the joint not to cause capsular disruption and spillage of the injected mixture into the epidural space and adjacent soft tissues.

Answers

1. Facet joint injection is a spinal interventional procedure used for both treatment and diagnosis of radicular pain syndromes.

   The procedure has a high diagnostic accuracy and reproducibility. The long-term clinical outcome is, however, variable.

   Facet joints are a common cause of chronic pain and were proven to be responsible for up to 45% of lower back pains. Facet joints are synovial joints and inflammation or trauma may lead to painful back movement. This may initiate a vicious cycle of physical deconditioning with irritation of the facet nerves and muscular spasm. The joints are richly innervated by the dorsal ramus of spinal nerves.

2. Indications for facet joint infiltrations are multiple and include clinical suspicion of facet syndrome, chronic low back pain with negative radiology, tenderness over the facet joints, and persistent low back pain postsurgery.

3. Although there are no absolute contraindications, the procedure is often avoided in patients with bleeding diathesis, allergy to contrast or to the injectates, infection particularly if affecting the puncture site, and pregnancy.

Pearls

- Facet joint injection is used for both treatment and diagnosis of radicular pain syndromes.
- The joint is infiltrated with a long-acting steroid depot preparation and a long-acting local anesthetic agent via a spinal needle inserted percutaneously.
- Complications are rare and include septic arthritis, spondylodiscitis, and allergy to the injectates.

Suggested Readings

Boyajian SS. Using image-guided techniques for chronic low back pain. *J Am Osteopath Assoc.* 2007 Nov;107(10 suppl 6):ES3-ES9.

Peh W. Image-guided facet joint injection. *Biomed Imaging Interv J.* 2011 Jan-Mar;7(1).

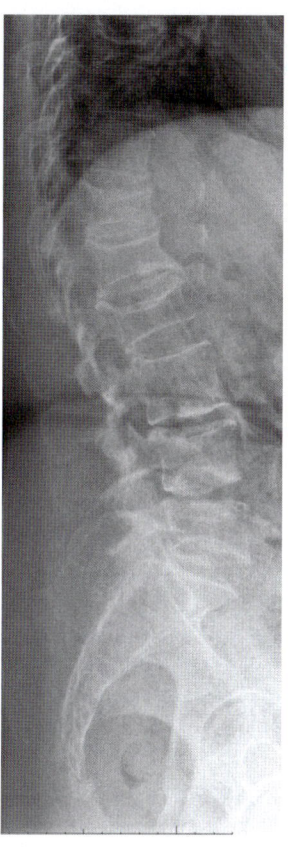 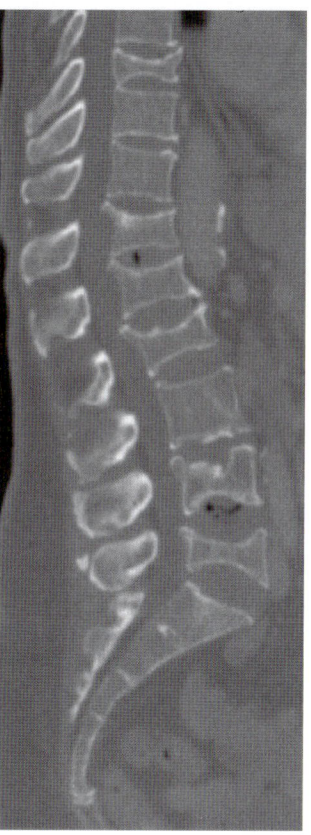

1. What are the major radiographic findings?

2. What determines the severity of the condition?

3. What are the types of vertebral osteoporotic compression fractures?

4. What are some of the radiographic pitfalls when diagnosing these fractures?

5. When is vertebral augmentation therapy indicated?

Case ranking/difficulty:

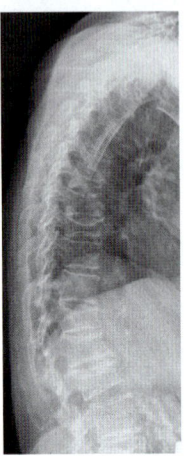

Similar findings in the thoracic spine.

Answers

1. The bones are diffusely osteopenic, with cortical thinning and accentuated vertical trabeculae. Multiple biconcave and wedge deformities are seen. Minimal retropulsion is seen at T12 and L2.

2. Although many factors are taken into consideration when determining severity, osteoporotic vertebral fractures are generally classified as mild, moderate, or severe depending on the degree of height loss.

3. Fractures are classified depending on which part of the vertebral body is involved: wedge (anterior), biconcave (middle), or crush (posterior).

4. Several entities may mimic osteoporotic compression fractures. These include a lateral film that is not a true lateral, ie, an oblique film, scoliosis, cupid's bow (a developmental variant), limbus vertebra, multiple Schmorl nodes (Scheuermann disease), and H-shaped vertebrae in sickle cell disease.

5. Failure to respond to medical therapy and intractable pain are the most important reasons for vertebral augmentation. These procedures include vertebroplasty where cement (polymethylmethacrylate or PMMA) is injected into the vertebral body percutaneously, or kyphoplasty where there is balloon inflation to restore vertebral height prior to injection of the cement. Kyphoplasties are performed in patients with vertebral fractures and associated kyphosis.

   Complications include those related to needle placement, iatrogenic fractures, cement extravasation, infection, and bleeding.

Pearls

- Osteoporotic vertebral compression fractures are extremely common, occurring in up to 50% of the US population after 50 years of age.
- Radiologic signs of osteoporosis include loss of bone density, cortical thinning, and accentuation of the vertical trabeculae.
- Fracture patterns include wedge fracture, biconcave fracture, and crush fractures. Severity is determined by the degree of height loss:
  - Mild: 20%-25%
  - Moderate: 26%-40%
  - Severe: 40%
- Acute fractures can demonstrate a cortical break and trabecular impaction, but these are often difficult to see especially on radiographs.
- Fractures are most common in the lower thoracic and upper lumbar spine (T12-L1), where a kyphotic deformity may occur.
- Radiologic pitfalls include simulation of endplate depression by an oblique lateral projection, scoliosis and the presence of multiple Schmorl nodes.

Suggested Readings

Kondo KL. Osteoporotic vertebral compression fractures and vertebral augmentation. *Semin Intervent Radiol.* 2008 Dec;25(4):413-424.

Lenchik L, Rogers LF, Delmas PD, Genant HK. Diagnosis of osteoporotic vertebral fractures: importance of recognition and description by radiologists. *AJR Am J Roentgenol.* 2004 Oct;183(4):949-958.

Motor vehicle accident

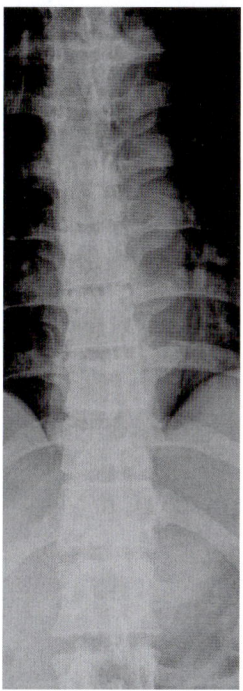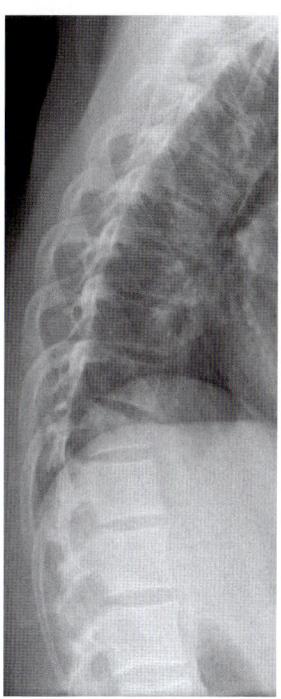

1. What are the major radiographic findings?

2. What is the diagnosis?

3. MRI is usually indicated in the workup of these individual. True or False?

4. What is the most commonly affected level?

5. Which patients are prone to this injury?

Case ranking/difficulty:

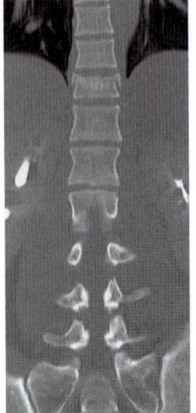

Horizontal component
well demonstrated.

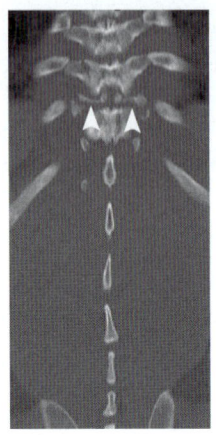

Posterior element
involvement.

Fracture well demonstrated.

Answers

1. There is anterior compression of the T11 vertebral body, with a horizontal split fracture involving the body and extending into the posterior elements.

2. The findings are compatible with a Chance fracture.

3. False. Neurological compromise is rare, and MRI is only indicated in the patient with unexplained neurological symptoms or in the polytrauma patient. Findings may include contusion of the conus medullaris, or cauda equina compression.

4. The most commonly affected level is L2. In children, where the center of gravity is lower, the fracture is usually in the midlumbar spine.

5. Patients using lap seatbelts alone in a motor vehicle accident are prone to this fracture. Fall from a height is another common mechanism. In addition, those with a rigid spine, eg, patients with ankylosing spondylitis are more susceptible to a Chance fracture.

Pearls

- Chance fractures are a result of a flexion distraction injury.
- The use of lap seatbelts alone is implicated. With the advent of combined lap and shoulder belts, the incidence is falling.
- The thoracolumbar junction, especially L2, is most commonly affected.
- Associated abdominal injuries are common, occurring in up to 50% of the pediatric population.
- Concomitant neurological compromise is rare.
- Treatment is usually conservative with reduction in extension, and placement of a cast. However, surgical fusion may be indicated where body habitus precludes adequate reduction, or in the polytrauma patient.

Suggested Readings

Bernstein MP, Mirvis SE, Shanmuganathan K. Chance-type fractures of the thoracolumbar spine: imaging analysis in 53 patients. *AJR Am J Roentgenol.* 2006 Oct;187(4):859-868.

Daffner RH. Chance fracture of the upper thoracic spine. *AJR Am J Roentgenol.* 2005 Aug;185(2):555.

Davis JM, Beall DP, Lastine C, Sweet C, Wolff J, Wu D. Chance fracture of the upper thoracic spine. *AJR Am J Roentgenol.* 2004 Nov;183(5):1475-1478.

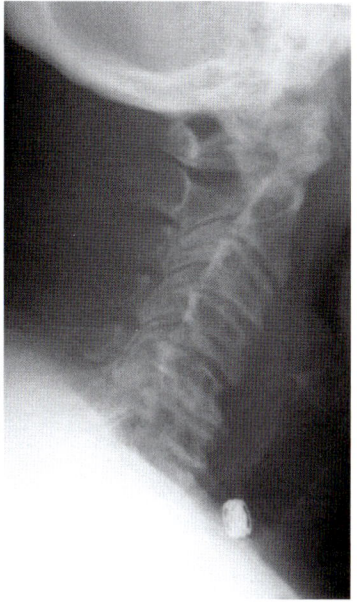 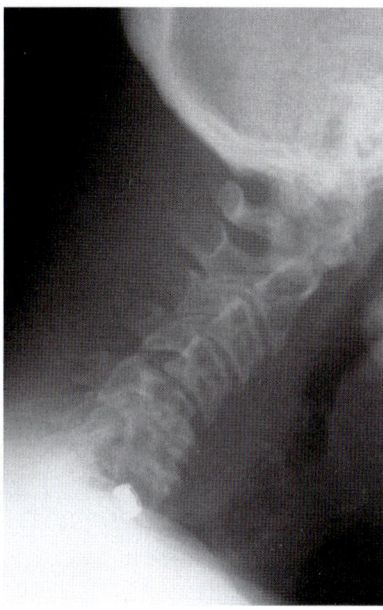 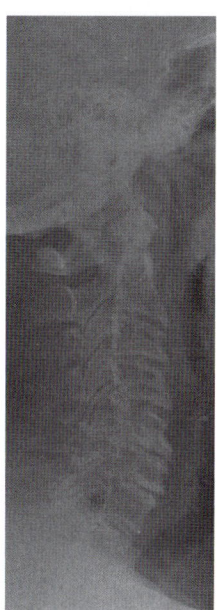

1. What is the major radiographic finding?

2. What is the diagnosis?

3. What measurement typically constitutes longitudinal instability?

4. What measurement typically constitutes rotational instability?

5. At what level in the pediatric cervical spine is anterolisthesis considered normal?

Case ranking/difficulty:

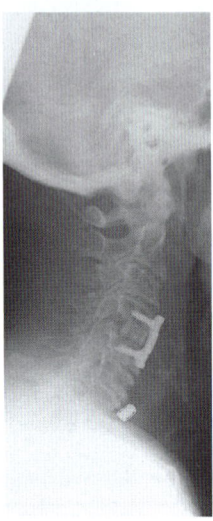

Treated with an anterior cervical fusion.

Answers

1. There is significant anterolisthesis of C4 on C5 on flexion, as well as an increase in angulation.

2. The findings are consistent with ligamentous instability.

3. Longitudinal instability in the cervical spine is implied if the total translational motion exceeds 3.5 mm. The total translational motion includes adding any retrolisthesis on extension to the anterolisthesis on flexion.

4. Sagittal rotational instability refers to the angular change at the level of the disc on flexion and extension, and is considered abnormal if greater than 11°.

5. There can be up to 3 mm of anterolisthesis of C2 on C3 in the pediatric cervical spine (patients less than 8 years old) as a normal finding, due to ligamentous laxity and more horizontal facets. Care must be taken when evaluating the pediatric trauma patient, as placement on a standard trauma board may cause the neck to flex due to the large head size, accentuating this pseudosubluxation. A trauma board that allows slight extension should be used.

   Pseudosubluxation may also occur to a lesser extent at C3-4.

Pearls

- Ligamentous instability of the spine has numerous etiologies, most commonly traumatic, degenerative, or related to ligamentous laxity.
- Instability can be longitudinal or rotational.
- In the cervical spine, anterior translation of more than 3.5 mm between flexion and extension implies longitudinal instability.
- Rotational instability is implied if sagittal rotation is greater than 11°.
- White and Panjabi proposed a checklist system for each region (cervical, thoracic, and lumbar).
- White and Panjabi criteria:
  - Anterior elements = 2
  - Posterior elements = 2
  - Sagittal translation 3.5 mm or 20% of vertebra = 2
  - Sagittal rotation greater than 11° = 2
  - Positive stretch test = 2
  - Cord damage = 2
  - Root damage = 1
  - Abnormal disc narrowing = 1
  - Dangerous loads anticipated = 1
- Unstable if total score greater than 5.
- Denis proposed a three-column concept for the spine (anterior, middle, and posterior), with injury to two or more columns implying instability.
- Treatment is usually with surgical fusion.

Suggested Readings

Denis F. Spinal instability as defined by the three-column spine concept in acute spinal trauma. *Clin Orthop Relat Res*. 1984 Oct;65-76(189):65-76.

White AA, Panjabi MM. *Clinical Biomechanics of the Spine*. 2nd ed. Philadelphia, PA: Lippincott; 1990:30-342.

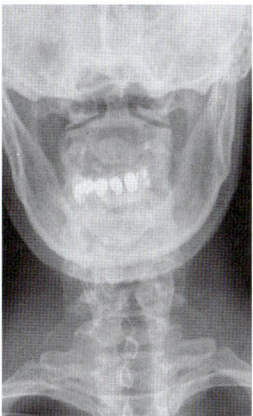 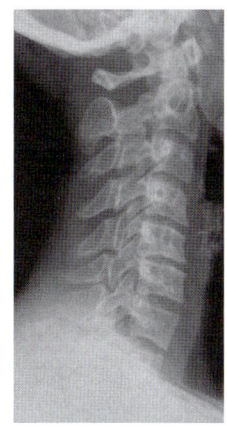 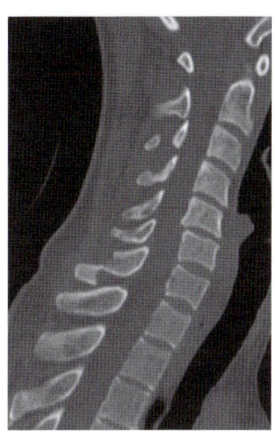 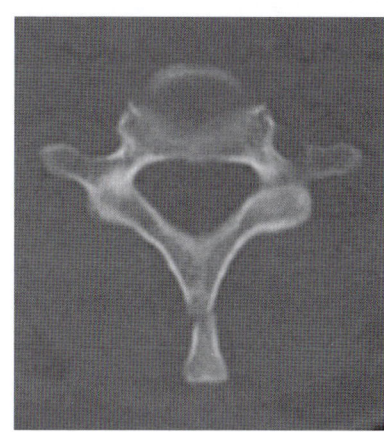

1. What is the main radiographic finding?

2. What is the double spinous process (or ghost) sign?

3. What is the proposed mechanism of injury?

4. Which vertebral level is most commonly affected?

5. The injury is unstable. True or False?

Case ranking/difficulty:

Category: Vertebral body

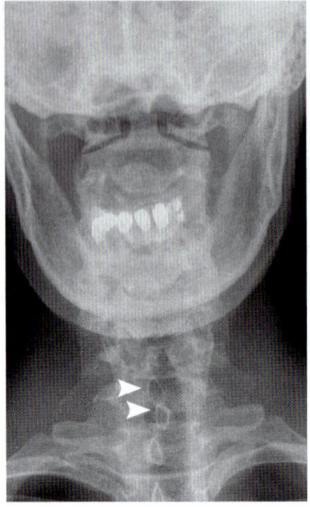

"Double spinous process" sign at C7.

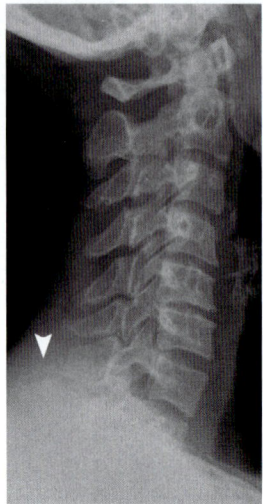

Displaced C7 spinous process fracture.

Answers

1. There is a displaced C7 spinous process fracture, a "clay shoveler" fracture.

2. The displaced fracture fragment and the native intact base give the appearance of two spinous processes at the affected level on the AP film. There are several described "ghost" signs, eg, meniscal radial tear, osteomyelitis of the Charcot foot etc, but there is only one described in the spine!

3. This fracture is believed to be an avulsion fracture of the spinous process by the powerful supraspinous ligament.

4. C7 is most commonly affected, although C6 and T1 are not uncommon. Other levels are much less common.

5. False. This avulsion fracture affects only the posterior column of the spine, and is considered a stable fracture.

Pearls

- Clay shoveler fracture was originally described in clay shovelers in Australia in the 1930s.
- It is an avulsion fracture of the spinous process of C7, and less commonly C6 or T1.
- The supraspinous ligament is believed to be responsible for the avulsion injury.
- AP film may show a "ghost" or "double spinous process" sign, representing the fracture fragment and the intact base.
- Lateral film shows that the fracture fragment is inferiorly displaced.
- Treatment is conservative with immobilization using an orthotic device.

Suggested Reading

Tehranzadeh J, Bonk RT, Ansari A, Mesgarzadeh M. Efficacy of limited CT for nonvisualized lower cervical spine in patients with blunt trauma. *Skeletal Radiol.* 1994 Jul;23(5):349-352.

Back pain and stiffness

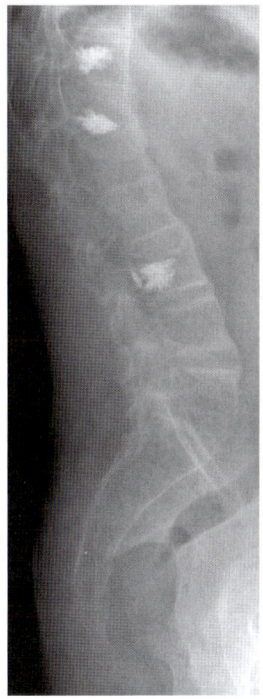
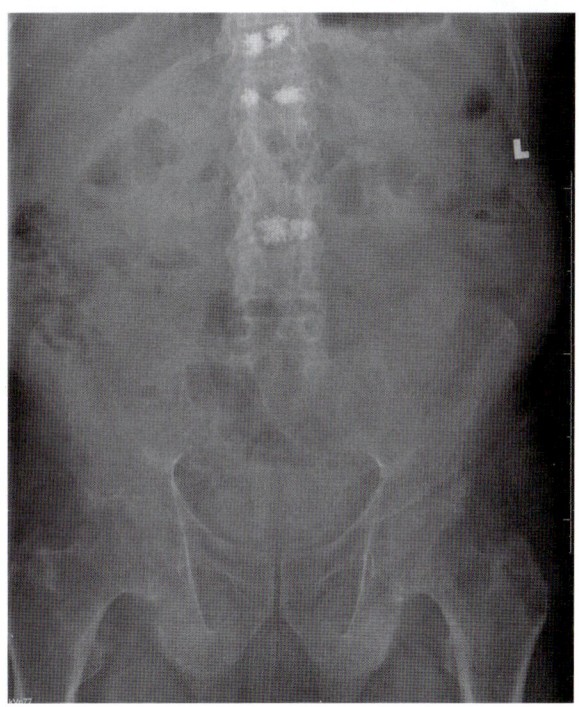

1. What are classical features of this condition?

2. Which diseases are associated with HLA-B27 positivity?

3. What are the possible treatments of this condition?

4. What are the local and systemic complications of this condition?

5. Which groups of patients have the highest levels of HLA- B27 concordance?

Case ranking/difficulty:

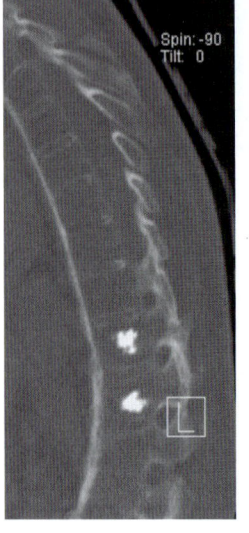

"Bamboo" spine.

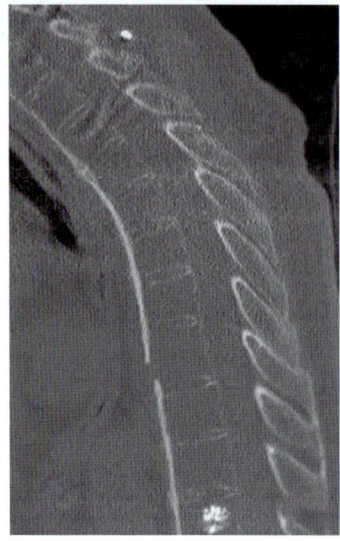

Subsequent fracture through the rigid immobile spine.

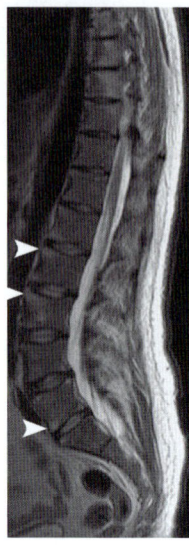

Another patient with Romanus lesions.

Answers

1. Entheseal inflammation is the basic pathology of ankylosing spondylitis. Atlantoaxial subluxation is a feature of rheumatoid arthritis. Sacroiliitis is usually bilateral and classically symmetric, although frequently asymmetric: if sacroiliitis is unilateral, infection must always be excluded. Peripheral joint ankylosis is not a feature.

2. Seronegative spondyloarthropathies include ankylosing spondylitis, psoriasis, inflammatory bowel disease, and reactive disease.

3. Treatment for ankylosing spondylitis is generally directed at symptom control. Surgical correction of a kyphotic deformity is not generally performed. Novel approaches include anti-TNF therapy, which is intended to treat active inflammation mediated by TNF-alpha cytokines.

4. Ankylosing spondylitis can predispose to spinal fracture and cord compression. Plantar fascitis is another association.

   Only 1% of cases are associated with an apical lung fibrosis.

5. Over 90% of Caucasians with ankylosing spondylitis are HLA-B27 positive. The male:female ratio is 3:1.

Pearls

- Bilateral symmetrical sacroiliitis is highly suggestive of ankylosing spondylitis.

- Due to the high relative incidence of the condition relative to other causes of sacroiliitis, unilateral or asymmetric sacroiliitis is still more likely to be due to ankylosing spondylitis than due to other disorders.
- Classical features include syndesmophytes, Romanus lesions, squaring of vertebral bodies, Andersson lesions, and bamboo spine.
- Syndesmophyte formation is due to ossification of the outer fibers of the annulus fibrosus. It is best assessed on a frontal radiograph.
- Chance fractures can occur through ossified intervertebral discs with relatively little trauma, as these are the sites of mechanical weakness.
- Early spinal features include inflammation at costovertebral and costotransverse joints, which is best assessed on a fluid-sensitive MRI sequence.
- It is important to look for extraarticular features and associated features of HLA-B27 disorders, eg, apical lung fibrosis and enthesitis. Also inflammatory bowel disease and psoriasis may be difficult to differentiate, so features of these conditions should be sought after.

Suggested Readings

Braun J, Baraliakos X. Imaging of axial spondyloarthritis including ankylosing spondylitis. *Ann Rheum Dis.* 2011 Mar;(70 suppl 1):i97-i103.

Ostergaard M, Poggenborg RP, Axelsen MB, Pedersen PJ. Magnetic resonance imaging in spondyloarthritis—how to quantify findings and measure response. *Best Pract Res Clin Rheumatol.* 2010 Oct;24(5):637-657.

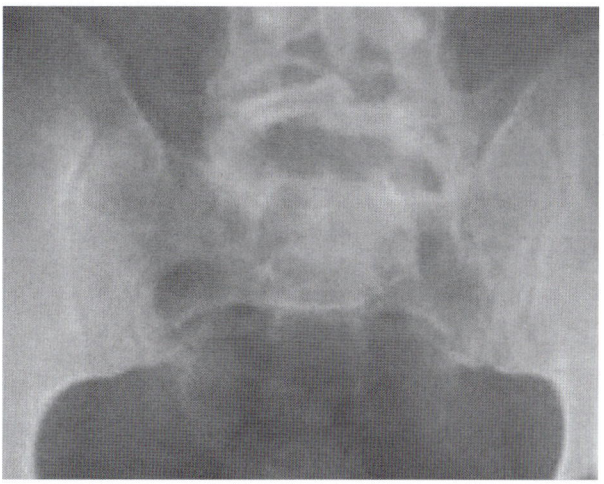 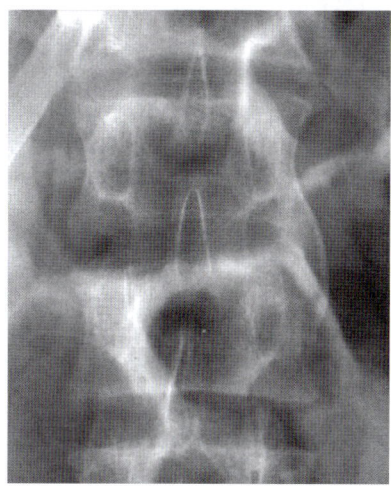

1. What are the radiographic findings?

2. What is the most likely diagnosis?

3. What are other spinal features of this entity?

4. What proportion of patients with cutaneous disease have an inflammatory arthritis?

5. What are the possible treatments of this condition?

Case ranking/difficulty:

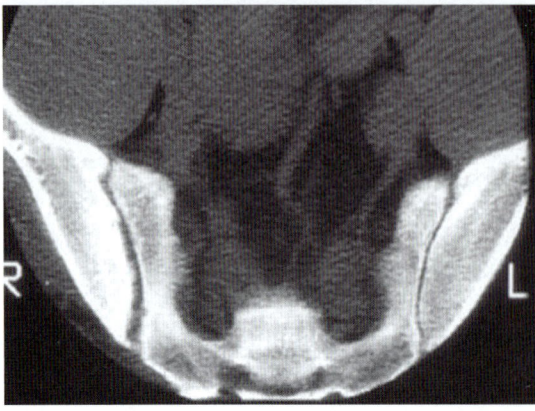

Erosions in the anterior vertebral body in another patient.

Right erosive sacroiliitis. No definite erosive changes in the left SI joint; however, MRI would be more sensitive in detecting early changes.

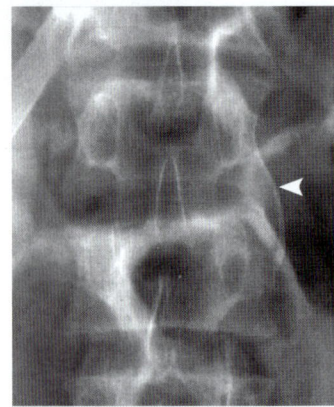

Bulky asymmetric lateral syndesmophyte.

Answers

1. There are bulky asymmetric syndesmophytes, with erosions in the right sacroiliac joint consistent with sacroiliitis.

2. Bulky and asymmetric syndesmophytes, ie, paraspinal ossification that flows from one vertebral body to the next (unlike the thin symmetric annular ossification seen in ankylosing spondylitis), along with an asymmetric sacroiliitis, is characteristic of the seronegative spondyloarthropathies. The presence of a chronic skin condition suggests psoriasis is the diagnosis.

3. Along with thick asymmetric syndesmophytes and an asymmetric sacroiliitis, psoriatic spondylitis may manifest as vertebral erosions and periostitis with eventual ankylosis. The ankylosed spine is prone to fractures.

4. Psoriatic arthritis is a relatively common generalized manifestation of psoriasis, occurring in up to one-third of patients with the skin condition. It is possible, however, to have arthritis as the first presentation of the disease, prior to the development of any skin lesions. Approximately 20% of psoriatic arthritis patients will develop a spondylitis.

5. Methotrexate and azathioprine are classic disease-modifying steroid-sparing antirheumatic drugs (DMARDs). Intra-articular injections have the benefit of avoiding or minimizing severe systemic corticosteroid side effects. Surgery is reserved for severe functionally limiting cases.

Pearls

- Psoriatic arthritis is one of the most common spondyloarthropathies, after primary ankylosing spondylitis.
- It may have many forms, but the most common manifestations are an asymmetric arthritis affecting a few joints, and a seronegative symmetric arthritis, clinically indistinguishable from rheumatoid arthritis.
- The most severe form of peripheral psoriatic arthritis is termed *arthritis mutilans*. Characteristic features of arthritis mutilans are severe erosions in a "pencil-in-cup" pattern, "sausage digits," and a distribution more distal than a typical rheumatoid pattern.
- Enthesitis (eg, Achilles) and dactylitis are characteristic of psoriatic arthritis.
- In the spine, it is characterized by bulky asymmetrical syndesmophytes unlike the smooth thin symmetric syndesmophytes of ankylosing spondylitis.
- Erosions and periostitis in the vertebral bodies may be seen.
- There is often a bilateral asymmetric sacroiliitis.
- Patients are frequently HLA-B27 positive.

Suggested Readings

Amrami KK. Imaging of the seronegative spondyloarthopathies. *Radiol Clin North Am.* 2012 Jul;50(4):841-854.

Paparo F, Revelli M, Semprini A, et al. Seronegative spondyloarthropathies: what radiologists should know. *Radiol Med.* 2013 Nov.

Sudoł-Szopinska I, Urbanik A. Diagnostic imaging of sacroiliac joints and the spine in the course of spondyloarthropathies. *Pol J Radiol.* 2013 Apr;78(2):43-49.

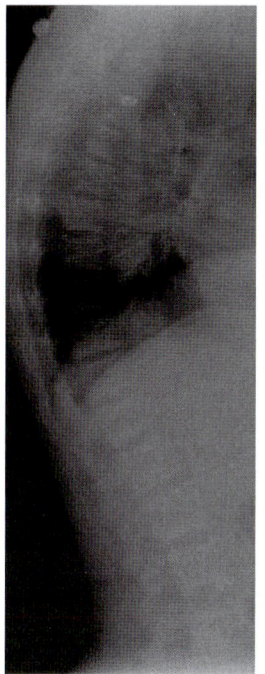 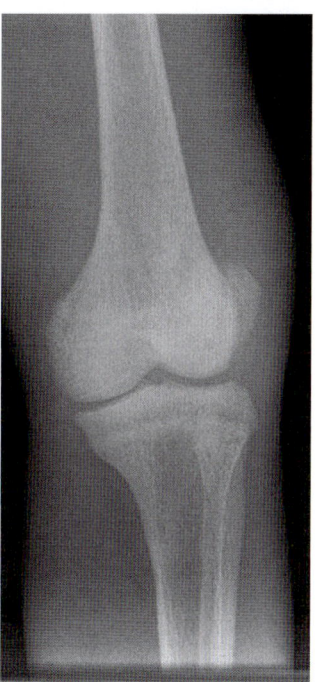

1. What is the major vertebral finding?

2. What is the differential diagnosis?

3. What is the presumed etiology?

4. What appearance may be seen in a radionuclide bone scan?

5. The changes are decreased after renal transplantation. True or False?

Case ranking/difficulty:

Category: Vertebral body

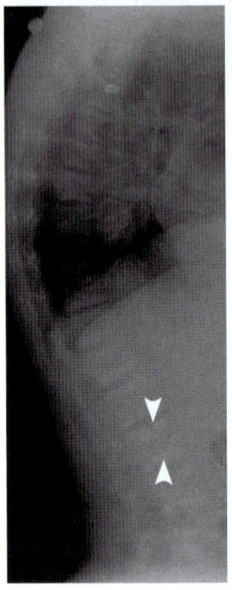

Sclerosis of the endplates of numerous vertebral bodies.

Answers

1. Alternating sclerotic endplates with more lucent central vertebral bodies is consistent with a "rugger jersey spine" appearance, typical of renal osteodystrophy.

2. A "sandwich vertebra" appearance is seen in osteopetrosis, and can have a similar appearance; however, the age group and medical history will help differentiate. Paget disease can result in a "picture–frame" appearance; however, the disease is usually not generalized, and the bones are typically expanded.

   Metastatic disease shows generalized osteosclerosis. Fluorosis and myelofibrosis can have a similar appearance, but there is usually vertebral/paraspinal calcification/ossification in fluorosis, and the spleen is enlarged in myelofibrosis.

3. An increase in the amount of cancellous bone, and an increase in the thickness and number of trabeculae are typically seen. There is also increased deposition of amorphous calcium phosphate.

4. A "superscan" appearance with increased bone uptake and soft tissue uptake (in extraskeletal calcification), but no renal excretion of radiopharmaceutical can be seen in renal osteodystrophy. The soft tissue uptake will help differentiate this superscan appearance from generalized metastatic disease.

5. False. The osseous changes of renal osteodystrophy are often paradoxically increased after renal transplantation.

Pearls

- A rugger jersey spine appearance is seen in patients with renal osteodystrophy. It refers to the appearance of sclerotic endplates with central lucency.
- A similar appearance can be seen in Paget disease or osteopetrosis (sandwich vertebrae).
- The etiology is poorly understood, but there is usually an increase in cancellous bone in these patients, as well as an increase in number and thickness of the trabeculae within the cancellous bone.
- Bones with a high concentration of cancellous bone, such as the vertebrae, are therefore often affected.
- Deposition of amorphous calcium phosphate rather than calcium hydroxyapatite in bone may also be contributory.
- Changes of renal osteodystrophy are typically seen when more than 50% of renal function is lost.

Suggested Readings

Beladi Mousavi. Renal bone disease among patients with ESRD. *Nephrourol Mon.* 2013 Jul;5(3):849-850.

Liu Y. Super-superscan on a bone scintigraphy. *Clin Nucl Med.* 2011 Mar;36(3):227-228.

Wittenberg A. The rugger jersey spine sign. *Radiology.* 2004 Feb;230(2):491-492.

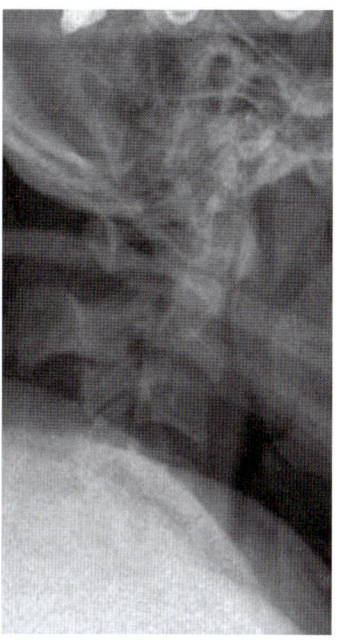 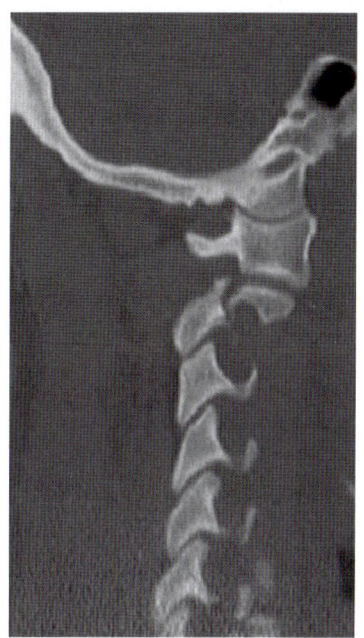

1. What are the imaging findings?

2. What is the diagnosis?

3. What is the typical mechanism of injury?

4. This injury is more common in young children.
   True or False?

5. Neurological compromise is very common.
   True or False?

Case ranking/difficulty: **Category:** Vertebral body

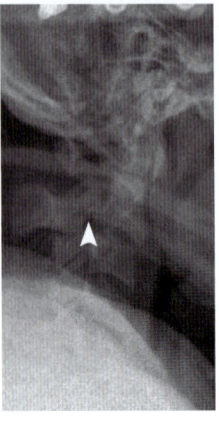

Fracture of the pars interarticularis of C2.

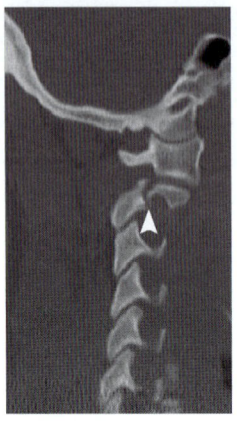

C2 pars fracture well demonstrated.

Bilateral C2 fractures, extending into the foramen transversarium bilaterally.

Answers

1. There are bilateral fractures of the pars inter-articularis of C2, with prevertebral soft tissue swelling and mild anterolisthesis of C2 on C3.

2. Bilateral pars or pedicle fractures of C2 is coined a "Hangman" fracture.

3. Extension and distraction are the typical mechanism of injury in "Hangman" fractures.

4. False. Injury in children under 8 years is uncommon because fractures preferentially occur through the unfused synchondrosis at the base of the dens. This synchondrosis usually fuses at 6-7 years.

5. False. The autodecompression of the spinal canal that occurs with bilateral C2 fractures reduces the incidence of spinal cord injury.

- Anterolisthesis of C2 on C3 and pre-vertebral soft tissue swelling are associated features. CT is indicated to assess the integrity of the foramen transversarium.
- If the fracture extends into the foramina, CT angiography is indicated to assess the condition of the vertebral arteries.
- MRI is mandatory in any patient with neurologic compromise. The soft tissues, discs, and spinal cord are readily assessed.
- Neurological deficit is not as common as one would expect because of the autodecompression of the spinal canal that occurs in bilateral pars interarticularis or pedicle fractures.
- Treatment is usually with a Halo-vest, and in some instances, with spinal fusion. When the mechanism involves extension and distraction, as in most cases, cervical traction should be avoided.

Pearls

- Hangman fracture is a fracture, typically bilateral, of the pedicles or pars interarticularis of C2.
- The injury is uncommon in children under 8 years, as fractures preferentially occur through the unfused synchondrosis at the base of the dens.
- Up to 33% of patients have additional cervical spine injury and 10% additional nonspinal injury.
- Craniofacial and vertebral artery injuries are quite common associated injuries.

Suggested Readings

Clark CR, Igram CM, el-Khoury GY, Ehara S. Radiographic evaluation of cervical spine injuries. *Spine (Phila Pa 1976).* 1988 Jul;13(7):742-747.

Hua Q, Ma WH, Zhao LJ, Fang Y. [Clinical application of multi-spiral CT thinner scanning and reconstruction in the diagnosis of atlantoaxial fracture and dislocation]. *Zhongguo Gu Shang.* 2009 May;22(5):349-352.

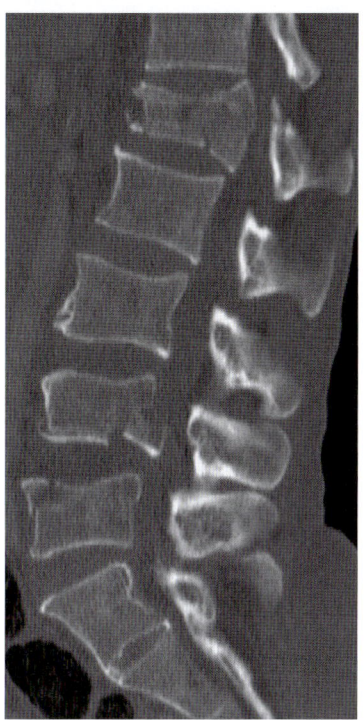
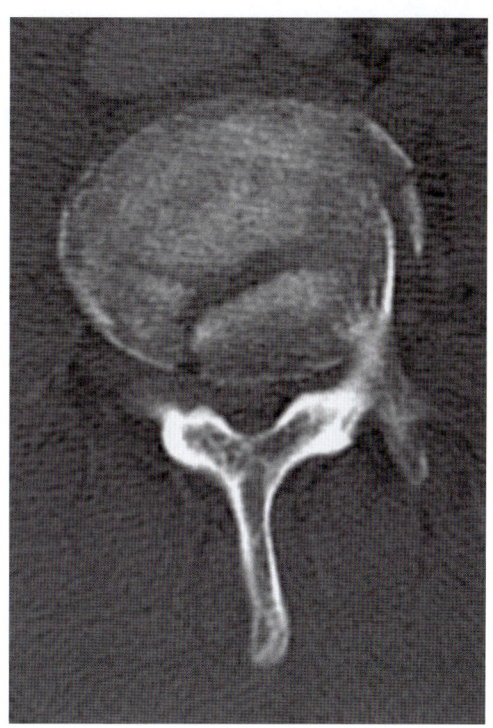

1. What are the major imaging findings?

2. What is the diagnosis at L1?

3. What is the most common location for these injuries?

4. What is the management for compression fractures of the spine?

5. Retropulsion into the spinal canal always requires surgical intervention. True or False?

Case ranking/difficulty:

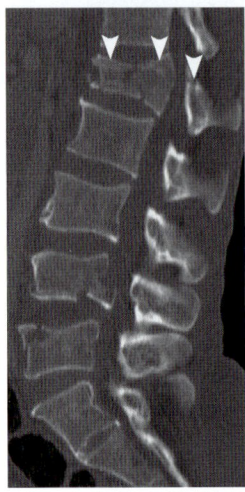

Marked comminution of the L1 vertebral body with retropulsion, similar changes at L4 and L5. The L1 fracture involves all three columns.

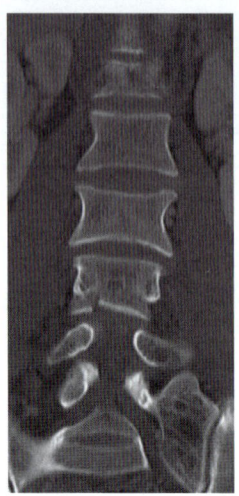

Similar findings.

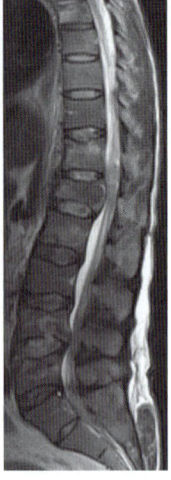

Multiple vertebral fractures, with the retropulsion at L1 causing compression and edema in the conus medullaris.

Answers

1. There are multiple thoracic and lumbar compression and burst fractures, with retropulsion and spinal canal compromise seen at L1 and L4.

2. Involvement of all three columns is seen; therefore, this is a burst fracture. Compression fractures involve only the anterior column; burst fractures involve the anterior and middle columns and sometimes the posterior column.

3. Most vertebral fractures occur at the thoracolumbar junction because this is the mechanical transition point between the rigid thoracic spine and the more mobile lumbar spine. T5-T8 is also a common location for burst fractures.

4. Compression fractures only involve the anterior column, unlike burst fractures. Therefore, the posterior ligamentous complex is typically intact and the fracture is deemed stable. However, if there is more than 50% anterior vertebral height loss or greater than 25% kyphosis, the posterior ligamentous complex is likely to be compromised and surgery is indicated.

5. False. If the retropulsed fragment involves less than 40% of the spinal canal and there is no neurologic compromise, then reabsorption and remodeling of up to 50% of the bone fragment may occur, and the patient can be treated conservatively.

Pearls

- Burst fractures occur after a fall from a height or motor vehicle accident.
- The mechanism of injury is axial loading, often with a flexion component.
- A compression fracture involves only the anterior column; however, a burst fracture involves the anterior and middle columns and sometimes all three columns.
- If there is neurologic compromise, more than 40% spinal canal compromise or greater than 25% kyphotic deformity, or greater than 50% vertebral height loss, the fracture will require surgical intervention.
- If the degree of spinal canal compromise is less than 40%, remodeling and reabsorption of the bony fragment occur and the patient can be treated with an orthosis.
- Follow-up radiographs should always be done in the standing position to assess for progression of kyphosis.

Suggested Readings

Atlas SW, Regenbogen V, Rogers LF, Kim KS. The radiographic characterization of burst fractures of the spine. *AJR Am J Roentgenol.* 1986 Sep;147(3):575-582.

Daffner RH, Deeb ZL, Rothfus WE. The posterior vertebral body line: importance in the detection of burst fractures. *AJR Am J Roentgenol.* 1987 Jan;148(1):93-96.

Shuman WP, Rogers JV, Sickler ME, et al. Thoracolumbar burst fractures: CT dimensions of the spinal canal relative to postsurgical improvement. *AJR Am J Roentgenol.* 1985 Aug;145(2):337-341.

Incidental finding

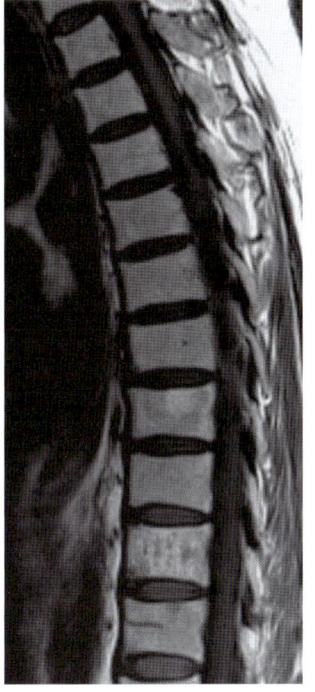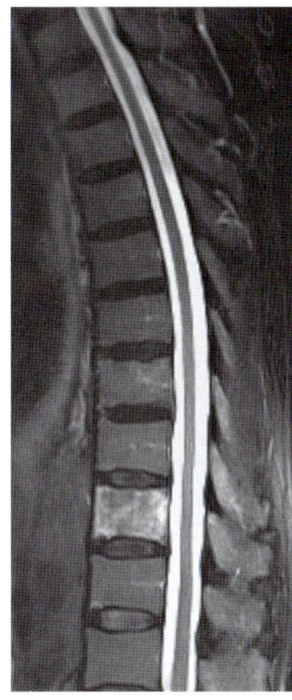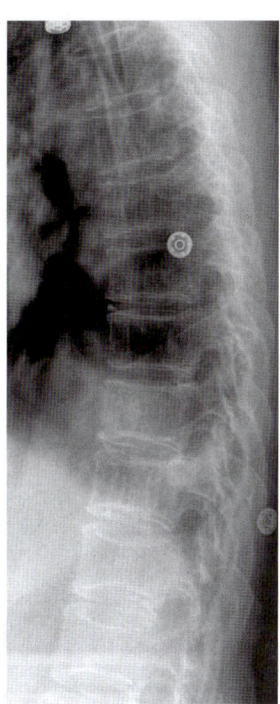

1. What is the name given to the plain radiographic appearance?

2. What is the likely diagnosis?

3. The lesions are never purely sclerotic. True or False?

4. What is the typical scintigraphic appearance?

5. What are the expected angiographic findings?

Case ranking/difficulty:

Category: Vertebral body

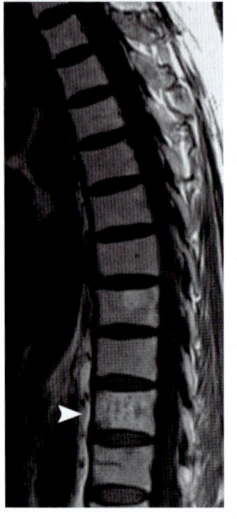

Increased fat within the T10 vertebral body (*arrowhead*), with coarse striations but no bony expansion. Similar smaller lesion at T8.

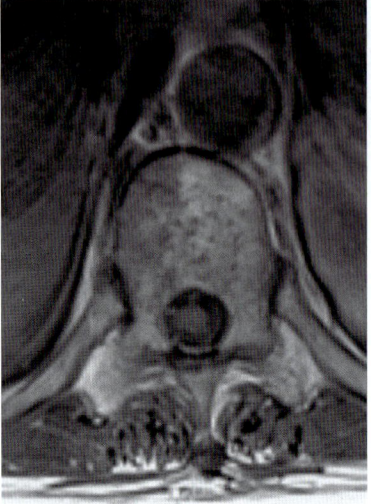

Increased fat and coarse striations well appreciated. No expansion or posterior element extension.

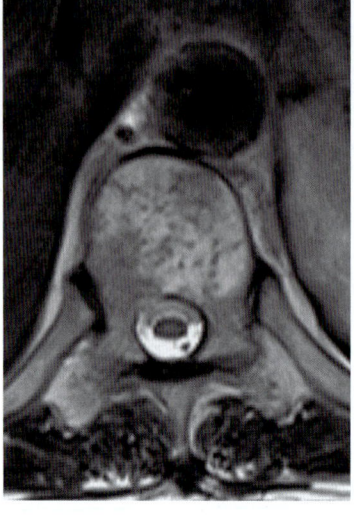

T2 hyperintensity. Coarse vertical trabeculae give a "polka dot" appearance.

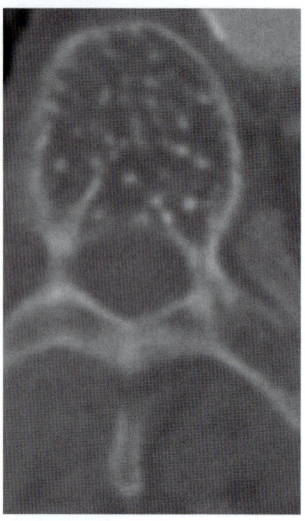

"Polka dot" appearance on CT (different patient).

Answers

1. The reinforced vertical trabeculae secondary to the resorbed horizontal trabeculae give the classic "corduroy" appearance.

2. Although lymphangioma, metastasis, and infection are in the differential, the appearance is classic for a vertebral hemangioma.

3. False. Vertebral hemangiomas may appear sclerotic with coarse vertical striations, giving an "ivory vertebra" appearance. The epithelioid subtype of hemangioma is typically lucent, although there are rare reported cases of diffuse osteosclerosis resembling metastases, lymphoma, or chronic infection.

4. The scintigraphic appearance is variable, with classically a photopenic lesion on Tc-99m MDP bone scanning. Lesions can, however, show normal or even increased activity especially if there is an associated pathologic fracture.

   Tc-99m RBC scan will show increased uptake.

5. Angiography will show increased vascularity, and is usually performed in conjunction with embolization of symptomatic lesions, prior to surgical removal.

Pearls

- Vertebral hemangiomas are extremely common, occurring in 10% of the adult population in one cadaver study. The most common location is the thoracic spine, followed by the lumbar spine.
- Plain radiographs show coarsened vertical trabeculae, giving a corduroy appearance.
- Axial CT scan shows the reinforced vertical trabeculae en face, leading to a polka dot appearance.
- T1 signal intensity is variable depending on the amount of adipose tissue. The T2 signal is usually increased. Lesions typically enhance after intravenous contrast.
- Most lesions are asymptomatic. Symptomatic lesions may be a result of bony expansion and posterior element involvement, with extension into the epidural space. Increased distention from activity, pregnancy, or menstruation may also lead to symptoms.

Suggested Readings

Friedman DP. Symptomatic vertebral hemangiomas: MR findings. *AJR Am J Roentgenol.* 1996 Aug;167(2):359-364.

Park HJ, Jeon YH, Rho MH, et al. Incidental findings of the lumbar spine at MRI during herniated intervertebral disk disease evaluation. *AJR Am J Roentgenol.* 2011 May;196(5):1151-1155.

Rodallec MH, Feydy A, Larousserie F, et al. Diagnostic imaging of solitary tumors of the spine: what to do and say. *Radiographics.* 2008 Jul-Aug;28(4):1019-1041.

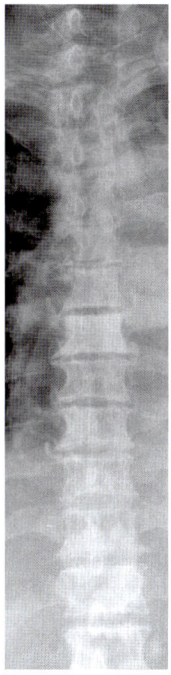 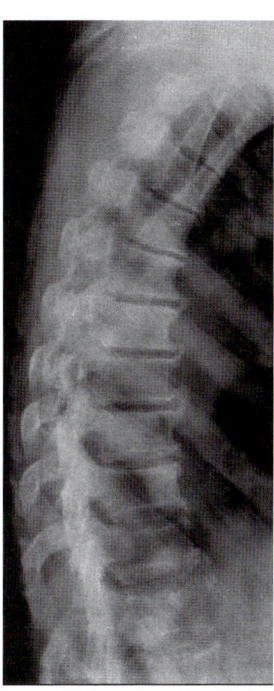

1. What is the most likely diagnosis in this patient?

2. What is the most appropriate initial management?

3. Which solid organ malignancies may present with this appearance?

4. What is the appropriate treatment for this condition?

5. What conditions can have an identical appearance?

Case ranking/difficulty:

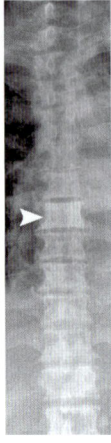

Numerous sclerotic vertebral lesions, with "ivory" vertebra (*arrowhead*).

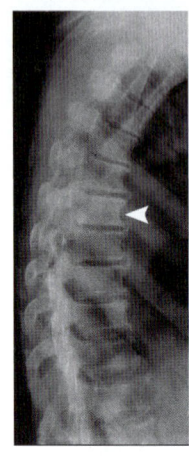

Similar findings.

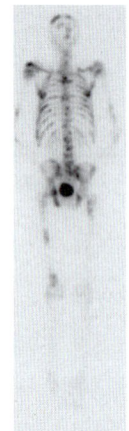

Numerous sclerotic vertebral lesions with "ivory" vertebrae (*arrowhead*s).

Multiple foci of increased radiopharmaceutical uptake.

Answers

1. Osteoblastic metastases. The common sclerotic metastases are from prostate, breast, colorectal, and lung carcinoma. There is no real differential in an elderly patient with a rising PSA other than prostatic carcinoma.

2. A bone scan with urological referral is most appropriate for a patient with diffuse sclerotic lesions and a rising PSA. A technetium bone scan is cheap and very sensitive in the detection of osteoblastic metastases. Other modalities, eg, SPECT or PET-CT, would be needlessly expensive when the diagnosis is in little doubt.

3. Breast, prostate, and colorectal carcinoma are the most common osteoblastic skeletal metastases. Lung and renal cell metastases are typically lytic.

4. Metastatic prostate cancer could be appropriately managed with palliation, radiotherapy for local or skeletal complications, hormonal therapy, or chemotherapy. However, radical curative surgery is not appropriate.

5. Breast and prostatic carcinoma metastases can have identical appearances. Other causes for diffuse sclerosis, eg, sickle cell disease, may look similar, although the patient demographics would be very different. Osteopetrosis has a more uniformly sclerotic appearance and is very rare in comparison.

Pearls

- Generalized osteosclerosis in an adult is often secondary to metastatic disease. In a male, this is usually from prostate carcinoma. In a female, this is usually from breast carcinoma.
- Other causes are rarer and are suggested by other imaging features, eg, fluorosis—enthesopathy; sickle cell disease—H-shaped vertebrae; osteopetrosis—age and Erlenmeyer flask deformity.
- The axial skeleton is involved first with prostatic metastases.
- Progressive sclerosis is not easy to monitor on imaging studies when comparison of treatment response is sought. For this purpose, serum PSA is an appropriate test, as changes from the baseline can be used to better monitor the response to therapy.
- Bone scans, plain radiographs, CT scans, and MRI scans can all be used to demonstrate the extent of disease. Technetium-99 radionuclide scans are still first-line investigations for mapping the extent of disease, although they may lack specificity, being positive in other instances, eg, post-trauma and infection.

Suggested Readings

Feydy A, Carlier R, Vallée C, et al. [Imaging of osteosclerotic metastases]. *J Radiol*. 1995 Sep;76(9):561-572.

Hackländer T, Scharwächter C, Golz R, Mertens H. [Value of diffusion-weighted imaging for diagnosing vertebral metastases due to prostate cancer in comparison to other primary tumors]. *Rofo*. 2006 Apr;178(4):416-424.

Spina bifida, status post myelomeningocele repair

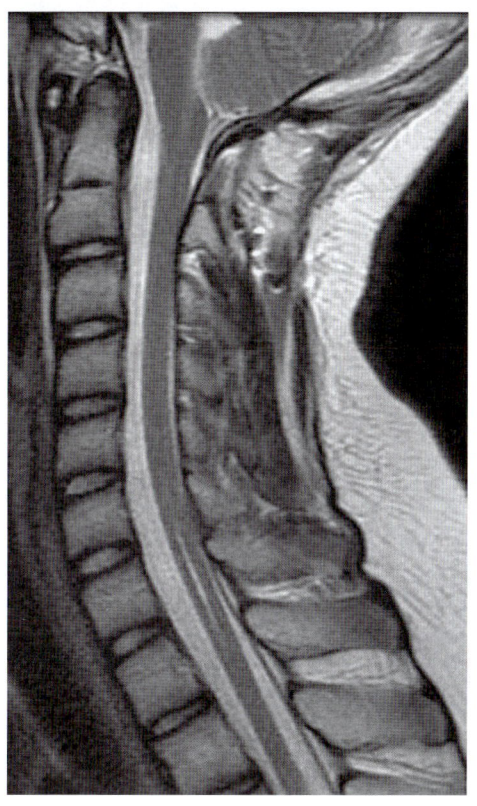 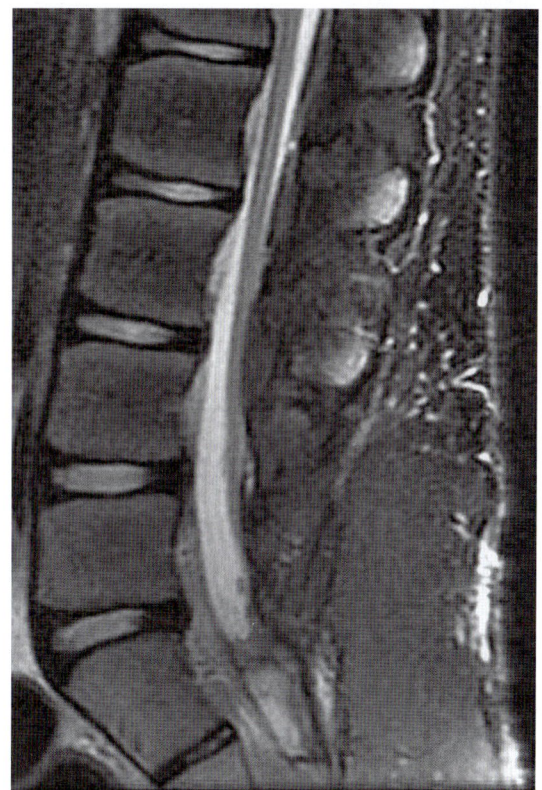

1. What is the most likely diagnosis?

2. What are associated maternal conditions?

3. What germ cell layers are involved?

4. What are associated cranial and brain malformations?

5. What are treatment options?

Case ranking/difficulty:

Category: More than one category

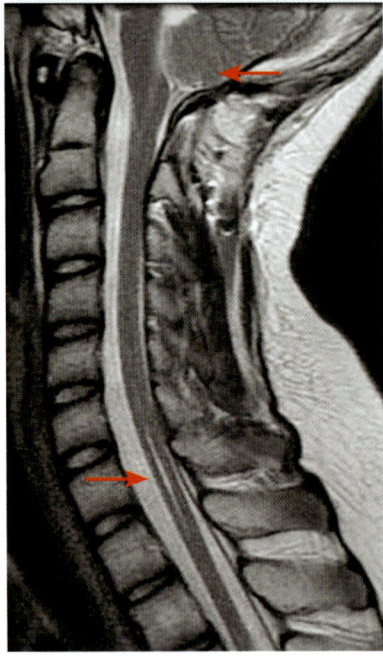

Sagittal T2 image demonstrates low-lying cerebellar tissue with small cervicothoracic syrinx.

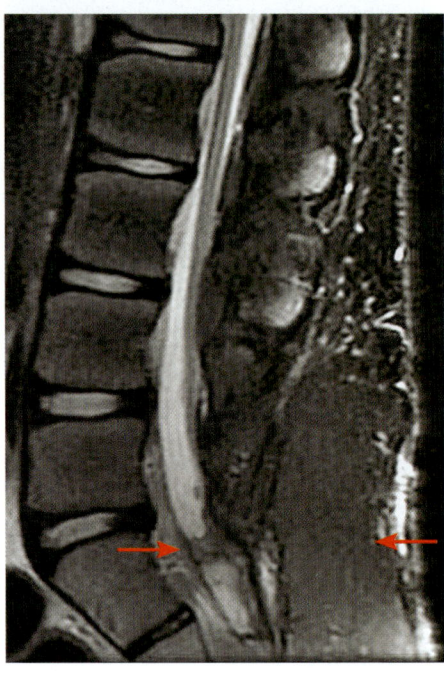

Sagittal T2 image demonstrates low-lying conus with complex fibrotic mass, consistent with postoperative change following myelomeningocele repair.

Answers

1. In this patient with a known history of myelomeningocele repair, the only differential possibility is Chiari II malformation.

2. Folate deficiency or defects in processing of folate can lead to Chiari II malformation. Folate supplementation is recommended prior to conception, through at least 6 weeks of gestational age.

3. Chiari II malformations involve abnormalities of the mesoderm (cranium) and neuroectoderm (both supra- and infratentorial).

4. Clivus shortening, beaking of the tectum, cervicomedullary kinking, dysgenesis of the corpus callosum, and a small posterior fossa may be seen in conjunction with Chiari II malformation.

5. All patients undergo myelomeningocele repair; others may require additional treatment, such as suboccipital craniectomy and ventriculoperitoneal or syringosubarachnoid shunt placement.

Pearls

- Chiari II malformation is universally present in patients with myelomeningoceles.
- Imaging of the brain and neuroaxis is necessary to document all associated abnormalities. Supratentorial abnormalities include dysgenesis of the corpus callosum, towering cerebellum, and interdigitation of the gyri.

Suggested Readings

McLone DG, Dias MS. The Chiari II malformation: cause and impact. *Childs Nerv Syst.* 2003;19:540-550.

Stevenson KL. Chiari type 2 malformation: past, present, and future. *Neurosurg Focus.* 2004;16:Article 5.

Left leg numbness

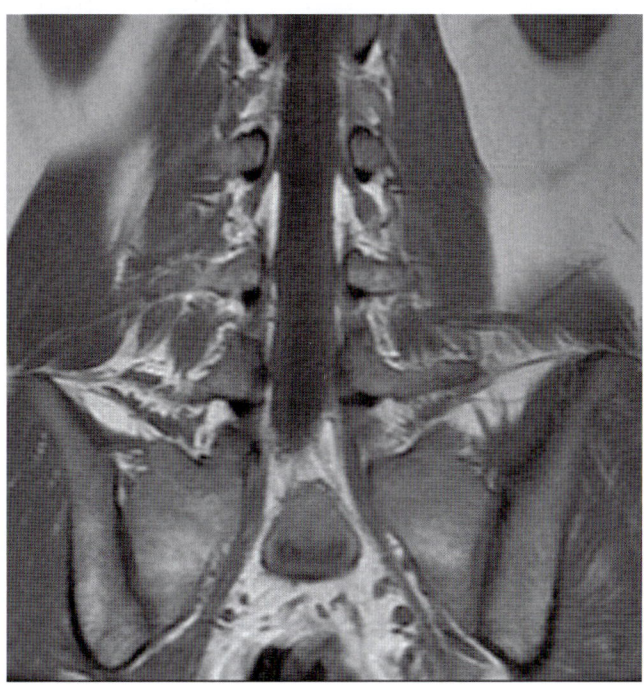

1. What should be included in the differential diagnosis?

2. What imaging findings can be seen in these patients?

3. What is the most common level where this occurs?

4. What are common presenting symptoms?

5. What are treatment options?

Case ranking/difficulty:

Category: Nerve roots/Nerve plexus/Peripheral nerves

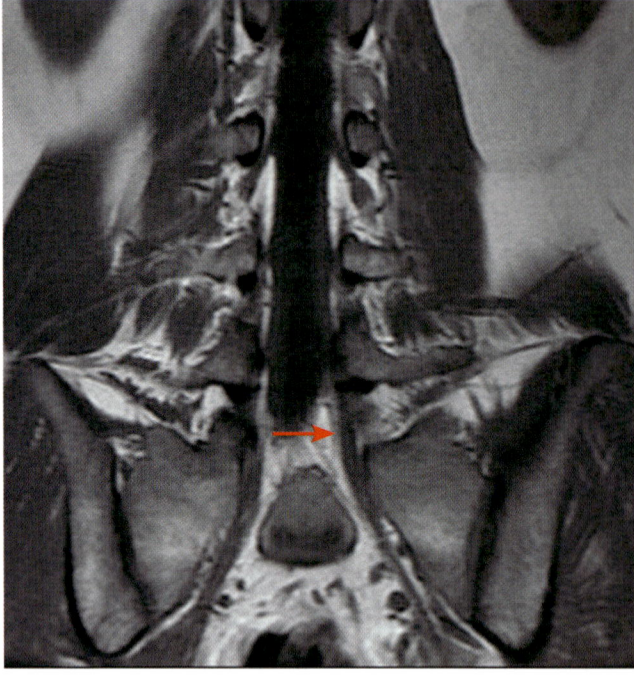

Coronal T1 image demonstrates a common origin of the left L5 and S1 nerve roots.

Answers

1. Nerve sheath tumor, synovial cyst, conjoined nerve root, and disc herniation can be included in the differential diagnosis.

2. Imaging findings can include enlargement of the neural foramen, soft tissue within the lateral recess, hypoplastic pedicles, and enlargement of the nerve sleeve. Spinal stenosis can be associated with conjoined nerve roots, particularly in the setting of hypoplastic pedicles.

3. Conjoined nerve roots most commonly occur at the L5-S1 level.

4. Radicular symptoms and pain are the most common presenting symptoms. Conjoined nerve roots are at a higher risk for compression in the lateral recess. Patients may also present with back pain.

5. Traditional diskectomy is often not sufficient in the setting of conjoined nerve roots and increased exposure via hemilaminectomy, foraminotomy, or pediculectomy may be required. Increased traction is contraindicated as conjoined nerve roots are often fixed in place and may result in dural leak or nerve root avulsion.

Pearls

- Conjoined nerve roots are relatively common abnormalities, which are frequently under-recognized.
- Conjoined nerve roots most commonly occur in the lumbar spine.
- Conjoined nerve roots can be clinically significant in the setting of radiculopathy resulting from compression.
- To identify conjoined nerve roots, search for the common nerve origin or enlargement of the surrounding nerve root sheath.

Suggested Readings

Scuderi GJ, Vaccaro AR, Brusovanik GV, Kwon BK, Berta SC. Conjoined lumbar nerve roots: a frequently underappreciated congenital abnormality. *J Spinal Disord Tech.* 2004;17:86-93.

Trimba R, Spivak JM, Bendo JA. Conjoined nerve roots of the lumbar spine. *Spine J.* 2012;12:515-524.

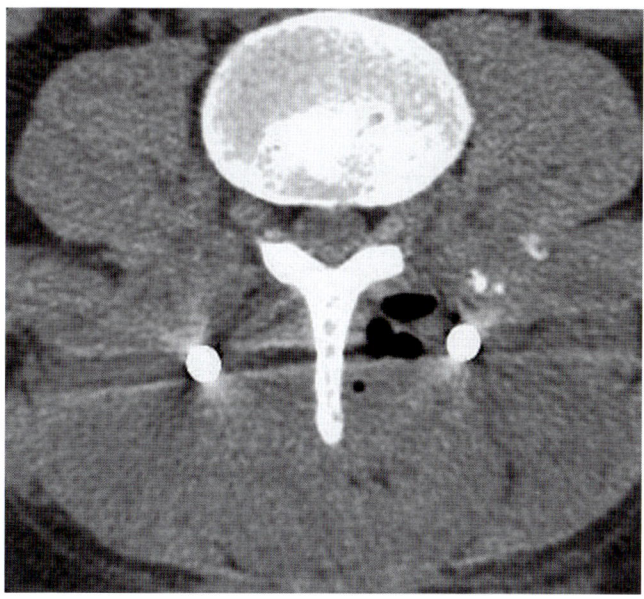

1. What should be included in the differential diagnosis?

2. What are common presenting symptoms?

3. What are risk factors?

4. What are the common organisms that are involved?

5. What are the treatment options?

Case ranking/difficulty:

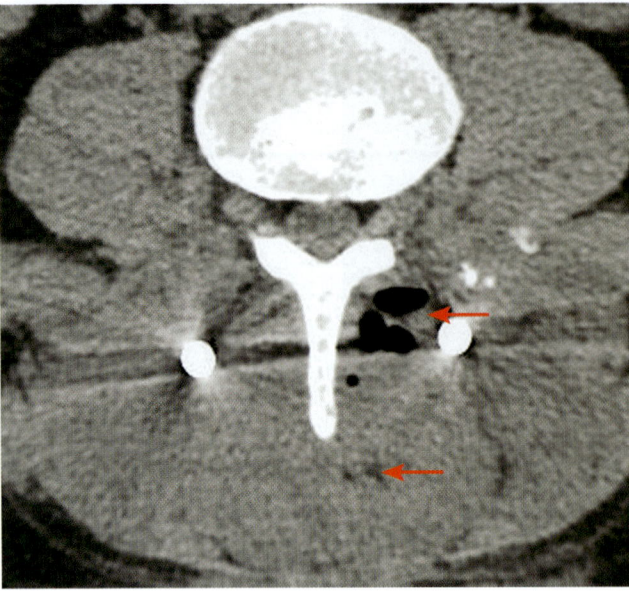

Axial CT image demonstrates postoperative changes of posterior spinal fusion from L3 to S1 with complex surrounding fluid collection and draining tract extending to posterior midline incision.

Answers

1. Focal soft tissue collection and gas can be seen in the setting of recent operative procedure, diskitis, cellulitis, and osteomyelitis.

2. Common presenting symptoms include fever, pain, cutaneous erythema, and incisional pus. Radicular symptoms may result from intraspinal extension of infection.

3. Risk factors for developing postoperative infection include diabetes, previous infection, and blood loss greater than 1 L. Anterior spinal approach decreases the risk of infection; multilevel fusion may increase the risk as it increased operative time.

4. The most common are *Staphylococcus* (both *aureus* and *epidermidis*) and *Enterococcus*.

5. Spinal infection is treated with antibiotics and consideration of percutaneous abscess drainage, open debridement, and hardware removal.

Pearls

- Postoperative infections are relatively uncommon in the setting of spinal instrumentation; however, they can occur over 2 years following surgery.
- Recent studies have shown obesity to be an independent risk factor for the development of infection.
- Clinical features that should raise concern for infection include cutaneous redness, pus drainage, or pain.
- Evaluation may include CT or CT myelography to evaluate for intraspinal extension. MRI may be used but can be limited by adjacent metal artifact.
- Superficial infections can be treated medically; however, extension below the fascia may necessitate surgical drainage/debridement and, in some cases, removal of infected hardware. This can be problematic in patients who may now have spinal instability.

Suggested Readings

Pull ter Gunne A, Cohen DB. Incidence, prevalence, and analysis of risk factors for surgical site infection following adult spinal surgery. *Spine*. 2009;34:1422-1428.

Young PM, Berquist TH, Bancroft LW, Peterson JJ. Complications of spinal instrumentation. *Radiographics*. 2007;27:775-789.

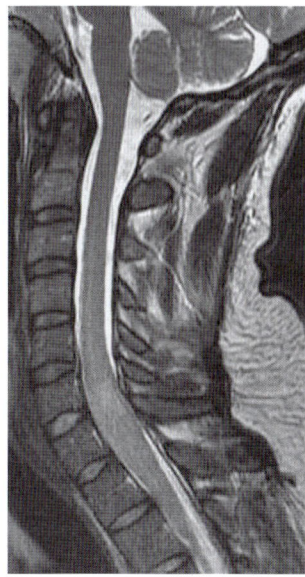 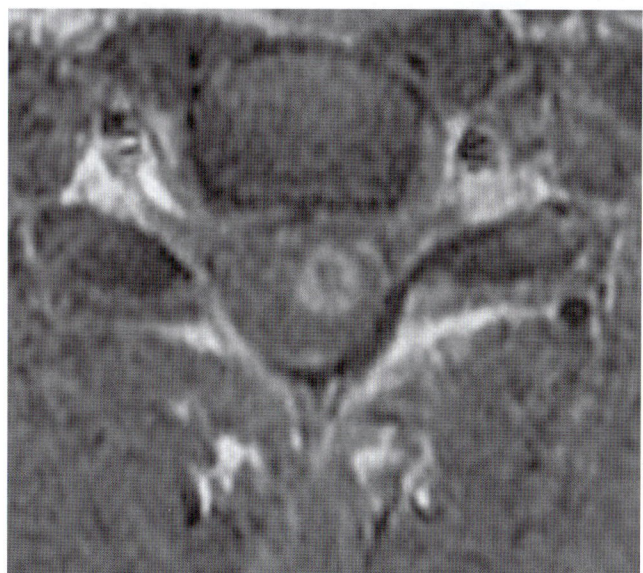

1. What should be included in the differential diagnosis?

2. What is the most common intramedullary spinal cord tumor in an adult?

3. What are common presenting symptoms?

4. What is the most common location within the cord?

5. What are the treatment options?

Case ranking/difficulty:

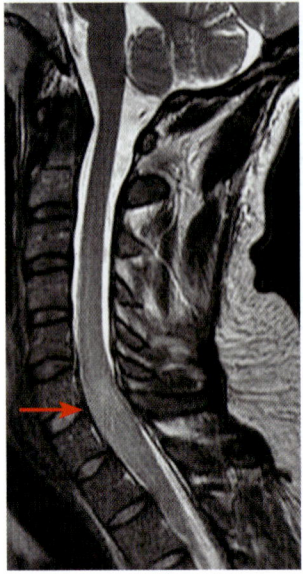

Sagittal T2 image demonstrates expansion and T2 hyperintensity within the spinal cord at the cervicothoracic junction.

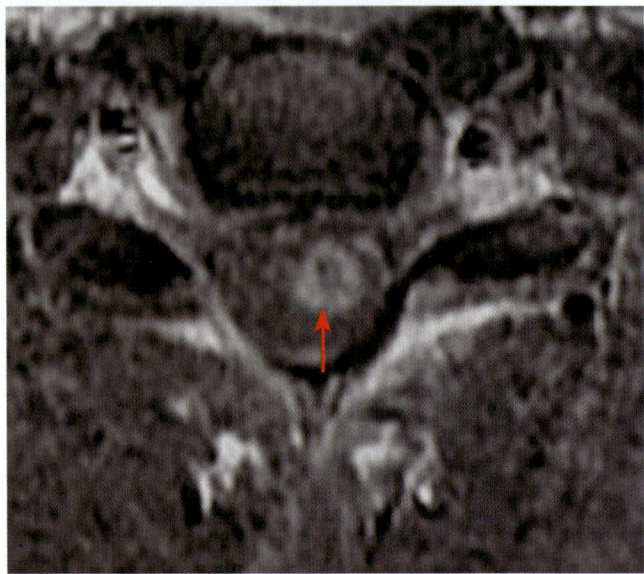

Axial T1 image following contrast administration demonstrates focal enhancement in the left cord.

Answers

1. T2 hyperintense expansion of the cord with focal enhancement can be caused by astrocytoma, hemangioblastoma, ependymoma, demyelinating disease, or metastasis. An atypical cord contusion could also present with a similar appearance.

2. Ependymomas are the most common intramedullary tumor in adults; astrocytomas are the most common intramedullary tumor in children.

3. Myelopathy is the most common presenting symptom; other symptoms include pain, radicular symptoms, sensory dysesthesia, and bowel/bladder incontinence.

4. The cervical spine is the most common site of most primary intramedullary tumors.

5. Biopsy is the first step to determine tumor pathology. For low-grade tumors, conservative management may be appropriate. In higher-grade tumors, chemotherapy and radiation have been shown to prolong survival. Resection is reserved for patients with progressive neurological symptoms.

Pearls

- Spinal cord astrocytomas are the second most common intramedullary neoplasm, but the most common in children.
- They tend to be low grade (WHO I-II); however, the rare high-grade tumors (WHO III-IV) have an extremely poor prognosis.
- Patients generally present with nonspecific symptoms of pain or myelopathy. Treatment is directed after tissue diagnosis is made.
- Oftentimes, the lower-grade tumors are subject to serial follow-up if the patient does not have symptoms.
- High-grade lesions are generally treated with chemotherapy and radiation with resection reserved for functional decline. Despite treatment, the survival is generally around 5 years.

Suggested Readings

Cohen AR, Wisoff JH, Allen JC, Epstein F. Malignant astrocytomas of the spinal cord. *J Neurosurg*. 1989:70:50-54.

Liu X, Germin BI, Ekholm S. A case of cervical spinal cord gliobastoma diagnosed with MR diffusion tensor and perfusion imaging. *J Neuroimaging*. 2011;21:292-296.

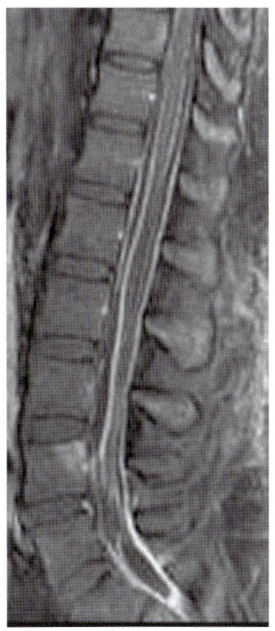 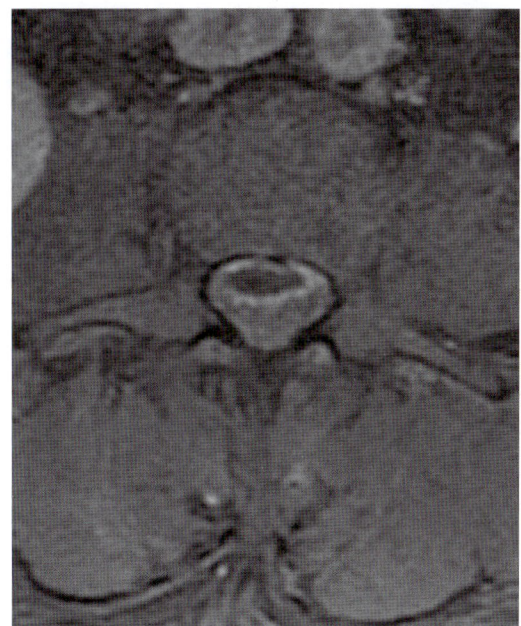

1. What should be included in the differential diagnosis?

2. What are common presenting symptoms?

3. What are the most common organisms in children?

4. What are the most common organisms in adults?

5. What are the treatment options?

Case ranking/difficulty:

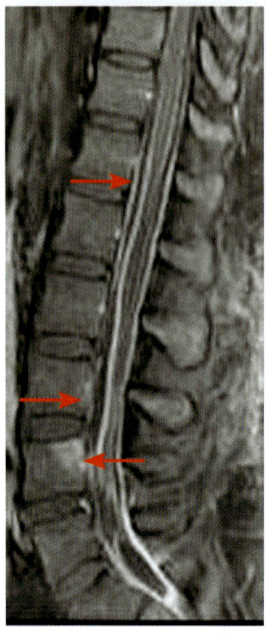

Sagittal T1 image following gadolinium administration demonstrates diffuse dural enhancement with enhancement along the conus and nerve roots. Note epidural abscess and enhancement of L4 vertebral body as well.

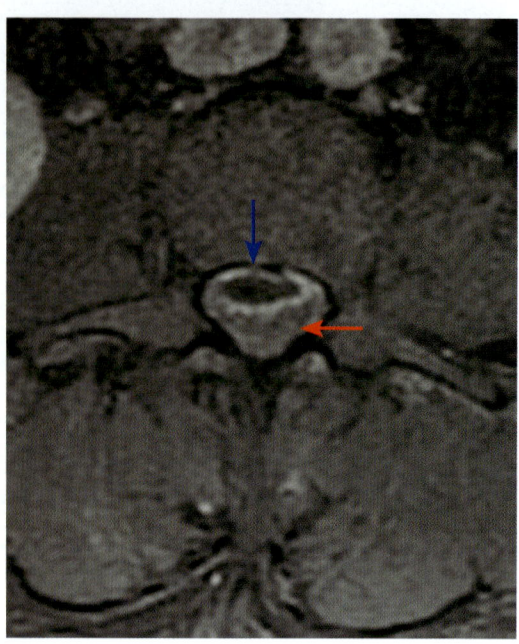

Axial T1 image following gadolinium administration demonstrates enhancement along the nerve roots (*red arrow*) and ventral epidural abscess (*blue arrow*).

Answers

1. Etiologies for abnormal spinal enhancement include bacterial meningitis, idiopathic hypertrophic pachymeningitis, leptomeningeal metastasis, Guillain Barre, and viral meningitis.

2. Common presenting symptoms include back pain, fever, and headache.

3. Group B *Streptococcus* predominates in neonates with *Haemophilus* in older children. Other etiologies include *Listeria*, *Neisseria meningitides*, and *Streptococcus pneumoniae*.

4. *Staphylococcus* is also seen in adult patients.

5. Antibiotics and comfort measures are the mainstays of treatment. While lumbar puncture is required for diagnosis, there is no benefit for therapeutic fluid removal.

- Organisms are generally spread hematogenously; however, contiguous spread or direct inoculation may be seen.
- Imaging demonstrates diffuse dural and pachymeningeal enhancement.
- Lumbar puncture is necessary to isolate an organism and differentiate other causes of enhancement (metastatic disease, viral infection, etc).
- Antibiotic and supportive therapy must be initiated as rapidly as possible, even before the performance of lumbar puncture.

Suggested Readings

Morris BJ, Fletcher N, Davis RA, Mencio GA. Bacterial meningitis after traumatic thoracic fracture-dislocation: two case reports and review of the literature. *J Orthop Trauma*. 2010;24:e49-e53.

Pai S, Welsh CT, Patel S, Rumboldt Z. Idiopathic hypertrophic spinal pachymeningitis: report of two cases with typical MR imaging findings. *AJNR*. 2007;28:590-592.

Pearls

- Spinal meningitis often presents with neck pain and stiffness, particularly in the setting of fever and headache.
- Patients may rapidly progress to mental status changes and seizures.

Back pain following posterior fusion

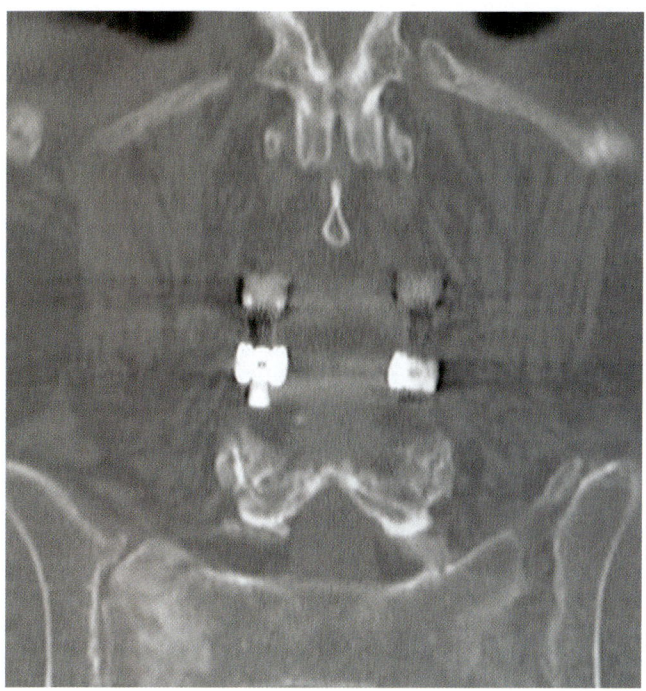

1. What should be included in the differential diagnosis?

2. What are risk factors?

3. What associated abnormalities are seen?

4. What are common presenting symptoms?

5. What are the treatment options?

Case ranking/difficulty:

Category: Vertebral body

4. Back, buttock, and groin pain, as well as palpable tenderness and radiculopathy, are all potential presenting symptoms; however, pain is most common.

5. Treatment options include analgesia, conservative management, physical therapy, and sacroplasty. Surgical fixation is generally not employed given the underlying osteoporosis.

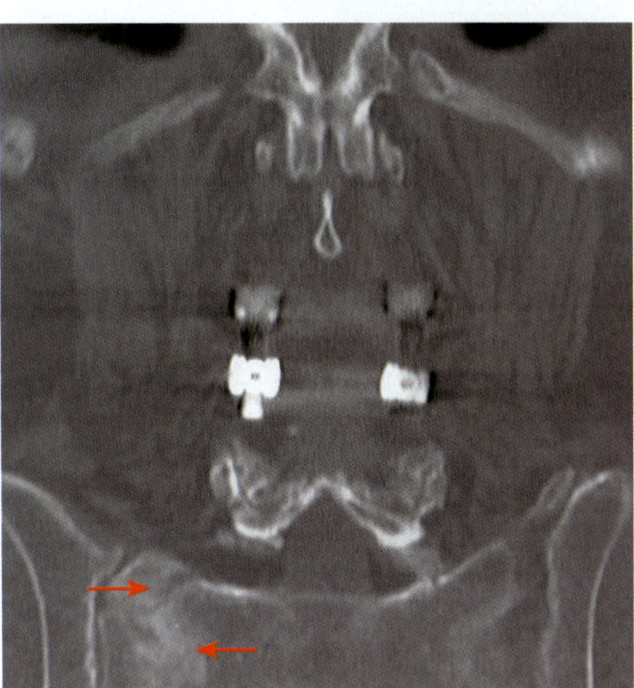

Coronal CT image demonstrates vertically oriented right sacral sclerosis, surrounding a linear lucency.

Pearls

- Sacral insufficiency fractures are important to recognize as they have a significant association with increased morbidity and mortality.
- It is important to evaluate for associated injuries, such as vertebral body compression fractures and hip fractures.
- The classic distribution of insufficiency fractures is the H-shaped fractures with vertical components through the sacral ala in conjunction with a transverse fracture across the sacral body. However, any variation of this configuration may be seen.
- Treatment is generally conservative with immobility and pain management, progressing to physical therapy and treatment of cause for osteopenia.
- Sacroplasty may be performed for pain management.

Answers

1. Mixed lucent and sclerotic sacral lesions include insufficiency fracture, metastasis, osteomyelitis, sacroiliitis, and traumatic fracture.

2. Osteoporosis, hyperparathyroidism, multiple myeloma, Paget disease, renal osteodystrophy, and rheumatoid arthritis all increase the risk of developing sacral insufficiency fractures. In addition, sacral insufficiency fractures may also occur following hip arthroplasty as patients begin to bear weight.

3. Sacral insufficiency fractures can be associated with other osteoporotic fractures, including femur and vertebral body compression fractures.

Suggested Readings

Lyders EM, Whitlow CT, Baker MD, Morris PP. Imaging and treatment of sacral insufficiency fractures. *AJNR*. 2010;31:201-210.

Odate S, Shikata J, Kimura H, Soeda T. Sacral fracture after instrumented lumbosacral fusion. *Spine*. 2013;38:E223-E229.

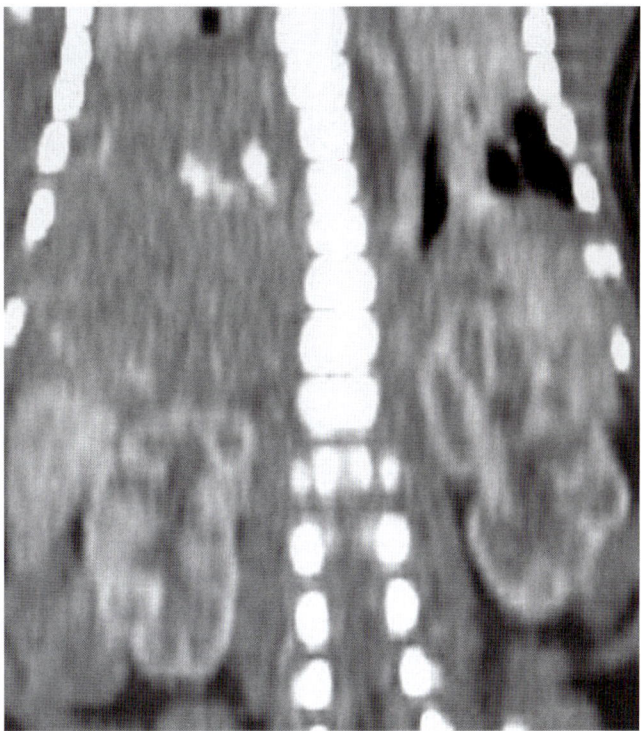

1. What should be included in the differential diagnosis?

2. What are associated clinical syndromes?

3. What are common presenting symptoms?

4. What are the components of the Evans anatomic staging system?

5. What are the treatment options?

Case ranking/difficulty:

Category: Paraspinal soft tissue

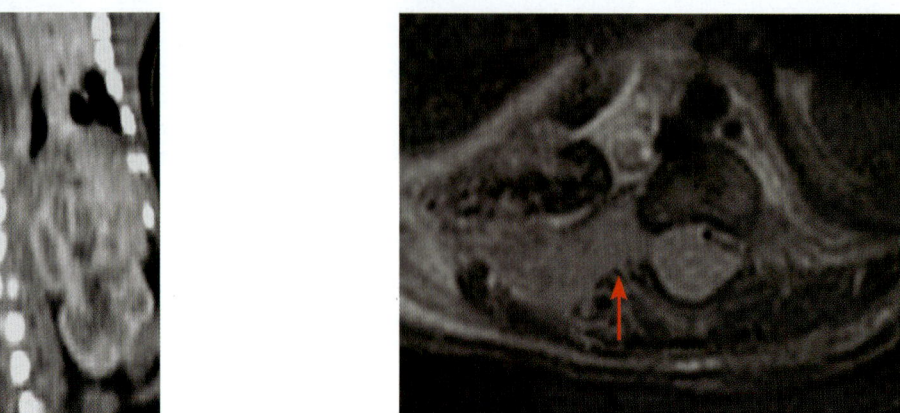

Coronal CT image demonstrates partially calcified (*arrowhead*) right paraspinal mass.

Axial T2 weighted image post-primary tumor resection demonstrates extension through the right T9-T10 neural foramen.

Answers

1. Etiologies for a paraspinal mass in a child include neuroblastic tumor, adrenal hemorrhage, lymphadenopathy, lymphoma, and adrenocortical tumor.

2. Blueberry muffin syndrome, Horner syndrome, Hutchinson syndrome, Kerner-Morrison syndrome, and Pepper syndrome are all syndromes associated with neuroblastoma.

3. Diarrhea results from increased VIP secretion (Kerner-Morrison syndrome). Opsoclonus-myoclonus and ataxia result from reaction of antineuroblastoma antibodies with cerebellar Purkinje cells. Myelopathy can occur from intraspinal extension.

4. Stages 1-3 are considered "locoregional" disease. (1—confined to organ; 2—extraorgan extension; 3—extraorgan extension, crossing midline). Stage 4 is systemic or metastatic disease. There is a subtype of Stage 4—Stage 4S—which is seen in patients less than 12 months at diagnosis with metastatic disease limited to skin, liver, and bone marrow. Stage 4S patients have an excellent prognosis versus Stage 4 patients who have approximately 10% chance of survival.

5. Primary treatment is surgery, chemotherapy, and radiation; steroids may be used to treat symptoms of adrenal insufficiency.

Pearls

- Neuroblastoma is a common solid malignancy of infancy and childhood, with most cases presenting before the age of 5.
- The classic imaging appearance is a paraspinal mass, often demonstrating extension into the spinal canal through multiple neural foramina.

- There are several clinical syndromes that patients may present with—or these lesions are occasionally diagnosed antenatally with ultrasound.
- Treatment includes surgery, chemotherapy, and radiation.
- Prognosis is based on Evans anatomic staging system.
- Stages 1-3 are considered "locoregional" disease. (1—confined to organ; 2—extraorgan extension; 3—extraorgan extension, crossing midline).
- Stage 4 is systemic or metastatic disease.
- Stage 4S, which is seen in patients less than 12 months at diagnosis, with metastatic disease limited to skin, liver, and bone marrow. Stage 4S patients have an excellent prognosis versus Stage 4 patients who have approximately 10% chance of survival.
- Neuroblastoma is along the spectrum of neuroblastic tumors, which includes ganglioneuroma and ganglioneuroblastoma (which are more benign).
- Ganglioneuroma patients often have complete cure following resection.
- Ganglioneuroblastoma patients have a prognosis based on the percentage of ganglioneuroma and neuroblastoma within their tumor.
- There are cases of extension both ways along the spectrum, with malignant degeneration and spontaneous differentiation.

Suggested Readings

Fisher JPH, Tweddle DA. Neonatal neuroblastoma. *Semin Fetal Neonatal Med*. 2012;17:207-215.

Wilne S, Walker D. Spine and spinal cord tumors in children: a diagnostic and therapeutic challenge to healthcare systems. *Arch Dis Child Educ Pract Ed*. 2010;95:47-54.

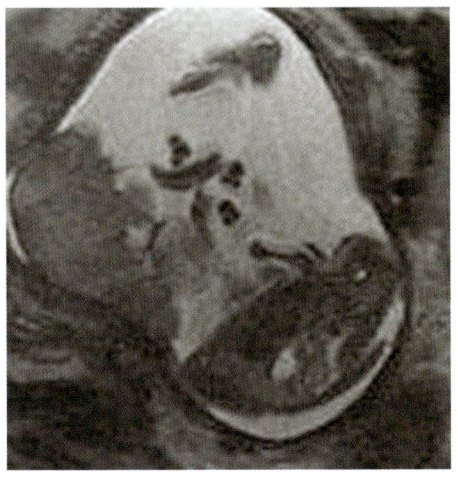 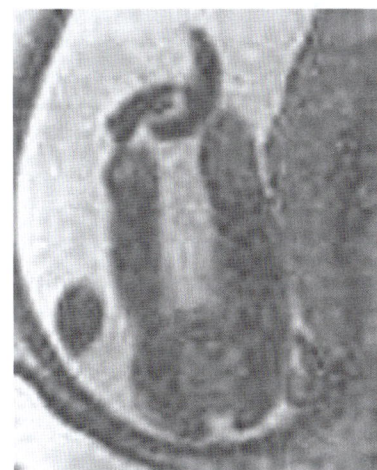

1. What should be included in the differential diagnosis?

2. What are risk factors?

3. What associated abnormalities are seen?

4. What portion of the spine is most commonly affected?

5. What are the treatment options?

Case ranking/difficulty:

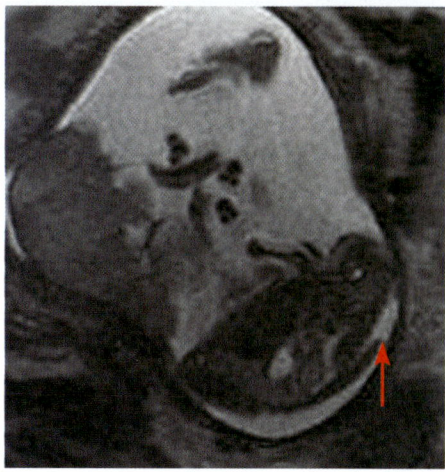

Sagittal T2 SSFSE image demonstrates an open neural tube defect in the lumbosacral spine with herniation of meninges.

Axial T2 SSFSE image demonstrates an open neural tube defect in the lumbosacral spine with herniation of meninges.

Answers

1. Etiologies for a cystic lumbosacral lesion seen on prenatal ultrasound include anterior sacral meningocele, closed spinal dysraphism, myelocele, myelocystocele, and sacrococcygeal teratoma.

2. Risk factors include Chiari II malformation, maternal folate deficiency, trisomy 13, and trisomy 18.

3. Associated abnormalities include clubfoot, dermal sinus, hydrocephalus, scoliosis, and syrinx.

4. Nearly half of myelomeningoceles are lumbosacral in location.

5. Primary myelomeningocele closure is the first treatment with untethering of spinal cord. Ventriculoperitoneal shunt placement may be needed in the setting of associated hydrocephalus.

- There is an association with osseous spinal abnormalities as well.
- The incidence of open neural tube defects has decreased with folate supplementation.
- Postnatal imaging is not routinely indicated with surgical repair of the open neural tube defect within the first days of life.
- Some centers perform in utero repair, which may help decrease hydrocephalus in patients with Chiari II.
- Per the MOMS (Management of Myelomeningocele Study) trial, the best chance for improved outcome arises with repair prior to 25 weeks' gestational age.
- Postoperative imaging focuses on identifying cases of retethering.

Pearls

- Meningomyelocele arises secondary to failure of closure of the neural tube.
- Meningomyelocele is often picked up on routine screening ultrasound with additional imaging performed using MRI.
- Evaluation should include images of the posterior fossa and supratentorial compartment to evaluate for associated Chiari II malformation and/or hydrocephalus.

Suggested Readings

Bulas D. Fetal evaluation of spine dysraphism. *Pediatr Radiol.* 2010;40:1029-1037.

Peruzzi P, Corbitt RJ, Raffel C. Magnetic resonance imaging versus ultrasonography for the in utero evaluation of central nervous system anomalies. *J Neurosurg Pediatrics.* 2010;6:340-345.

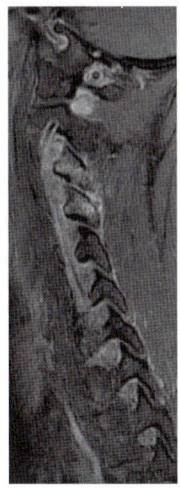
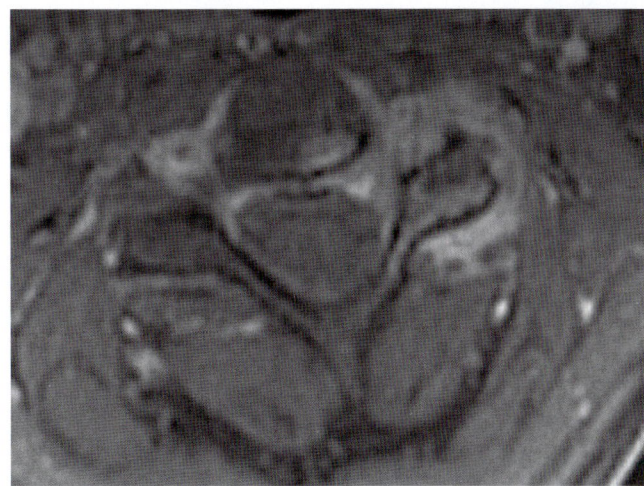

1. What should be included in the differential diagnosis?

2. What are common presenting symptoms?

3. What are common etiologies?

4. What are the common organisms that are involved?

5. What are the treatment options?

Case ranking/difficulty: **Category:** More than one category

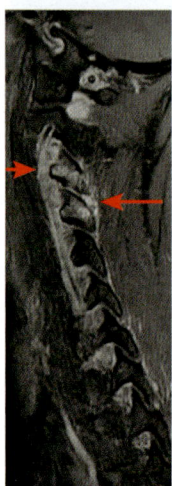

Parasagittal T1 image following contrast administration demonstrates enhancement surrounding the C3-C4 left facet joint.

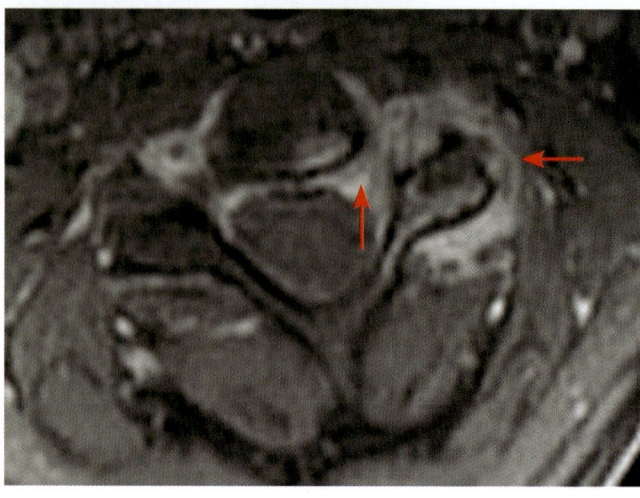

Axial T1 image following contrast administration demonstrates enhancement surrounding the C3-C4 left facet joint with epidural extension.

Answers

1. The differential diagnosis should include metastatic disease, osteoarthritis, rheumatoid arthritis, and synovial cyst.

2. Fever and pain are the most common presenting symptoms; variable radiculopathy and myelopathy can be seen depending on extent of infection.

3. Hematogenous spread is the most common etiology. Other etiologies include contiguous spread from meningitis, diskitis, or appendicitis, as well as direct inoculation.

4. *Staphylococcus aureus* accounts for over 80% of cases. *Streptococcus* is the second most common organism.

5. These lesions are primarily treated medically with analgesia, antibiotics, and/or percutaneous drainage of soft tissue abscess; surgical intervention is indicated in cases of spinal instability or spinal cord compromise.

Pearls

• Facet joint septic arthritis is rare and may be the result of hematogenous or contiguous spread. In addition, it can rarely be seen after therapeutic injections.

• Classically, patients present with pain and symptoms of infection; however, there may be associated radicular or myelopathic symptoms depending on spread.

• In addition to the findings of arthritis at the facet joint, the presence of enhancement raises the question of infection.

• It is important to evaluate for epidural and paraspinal extension.

• Treatment is usually medical; however, aggressive infections may lead to osseous destruction and instability requiring surgical intervention and stabilization.

Suggested Readings

Jones JL, Ernst AA. Unusual cause of neck pain: septic arthritis of a cervical facet. *Am J Emer Med.* 2012;30:2094.1-2094.4

Weingarten TN, Hooten WM, Huntoon MA. Septic facet joint arthritis after a corticosteroid facet injection. *Pain Med.* 2006;7:52-56.

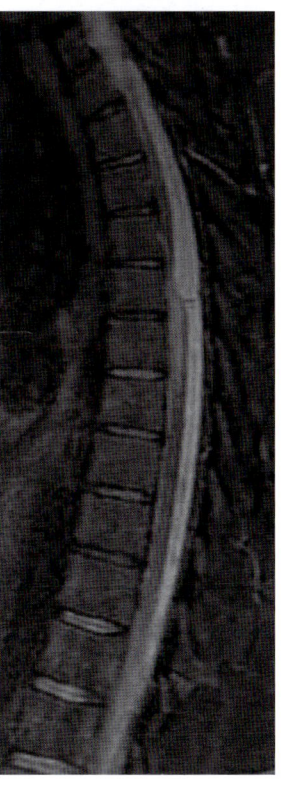

1. What should be included in the differential diagnosis?

2. What are common presenting symptoms?

3. What are the stages of this abnormality within the cord?

4. What are treatment options for spinal arachnoid cyst?

5. What are the treatment options for myelomalacia?

Case ranking/difficulty: **Category:** More than one category

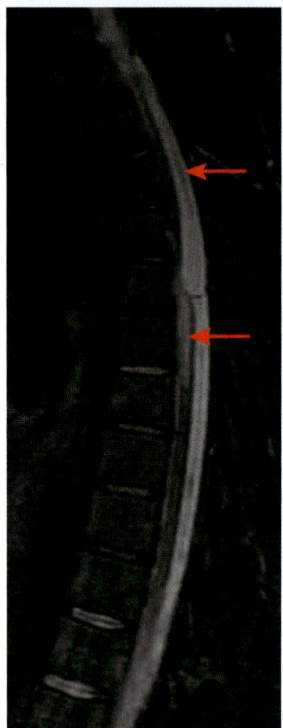

Sagittal T2 image demonstrates dorsal cystic lesion (*cephalad arrow*) with compression of the spinal canal and compression and increased T2 signal within the spinal cord (*caudal arrow*).

Answers

1. Etiologies of intramedullary T2 hyperintensity include astrocytoma, ependymoma, multiple sclerosis, acute disseminated encephalomyelitis, and Wallerian degeneration from a proximal lesion.

2. Myelopathic symptoms predominate in presentation, including distal weakness and numbness, and bowel and bladder dysfunction.

3. There are four stages of Wallerian degeneration:

   Stage 1—axonal destruction

   Stage 2—myelin protein breakdown

   Stage 3—myelin lipid breakdown and gliosis

   Stage 4—volume loss

4. Asymptomatic lesions do not require treatment. Symptomatic lesions are preferentially treated with resection; however, if this is not possible, fenestration or marsupialization of the cyst can be performed. Alternative options include placement of a cyst-subarachnoid space shunt.

5. In chronic myelomalacia, conservative management and physical therapy are the best treatment options. Surgery is reserved for relieving compressive lesions.

Pearls

- Myelomalacia is a generic term that refers to gliosis within the spinal cord.
- It can be the result of external compression (as in this case), secondary to trauma with cord contusion or the result of a proximal lesion with subsequent Wallerian degeneration.
- It is important to differentiate high T2 signal from gliosis from edema related to underlying lesion. Myelomalacia will progress to volume loss in the chronic phase.
- Patients will generally present with myelopathic symptoms related to the level of insult.
- Treatment is aimed at primary etiology, if possible, or supportive.

Suggested Readings

Ergun T, Lakadamyali H. Multiple extradural spinal arachnoid cysts causing diffuse myelomalacia of the spinal cord. *Neurologist*. 2009;15:347-350.

Kumar A, Sakia R, Singh K, Sharma V. Spinal arachnoid cyst. *J Clin Neurosci*. 2011;18:1189-1192.

Back pain

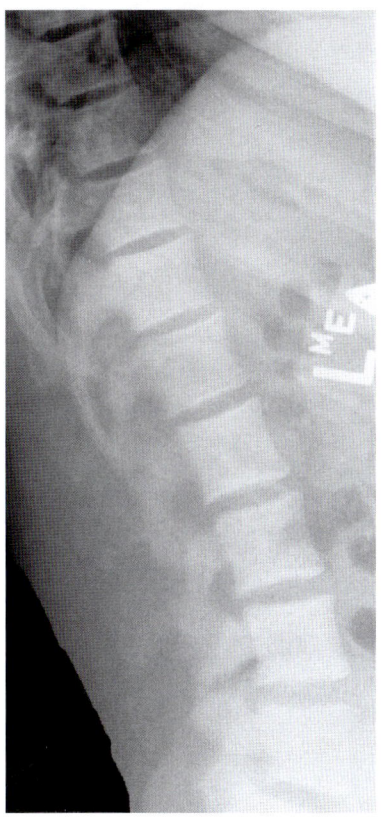

1. What should be included in the differential diagnosis?

2. What are common presenting symptoms?

3. What are associated complications?

4. What portion of the spine is most commonly affected?

5. What are the treatment options?

Case ranking/difficulty:

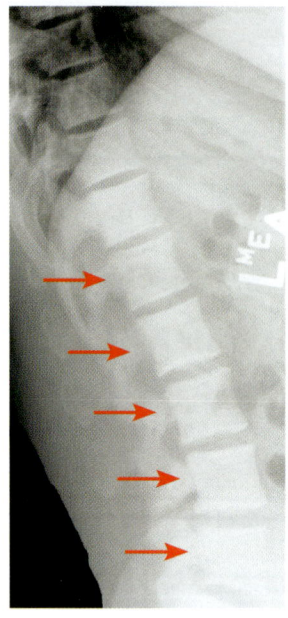

Lateral radiograph demonstrates sclerosis, expansion, cortical thickening and trabecular coarsening within the affected thoracolumbar vertebral bodies.

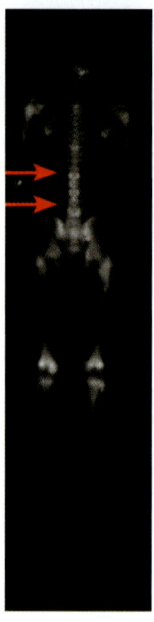

Whole-body bone scan demonstrates increased radiotracer uptake in the thoracolumbar spine, as well as femurs, pelvis, and humeral heads.

Answers

1. Etiologies for increased density within a vertebral body include metastasis, hemangioma, osteopetrosis, lymphoma, and osteosarcoma.

2. Pain and pathologic fracture are most common; however, osseous expansion can lead to scoliosis and radicular symptoms. Myelopathy can occur secondary to cord ischemia from shunting.

3. Potential complications include basilar impression, compression fracture, kyphosis, scoliosis, and spondylosis.

4. The lumbar spine is more commonly involved than the thoracic spine, which is more commonly involved than the cervical spine.

5. Potential treatments include conservative management, bisphosphonate therapy, calcitonin therapy, and arthroplasty. There is no role for radiation in the treatment of Paget disease.

Pearls

- Paget disease affects up to 1 out of every 10 patients over 80 years of age with spinal involvement in up to half of all affected patients.
- Patients most commonly present with asymmetric multifocal involvement; however, occasionally there may be a solitary site of involvement.
- In the spine, vertebral body involvement is the rule with variable extension to the posterior elements.
- Radiographic presentations include the ivory vertebra and the picture frame vertebra.
- Patients often present with pain or pathologic fracture; however, there may be serious sequelae secondary to basilar invagination, cord ischemia, or compression.
- Treatment is primarily medical, using bisphosphonates and calcitonin; however, surgery may be used to relieve spinal cord compression or stabilize fractures.

Suggested Readings

Cortis K, Micallef K, Mizzi A. Imaging Paget's disease of bone—from head to toe. *Clin Radiol*. 2011;66:662-672.

Theodorou DJ, Theodorou SJ, Kakitsubata. Imaging of Paget disease of bone and its musculoskeletal complications: review. *AJR*. 2011;196:S64-S75.

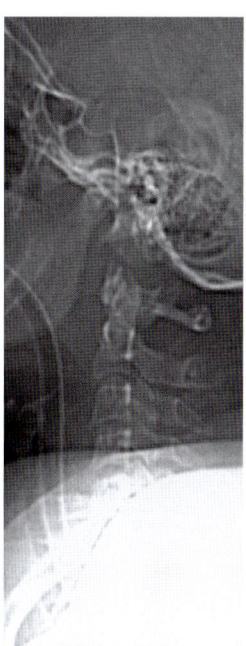

1. What should be included in the differential diagnosis?

2. What is the definition of Wachenheim line?

3. What is Powers ratio?

4. What underlying disorders are associated with a higher incidence of this abnormality?

5. What are the treatment options?

Case ranking/difficulty:

Category: Vertebral body

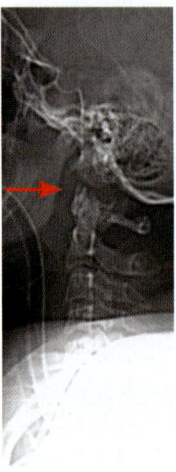

Lateral CT scout image demonstrates prevertebral soft tissue swelling and inferior displacement of the dens.

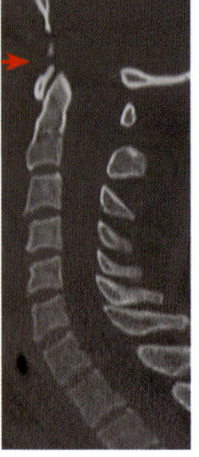

Sagittal CT reconstruction confirms atlantooccipital dislocation with inferior displacement of the dens. An additional fracture fragment is noted cephalad to the C1 anterior arch.

Answers

1. Atlantooccipital dislocation is identified by disruption of Wachenheim line and increased atlantooccipital condyle distance. While commonly fatal, this can be a survivable injury; however, death is usually secondary to brain stem injury.

2. Wachenheim line is drawn along the dorsal surface of the clivus and should intersect the odontoid tip. It is used to assess for anterior or posterior subluxation based on the position of the odontoid relative to the line. It is independent of head positioning and does not vary based on patient age.

3. Powers ratio is used to determine anterior subluxation and is defined as the distance from the basion to the midvertical posterior lamina of the axis divided by the distance from the opisthion to the midvertical portion of the anterior atlas ring (BC/OA).

4. Down syndrome and rheumatoid arthritis have an increased incidence of atlantooccipital instability.

5. Rigid cervical collar should be maintained until the patient is taken to the operating room, for surgical fixation (generally from occiput to C2) and halo placement, which allows adjustment to obtain reduction. Soft cervical collars do not provide enough stability and traction is contraindicated as it may increase the risk of vascular and spinal cord injury.

Pearls

- Cervical spine injuries are commonly encountered in the setting of trauma.

- Upper cervical spine injuries are particularly worrisome given the potential instability and associated cord injury.
- Injuries above the level of C3 are potentially lethal, as the C3 through C5 spinal nerves give supply to the phrenic nerve and innervate the diaphragm.
- Imaging should be undertaken immediately upon arrival while the patient is immobilized if clinical concern exists.
- Prompt neurosurgical or orthopedic evaluation is recommended for consideration of surgical intervention in unstable cases.
- Atlantooccipital dislocation can also be associated with injury to the vertebral arteries at the skull base, leading to vertebrobasilar infarction or insufficiency. Consideration of vascular imaging is recommended.
- Atlantooccipital dislocation is defined using the Powers ratio, which determine anterior subluxation and is defined as the distance from the basion to the midvertical posterior lamina of the axis divided by the distance from the opisthion to the midvertical portion of the anterior atlas ring (BC/OA). Normal is less than 1.
- The basion is defined as the midpoint anterior foramen magnum; the opisthion is defined as the midpoint posterior foramen magnum.

Suggested Readings

Bucholz RW, Burkhead WZ. The pathological anatomy of fatal atlanto-occipital dislocations. *JBJS*. 1979;61-A:248-250.

Watanabe M, Sakai D, Yamamoto Y, Sato M, Mochida J. Upper cervical spine injuries: age-specific clinical features. *J Orthop Sci*. 2010;15:485-492.

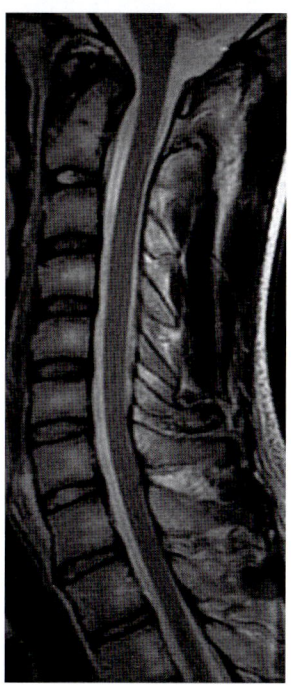

1. What should be included in the differential diagnosis?

2. What are common presenting symptoms?

3. Early radiation changes can be seen how long after radiation?

4. What is the threshold dose that leads to permanent fatty marrow replacement?

5. What are the treatment options?

Case ranking/difficulty:

Category: More than one category

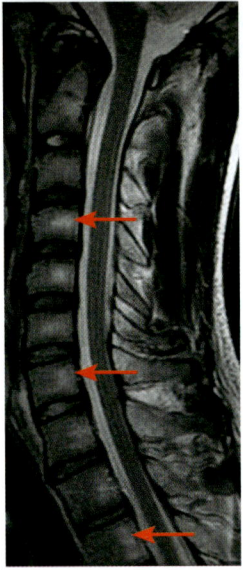

Sagittal T2 image demonstrates geographic hyperintensity throughout the posterior vertebral bodies and posterior elements, consistent with marrow edema related to proton beam radiation.

Answers

1. Focal lesions within the vertebral bodies include hemangioma, infection, metastasis, normal fatty marrow, and primary bone tumor; however, the key to diagnosis is the geographic distribution and T1 and T2 hyperintensity.

2. Fatty marrow replacement does not cause symptoms; however, extensive conversion of active marrow could produce anemia, leukopenia, and thrombocytopenia. Pathologic fractures have been reported in vertebral bodies that receive high doses.

3. Early changes can be seen as early as 2 weeks following radiation.

4. Above doses of 50 Gy, reconversion to active marrow is unlikely.

5. There is no indication to discontinue radiation as most patients require no treatment. Vertebroplasty could be considered in the setting of pathologic fracture.

Pearls

- Spinal irradiation causes characteristic changes within the vertebral bodies, with conversion of active marrow to fatty marrow.
- The key to diagnosis is recognizing the geographic pattern of involvement.
- This is particularly apparent in pediatric patients, but can be seen in adult patients, especially in those patients who have reactivation of bone marrow.
- There may be long-term recovery of the marrow with a reconversion to active marrow.

Suggested Readings

Hwang S, Lefkowitz R, Landa J, et al. Local changes in bone marrow at MRI after treatment of extremity soft tissue sarcoma. *Skeletal Radiol.* 2009;38:11-19.

Stevens SK, Moore SG, Kaplan ID. Early and late bone-marrow changes after irradiation: MR evaluation. *AJR.* 1990;154:745-750.

Numbness and macrocytic anemia

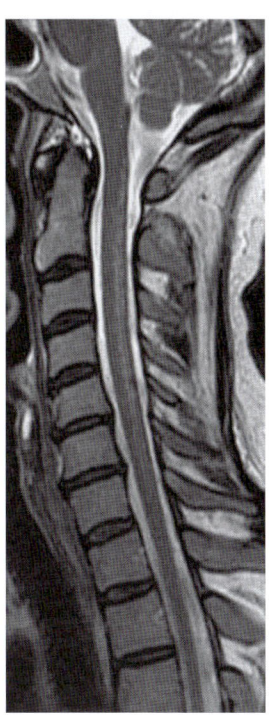

1. What should be included in the differential diagnosis?

2. What are common presenting symptoms?

3. What etiologies can lead to the development of this abnormality?

4. What is the prognosis?

5. What are the treatment options?

Case ranking/difficulty: **Category:** Spinal cord

Sagittal T2 image demonstrates hyperintensity within the dorsal and lateral columns.

Answers

1. Etiologies for intramedullary T2 hyperintensity include copper deficiency myelopathy, HIV vacuolar myelopathy, infarction, multiple sclerosis, and transverse myelitis; however, multiple sclerosis generally does not present with long segment involvement.

2. Common presenting symptoms are ataxia and parasthesias. Additional symptoms include loss of position and vibration sense, spasticity, and hyperreflexia.

3. Pernicious anemia is the most common cause in the United States. Other etiologies include ileal resection, nitrous oxide exposure, partial gastrectomy, and vegan diet.

4. Resolution of symptoms is related to severity and duration of symptoms; the longer and worse the symptoms, the less likely the complete resolution. Partial resolution following treatment is the general rule.

5. Parenteral B12 is the treatment, with treatment of underlying cause if present.

Pearls

- Subacute combined degeneration occurs in the setting of impaired B12 metabolism or deficiency.
- Nitrous oxide exposure can also result in subacute combined degeneration; however, the pathway is poorly understood.
- B12 is a critical coenzyme in pathways responsible for myelin maintenance, and deficiency leads to demyelinization, vacuolization, and eventually axonal loss.
- There is significant crossover with copper deficiency myelopathy.
- There is preferential involvement of the dorsal columns with the resultant presentation of loss of proprioception and vibration with paresthesias.
- Involvement of the lateral columns leads to spasticity and hyperreflexia.
- T2 hyperintensity and mild expansion are seen without significant enhancement.
- Treatment is aimed at B12 supplementation with general resolution of symptoms.

Suggested Readings

Naidich MJ, Ho SU. Case 87: Subacute combined degeneration. *Radiology*. 2005;237:101-105.

Tsang BK-T, Crump N, Macdonel RA. Subacute combined degeneration of the spinal cord despite prophylactic vitamin B12 treatment. *J Clin Neuroscience*. 2012;19:908-910.

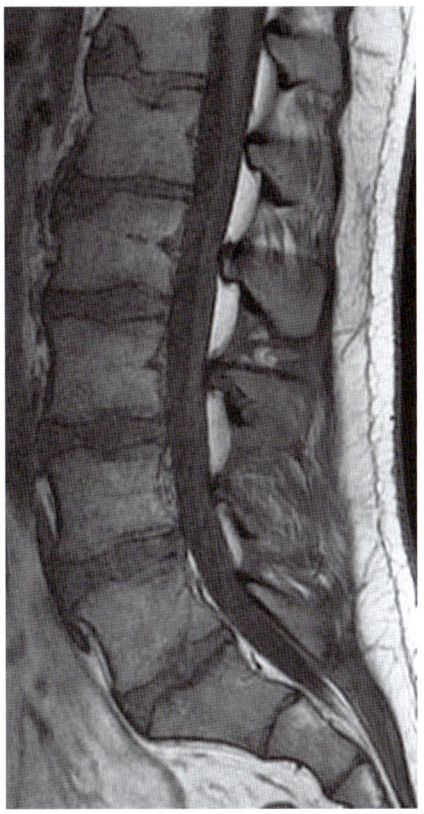 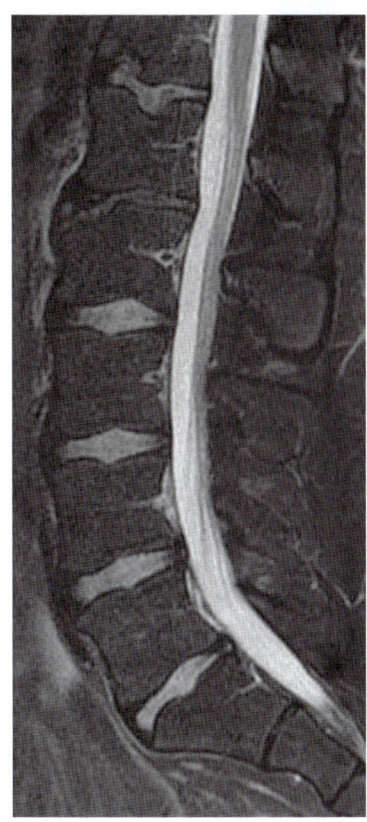

1. What should be included in the differential diagnosis?

2. This abnormality occurs from an insult before what age?

3. What portion of the spine is most commonly affected?

4. What are common presenting symptoms?

5. What are the treatment options?

Case ranking/difficulty:

Category: Vertebral body

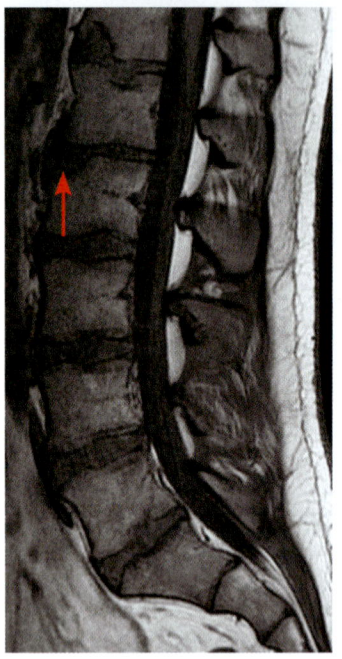

Sagittal T1 image demonstrates a small osseous fragment adjacent to the superior anterior corner of the L2 vertebral body.

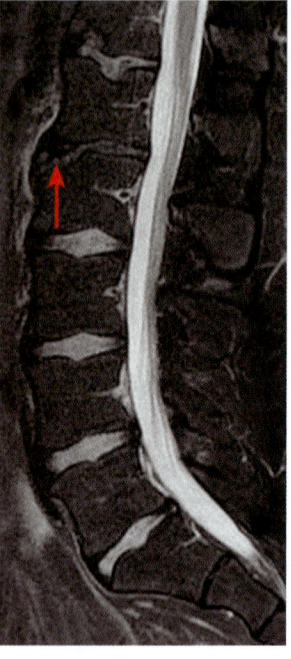

Sagittal T2 image demonstrates a small osseous fragment adjacent to the superior anterior corner of the L2 vertebral body. There is no adjacent edema to suggest fracture or instability.

Answers

1. Vertebral body fracture, osteophyte fracture, Schmorl node, diskitis/osteomyelitis, and limbus vertebra could all be considered; however, the lack of T2 hyperintense marrow would argue against most of these entities.

2. The rim apophysis usually fuses around 20 years of age; a limbus vertebra results from an injury prior to fusion.

3. The lumbar spine is most commonly involved, specifically, the anterosuperior endplates.

4. Pain, decreased range of motion, and kyphosis are the most common presenting symptoms; however, this may also be an incidental finding.

5. Treatment is conservative with physical therapy and analgesia. There is no indication for surgical intervention.

Pearls

- Limbus vertebrae are common incidental findings in spine imaging that result from incomplete fusion of the rim apophysis and vertebral body.
- The etiology is felt to be a traumatic insult during childhood, before 20 years old (when fusion is complete)—often the trauma is not significant enough to be remembered.
- It is important to differentiate this from a fracture, which can be done by noting the lack of adjacent edema.
- These lesions require no further imaging or management.

Suggested Readings

Carr RB, Tozer Fink KR, Gross JA. Imaging of trauma: Part I, pseudotrauma of the spine. *AJR*. 2012;199:1200-1206.

Runge M. Traps in spinal MR imaging. *Diagn Interv Imaging*. 2012;93:993-999.

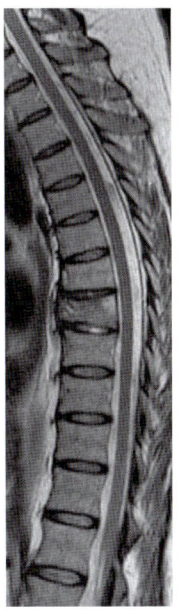 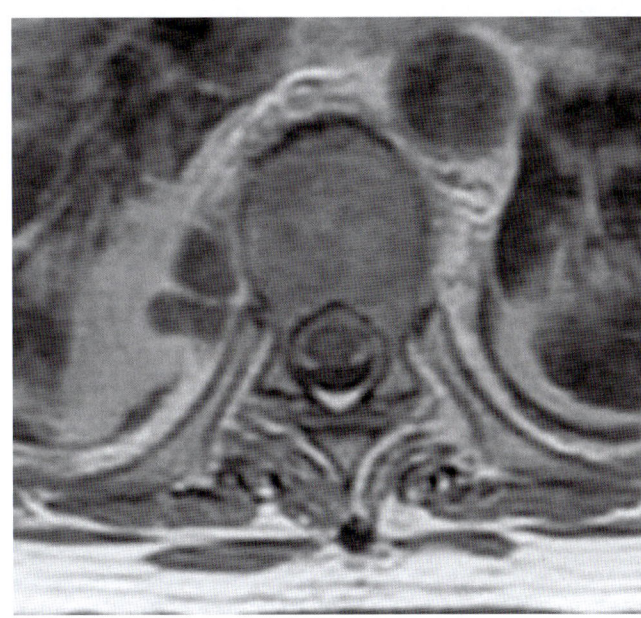

1. What should be included in the differential diagnosis?

2. What are common presenting symptoms?

3. What location within the spine is most commonly affected?

4. Which portion of the spine is most commonly affected?

5. What are the treatment options?

Case ranking/difficulty:

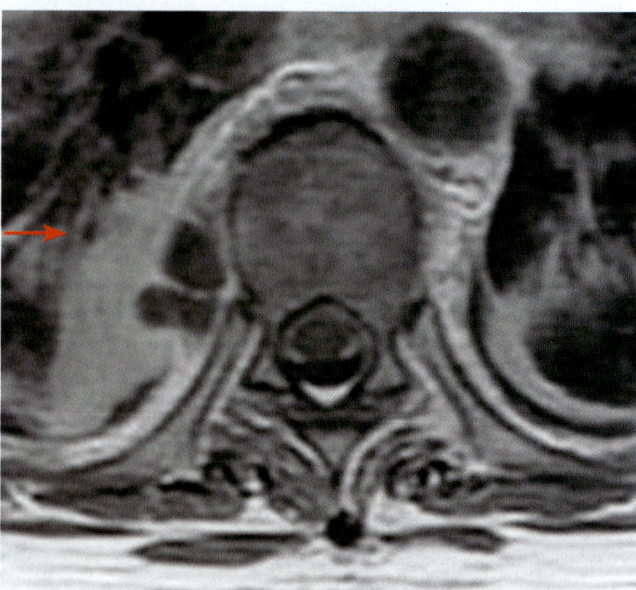

Sagittal T2 image demonstrates compression deformity of the T8 vertebral body with increased signal within the T8-T9 intervertebral disc.

Axial T1 image following gadolinium administration demonstrates enhancement of the lateral aspect of the T8 vertebral body with a peripherally enhancing right paraspinal collection.

Answers

1. Lesions that may involve the vertebral body, intervertebral disc, and paraspinal soft tissues include metastatic disease and infectious spondylitis (pyogenic, fungal, tubercular, Brucellar).

2. Presenting symptoms include fever, night sweats, back pain, radiculopathy, and myelopathy.

3. Most spinous involvement is centered at the thoracolumbar junction.

4. The vertebral body and intervertebral disc are commonly involved.

5. Long-term antituberculosis agents are the mainstay of treatment. Abscess drainage and surgical debridement may be considered in some cases.

- Spread is primarily hematogenous to the vertebral body endplates. From there, the infection can spread into the disc space and paraspinal soft tissues.
- Factors that can differentiate tuberculous spondylitis from other etiologies include calcification within paraspinal abscesses and lack of periosteal reaction.
- Tuberculosis also characteristically spares the posterior elements, helping differentiate it from metastatic disease.
- Treatment consists primarily of long-term multidrug regimens.
- Surgical resection and decompression may be indicated in up to one-fourth of patients if neurological compromise or spinal deformity is present.

Pearls

- Tuberculous spondylitis is increasing in frequency in developed nations, primarily within immunocompromised populations.
- The spine is involved in half of patients with osseous tuberculosis involvement, most commonly around the thoracolumbar junction.

Suggested Readings

Burrill J, Williams CJ, Bain G, Conder G, Hine AL, Misra RR. Tuberculosis: a radiologic review. *Radiographics*. 2007;27:1255-1273.

Harisinghani MG, McLoud TC, Shepard J-A O, Ko JP, Shroff MM, Mueller PR. Tuberculosis from head to toe. *Radiographics*. 2000;20:449-470.

Acute-onset paraplegia in patient with lupus

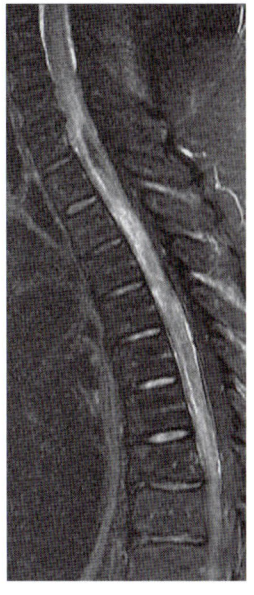 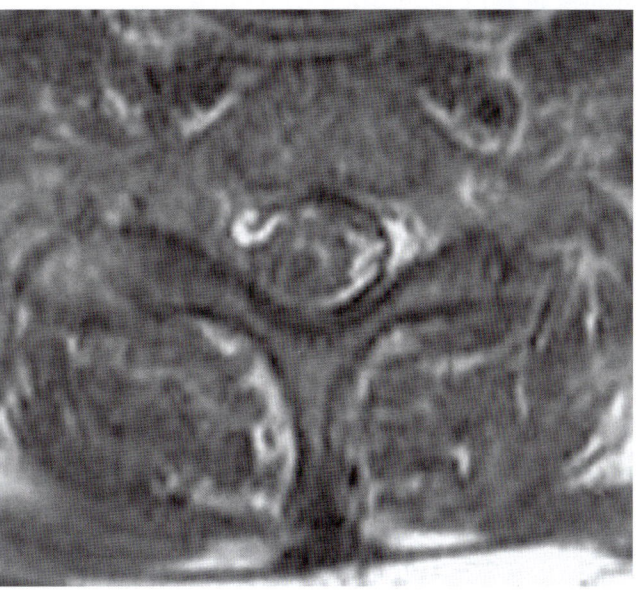

1. What should be included in the differential diagnosis?

2. What entities are associated with a higher incidence of this abnormality?

3. What is the best prognostic factor of recovery?

4. What is the most common location within the cord?

5. What are the treatment options?

Case ranking/difficulty:

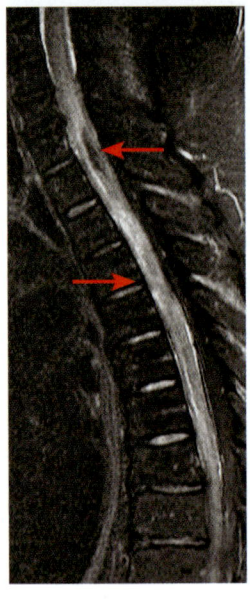

Sagittal T2 image demonstrates intramedullary low signal, consistent with hemorrhage, with surrounding T2 hyperintensity (*caudal arrow*), consistent with vasogenic edema.

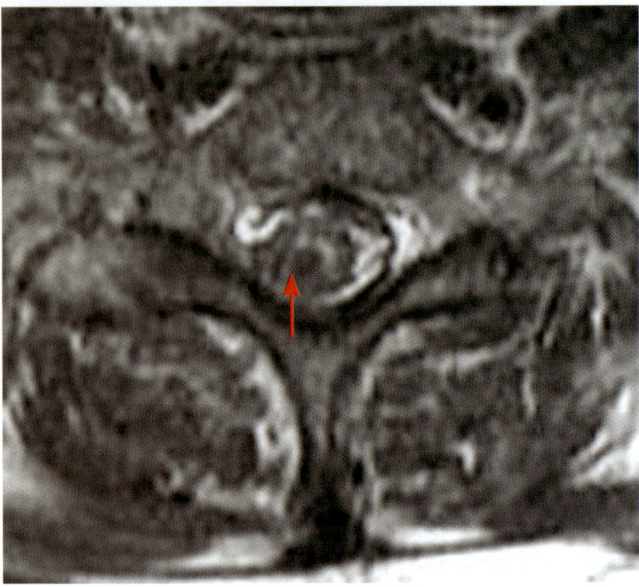

Axial T2 image demonstrates focus of signal dropout, consistent with hemorrhage.

Answers

1. Etiologies of T2 hyperintensity within the cord include astrocytoma, ependymoma, vascular malformation, infarction, and demyelinating disease; however, it would be unusual to see hemorrhage with demyelinating disease.

2. Thoracic aortic aneurysm and thoracic aortic aneurysm repair, atherosclerosis, vasculitis, and trauma are all associated with cord infarction.

3. The greater the symptoms are at presentation, the worse the prognosis.

4. The most common location is within the thoracic cord.

5. Treatment options include conservative management, physical therapy, and steroid and anticoagulant administration. There is no role for surgical resection, although hematoma evacuation could be considered in select cases.

Pearls

- Spinal cord infarction should be considered in a patient with the sudden onset of paralysis or myelopathic symptoms.
- Risk factors include the same risk factors for intracranial infarction, including atherosclerosis and vasculitis.

- The prognosis for spinal cord infarction is poor, generally with permanent loss of function.
- Diffusion-weighted imaging may help in diagnosis, particularly in the sagittal plane.
- Treatment is geared at restoring blood flow with anticoagulation (although this should be used judiciously in the setting of cord hemorrhage) and steroids to reduce edema.

Suggested Readings

Robertson CE, Brown RD, Wijdicks EFM, Rabinstein AA. Recovery after spinal cord infarcts: long-term outcome in 115 patients. *Neurology*. 2012;78:114-121.

Sang BK, Foster E, Kam A, Storey E. Diffusion weighted imaging with trace diffusion weighted imaging, the apparent diffusion coefficient and exponential images in the diagnosis of spinal cord infarction. *J Clin Neurosci*. 2013;20:1630-1632.

Tator CH. Update on the pathophysiology and pathology of acute spinal cord injury. *Brain Pathol*. 1995;5:407-413.

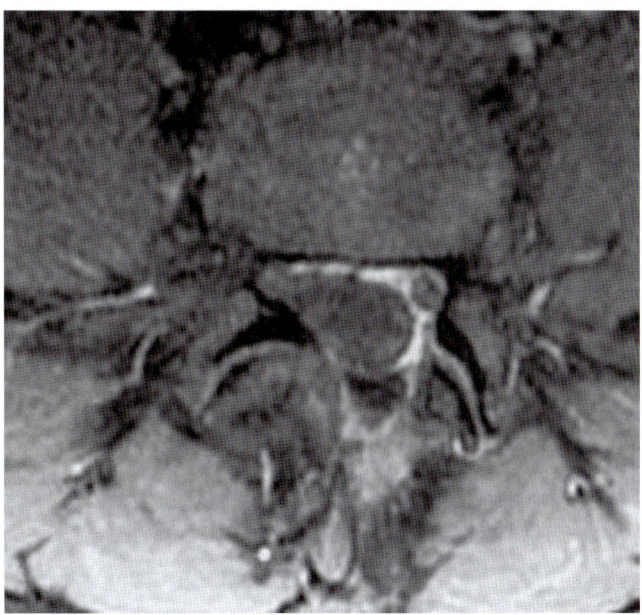

1. What should be included in the differential diagnosis?

2. What are common presenting symptoms?

3. What is the prognosis?

4. What portion of the spine is most commonly affected?

5. What are the treatment options?

Case ranking/difficulty:

Category: More than one category

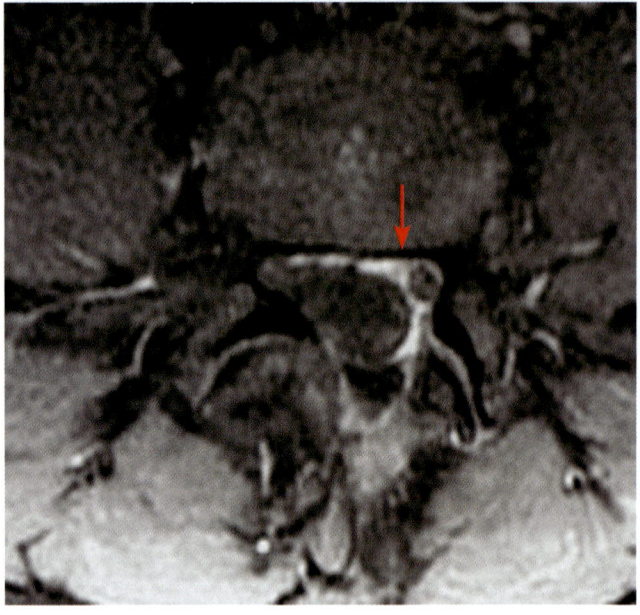

Axial T1 image following gadolinium administration demonstrates enhancement in the left lateral recess, surrounding the traversing S1 nerve root. Note the postoperative changes of prior left L5 hemilaminectomy.

Answers

1. Epidural soft tissue masses include epidural abscess, epidural fibrosis, epidural hematoma, epidural metastasis, and recurrent disc herniation.

2. Potential presenting symptoms of epidural fibrosis include back pain, radiculopathy, loss of reflexes, and dysesthesia. The key is the history of previous successful surgery and the onset of gradually progressive symptoms.

3. Generally, the symptoms are stable to slowly progressive. Approximately one-third of patients have improvement of symptoms following repeat surgery, while about half of patients have improvement following spinal cord stimulator placement.

4. Peridural fibrosis is most commonly seen in the lumbar spine.

5. Potential treatment options include physical therapy, analgesia, corticosteroid injection, spinal cord stimulation, and surgical resection; however, surgical resection is unlikely to be beneficial in cases of pure fibrosis. It can be helpful for removal of recurrent disc herniation and is more successful if no peridural fibrosis is present.

Pearls

- Peridural fibrosis can occur in up to 10% of patients following diskectomy.
- The classic presentation is progressive back pain/radicular symptoms in a patient with prior diskectomy with good results.
- This entity is one of the reasons that gadolinium administration is recommended in postoperative follow-up imaging of the lumbar spine.
- Imaging findings include soft tissue and enhancement surrounding a nerve root within the lateral recess.
- It is important to differentiate peridural fibrosis from recurrent or residual disc fragment.
- Repeat surgery is more successful if a recurrent or residual disc fragment is identified, particularly in the absence of associated fibrosis.

Suggested Readings

Hueftle MG, Modic MT, Ross JS, et al. Lumbar spine: postoperative MR imaging with Gd-DTPA. *Radiology.* 1988;167:817-824.

Lee YS, Choi ES, Song CJ. Symptomatic nerve root changes on contrast-enhanced MR imaging after surgery for lumbar disk herniation. *AJNR.* 2009;30:1062-1067.

Fixed torticollis

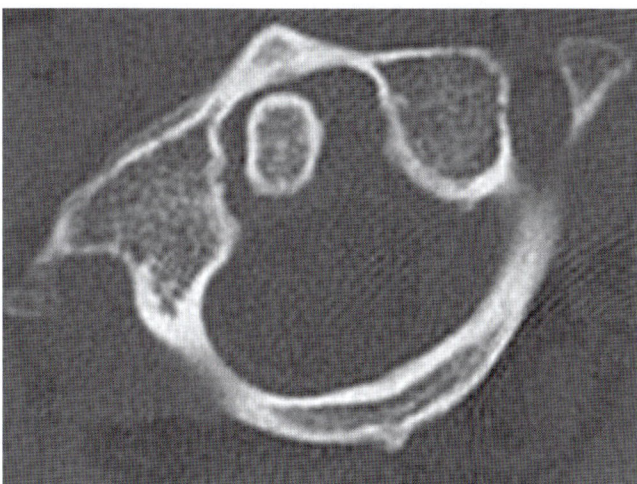 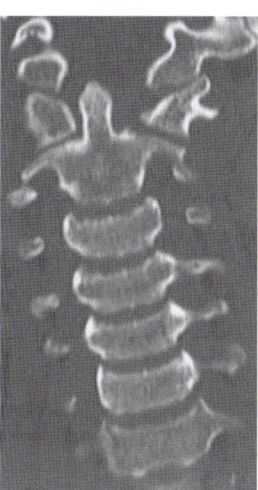

1. What are etiologies of this abnormality?

2. What is the classification system according to the Fielding and Hawkins system?

3. What syndromes are associated with increased incidence?

4. What ligaments are disrupted?

5. What are the treatment options?

Case ranking/difficulty:

Category: Vertebral body

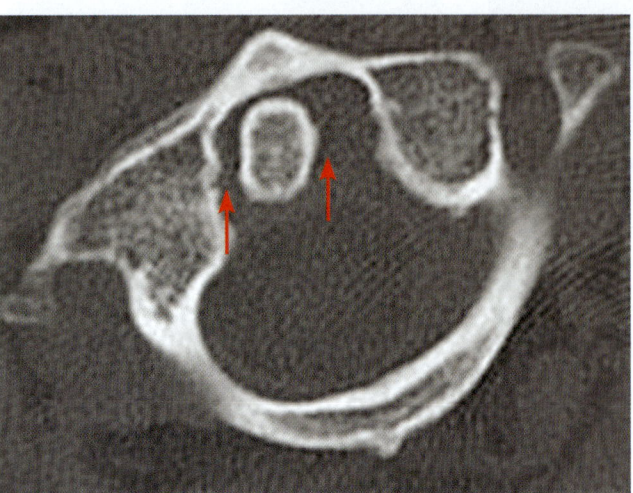

Axial CT image demonstrates asymmetry of the C1-C2 articulation.

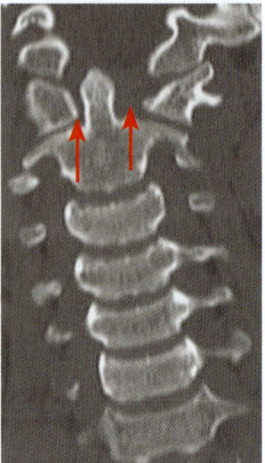

Coronal CT image demonstrates asymmetry of the C1-C2 articulation.

Answers

1. Trauma is the most common cause; however, prior surgery may lead to laxity and nasopharyngeal infection may spread to the craniocervical junction joints.

2. Fielding and Hawkins system:

   Type 1—anterior atlas displacement <3mm

   Type 2—anterior atlas displacement 3-5 mm

   Type 3—anterior atlas displacement >5 mm

   Type 4—posterior atlas displacement

   There has been a refinement with the Pang system based on three position CT.

3. Down syndrome, Marfan syndrome, Morqui syndrome, and rheumatoid arthritis all have a higher incidence of ligamentous laxity leading to increased incidence of rotatory subluxation.

4. The alar and transverse ligaments are disrupted; however, this may occur in the setting of other traumatic injuries and evaluation of the remaining ligaments is critical.

5. Initial treatment is bracing; patients who fail bracing may require traction and additional bracing, halo fixation, or posterior fusion.

Pearls

- Rotatory subluxation is the result of ligamentous disruption at the C1-C2 articulation.
- It is more common in children, secondary to the inherent ligamentous laxity, and relatively large head size with respect to the remainder of the body.
- On static imaging, this injury is suspected by the offset of C1 with respect to the dens and C2.
- If there is concern, consideration of dynamic three phase CT is recommended—including neutral and maximum head turning to each side. This should only be undertaken under advisement of neurosurgery to avoid permanent patient injury.

Suggested Readings

Beier AD, Vachhrajani S, Bayerl SH, et al. Rotatory subluxation: experience from the Hospital for Sick Children. *J Neurosurg Pediatrics*. 2012;9:144-148.

Haque S, Bin Bilal Shafi B, Kaleem M. Imaging of torticollis in children. *Radiographics*. 2012;32:557-571.

Pang D, Li V. Atlantoaxial rotatory fixation: Part 3—a prospective study of the clinical manifestation, diagnosis, management, and outcome of children with alantoaxial rotatory fixation. *Neurosurgery*. 2005;57(5):954-972.

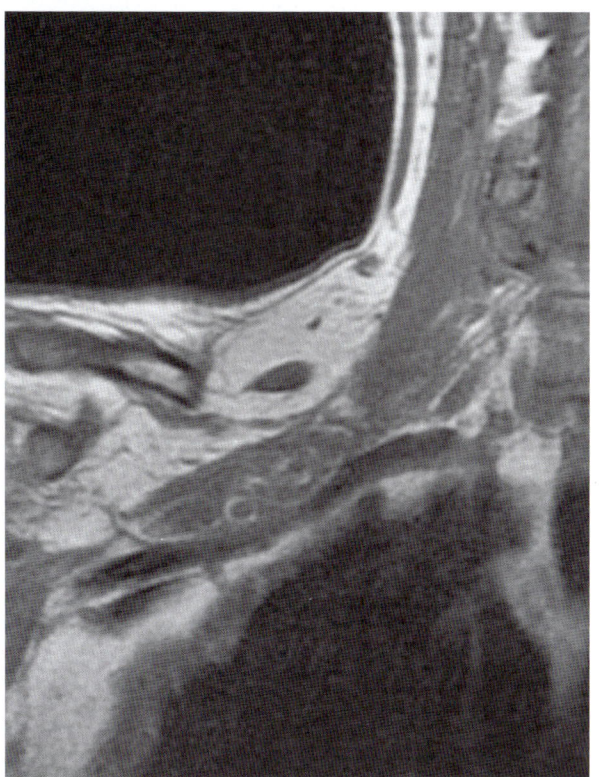 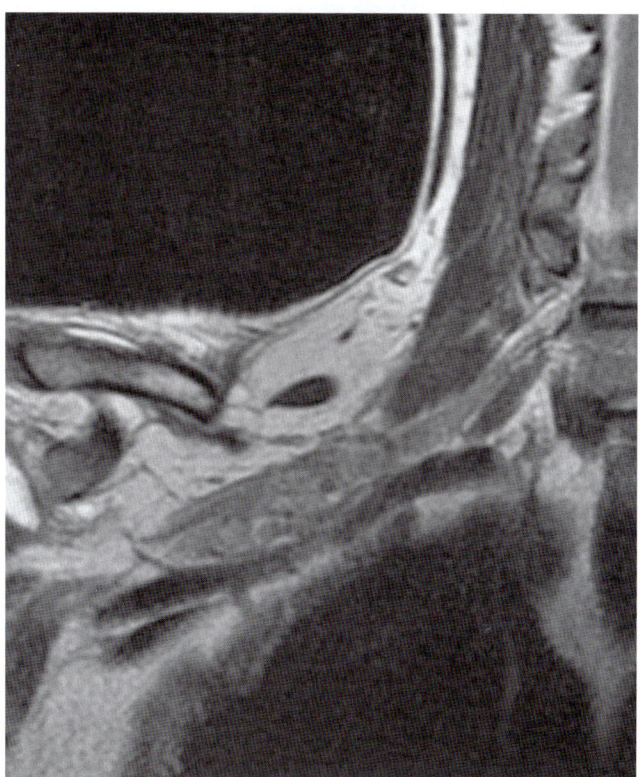

1. What is the motor innervation supplied by the brachial plexus trunks and cords?

2. What are the common presenting symptoms of compressive brachial plexopathy?

3. What are some of the common causes of compressive brachial plexopathy?

4. What are imaging landmarks used to evaluate the segments of the brachial plexus?

5. What is the next most appropriate step in management?

Case ranking/difficulty:

Category: Nerve roots/Nerve plexus/Peripheral nerves

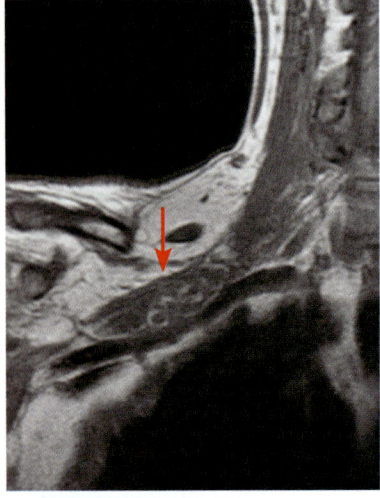

Coronal T1 image demonstrates mixed intensity mass, consistent with hematoma.

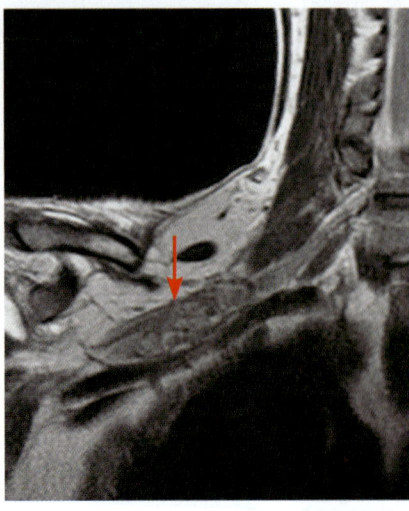

Coronal T2 image demonstrates mixed intensity mass, consistent with hematoma.

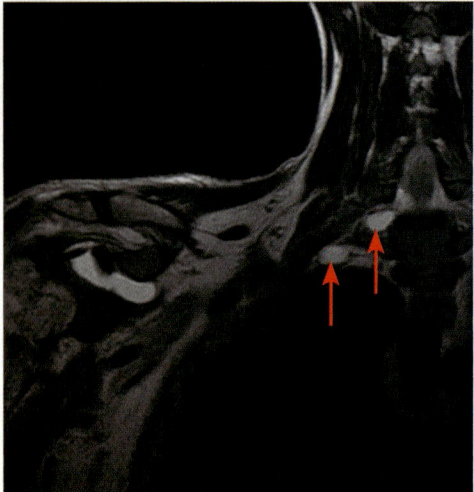

Coronal T2 image demonstrates pseudomeningoceles at C8 and T1.

Answers

1. The trunks and posterior cords innervate the shoulder, the medial cord innervates the hand, and the lateral cord innervates the upper chest.

2. Compressive plexopathies are generally more difficult to diagnose clinically as they present with mixed motor and sensory symptomatology.

3. Extrinsic compression of the brachial plexus by tumor is more common than primary tumors of the brachial plexus. The most common etiologies of compression include hematoma, lymphoma, leukemia, and metastatic lymphadenopathy.

4. Roots are located in the neural foramina; trunks are located between the scalene muscles; divisions are located posterior to the clavicle; cords are located inferior to the clavicle. Knowing the anatomic location is important for identifying abnormalities.

5. Evaluation for a vascular injury may be indicated depending on the clinical history. Analgesia and physical therapy are additional appropriate management steps in this patient, with the consideration of surgical reanastomosis if appropriate.

Pearls

- Traumatic brachial plexus injuries usually present with motor symptoms.
- The radiologist's role is to define the distance between avulsed nerve segments, if possible.
- In addition, it is important to describe the location of avulsion: the more proximal the avulsion, the more difficult the surgical reanastomosis.
- Evaluation should include mention of associated injuries, including to the cervical spine, spinal cord, or shoulder joint.

Suggested Readings

Castillo M. Imaging the anatomy of the brachial plexus: review and self-assessment module. *AJR*. 2005;185:S196-S204.

Sureka J, Cherian RA, Alexander M, Thomas BP. MRI of brachial plexopathies. *Clin Radiol*. 2009;64:208-218.

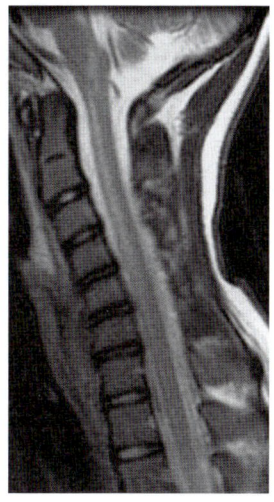 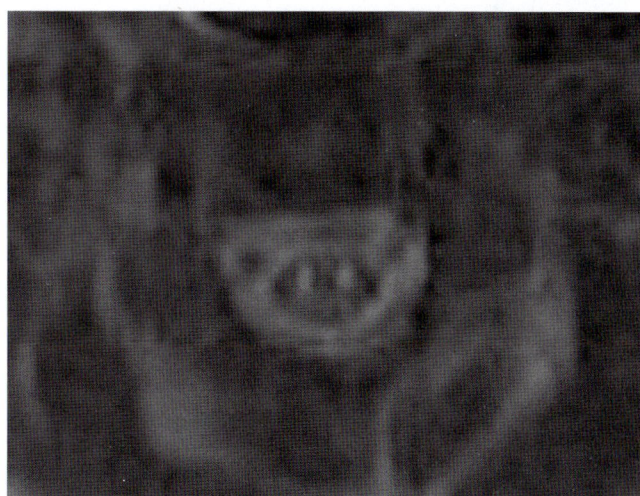

1. What should be included in the differential diagnosis?

2. What are common presenting symptoms?

3. What viruses are most commonly associated with this abnormality?

4. What part of the spinal cord is most commonly involved?

5. What are the treatment options?

Case ranking/difficulty:

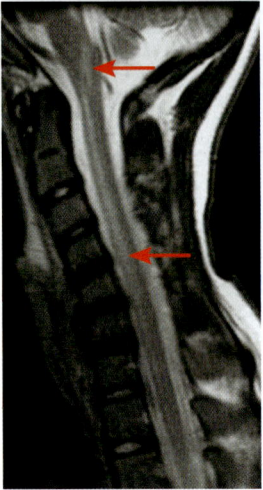

Sagittal T2 image demonstrates ventral T2 hyperintensity extending from the craniocervical junction through the cervical cord.

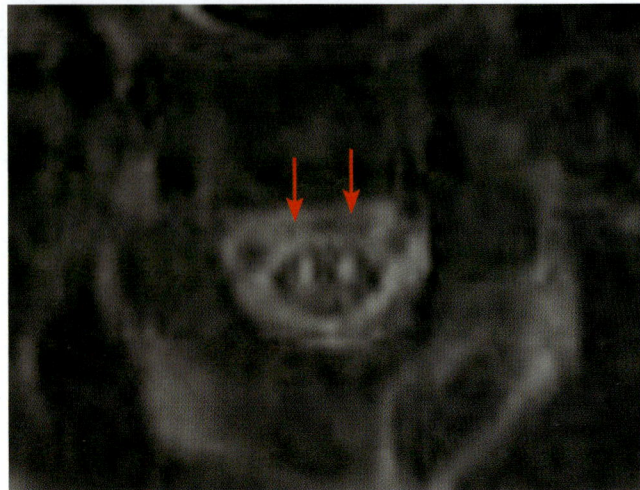

Axial T2 image demonstrates T2 hyperintensity within the ventral horns.

Answers

1. Etiologies for T2 hyperintensity within the cord include polio, idiopathic transverse myelitis, multiple sclerosis, viral myelitis, and acute disseminated encephalomyelitis.

2. Given the ventral horn distribution of the signal abnormality, it is not surprising that motor symptoms predominate. However, it is possible to have sensory symptoms as well.

3. The enteroviruses are the most common (coxsackie, echovirus, rubella, measles, mumps, hepatitis); other etiologies include herpes, West Nile, and human immunodeficiency viruses.

4. The cervical and thoracic cords are most often involved with extension to the craniocervical junction. Oftentimes the signal abnormality may even extend cephalad to the brainstem.

5. Treatment options include supportive management, antiviral agents, steroids, and intravenous immunoglobulin.

Pearls

- T2 hyperintense signal within the cord is seen in a variety of pathologies.
- The distribution can be helpful to differentiate diagnoses.

- In this case, there is long segment involvement of the bilateral ventral horns, typical of viral myelitis.
- Demyelinating disease tends to have a more patchy distribution and each individual lesion tends to be less than two vertebral body heights in length.
- Polio has a very similar appearance but is rarely encountered in the post-vaccine era.
- Gadolinium administration is rarely helpful as any of these etiologies may demonstrate enhancement.
- Patients with viral myelitis tend to present with weakness, which may progress to paralysis. Sensory disruption may also be seen.
- Lumbar puncture is key to diagnosis—the cerebrospinal fluid demonstrates a typical pattern for viral infection with elevated protein and mononuclear cells. Additionally, the fluid can be sent for viral PCR.

Suggested Readings

Ooi MH, Wong SC, Lewthwaite P, Cardosa MJ, Solomon T. Clinical features, diagnosis and management of enterovirus 71. *Lancet Neurol.* 2010;9:1097-1105.

Shen WC, Tsai C-H, Chiu H-H, Chow K-C. MRI of enterovirus 71 myelitis with monoplegia. *Neuroradiology.* 2000;42:124-127.

Neurofibromatosis, type 1

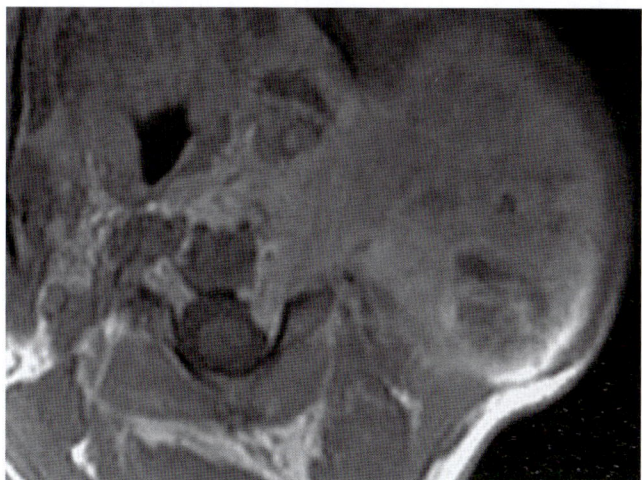

1. What should be included in the differential diagnosis?

2. What are common presenting symptoms?

3. What are risk factors for development?

4. What are common sites of metastases?

5. What are the treatment options?

Case ranking/difficulty:

Category: Nerve roots/Nerve plexus/Peripheral nerves

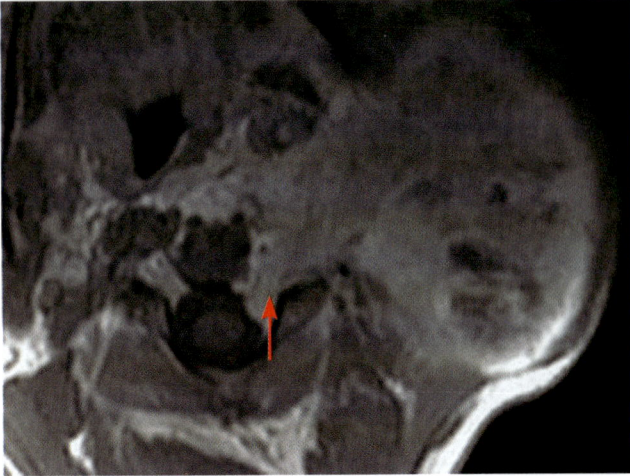

Axial T1 image following gadolinium administration demonstrates a large left paraspinal soft tissue mass with heterogeneous enhancement; note extension through the left C2-C3 neural foramen.

Answers

1. The differential diagnosis includes malignant peripheral nerve sheath tumor, lymphadenopathy, pleomorphic undifferentiated sarcoma, neurofibrosarcoma, and plexiform neurofibroma.

2. Common presenting symptoms include pain, rapid enlargement, radiculopathy, peripheral edema, and motor deficit.

3. Risk factors for developing malignant peripheral nerve sheath tumors include neurofibromatosis, type 1, neurofibromatosis, type 2, previous radiation of a ganglioneuroma or pheochromocytoma, and presence of a plexiform neurofibroma.

4. Common sites of metastases from malignant peripheral nerve sheath tumors include bone, brain, liver, lung, and lymph nodes.

5. Surgical resection is the mainstay of treatment with adjuvant chemotherapy and radiation; however, reconstruction and grafting are not routinely recommended.

Pearls

- Malignant peripheral nerve sheath tumors are uncommon in the general population with an incidence of approximately 0.001%; however, patients with neurofibromatosis, type 1, have a lifetime incidence of up to 10%.
- Half of all malignant peripheral nerve sheath tumors are diagnosed in patients with neurofibromatosis, type 1.
- Malignant degeneration of a neurofibroma should be suspected in the setting of a rapid increase in size or development of pain.
- MRI is the imaging study of choice for evaluation of the involved nerves; however, PET imaging can be helpful to differentiate benign from malignant tumors in select cases.
- The primary treatment is surgical resection; however, total resection can be problematic.
- Adjuvant radiation therapy is used for improved local control, but does not extend life.
- Chemotherapy can be added for distant metastatic disease; however, it has limited benefit.

Suggested Readings

Anghileri M, Miceli R, Fiore M, et al. Malignant peripheral nerve sheath tumors: prognostic factors and survival in a series of patients treated at a single institution. *Cancer.* 2006;107:1065-1074.

Gupta G, Maniker A. Malignant peripheral nerve sheath tumors. *Neurosurg Focus.* 2007;22:E12.

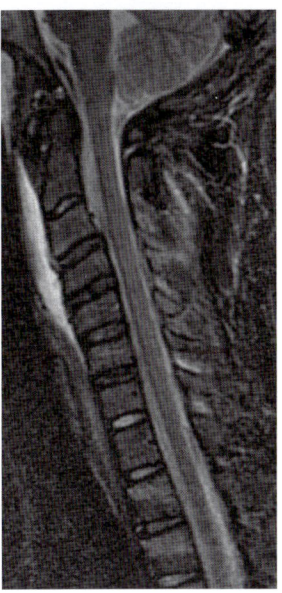

1. What should be included in the differential diagnosis?

2. What are common mechanisms of injury?

3. What structures should be evaluated during cervical spine imaging for trauma?

4. What are the indications for cervical spine MRI in the setting of trauma?

5. What are the treatment options?

Case ranking/difficulty:

Category: More than one category

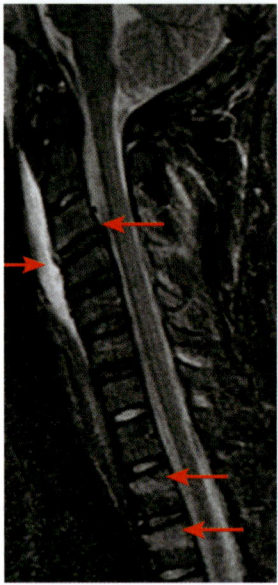

Sagittal STIR image demonstrates focal disruption of the anterior and posterior longitudinal ligaments and the ligamentum flavum with associated prevertebral edema. Also note hyperintensity within the T2 -T4 vertebral bodies, concerning for fractures.

Answers

1. Prevertebral soft tissue enlargement can be seen in ligamentous injury, prevertebral hematoma, longus colli tendonitis, and retropharyngeal abscess.

2. Hyperextension, hyperflexion, rotatory flexion, rotatory extension, and lateral flexion can lead to ligamentous disruption.

3. It is critical to evaluate osseous structures, ligaments, paraspinal musculature, vasculature, and spinal cord in the setting of cervical spine trauma.

4. Indications for MRI in the setting of trauma include fracture, persistent neck pain, weakness, altered sensation, and instability on dynamic imaging.

5. Cervical collar/immobilization is the first-line therapy for patients without malalignment or instability. Surgical fixation is reserved for unstable injuries. Steroids can be used to alleviate cord edema in selected patients.

Pearls

- Evaluation of the cervical spine in trauma is not complete without considering the soft tissues.
- While the ligaments are difficult to assess on CT, there are clues that there is injury, including prevertebral edema and epidural hematoma.
- Further evaluation in these patients should include MRI, including sagittal T2-weighted sequences with fat suppression (either T2 with fat saturation or STIR).
- Management in ligamentous injury depends on degree of disruption, as well as stability during dynamic imaging.
- Some of these injuries can be treated with bracing/ cervical collar, while some require surgical stabilization.

Suggested Readings

Duane TM, Cross J, Scarcella N, et al. Flexion-extension cervical spine plain films compared with MRI in the diagnosis of ligamentous injury. *Am Surg.* 2010;76:595-598.

Schoenfeld AJ, Bono CM, McGuire KJ, Warholic N, Harris MB. Computed tomography alone versus computed tomography and magnetic resonance imaging in the identification of occult injuries to the cervical spine: a meta-analysis. *J Trauma Inj Infect Crit Care.* 2010;68:109-114.

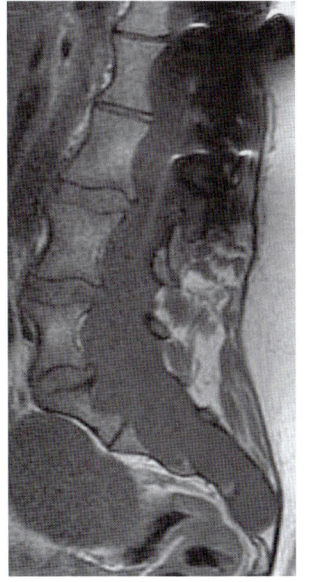 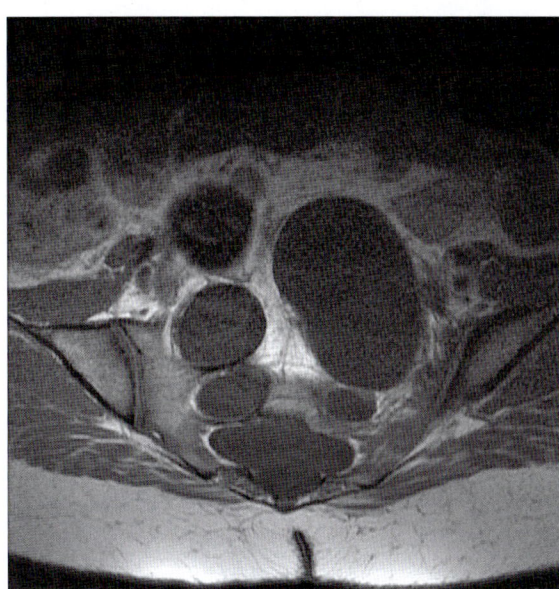

1. What should be included in the differential diagnosis?

2. What are common presenting symptoms?

3. What factors should be evaluated in order to assess for the presence of this abnormality?

4. What are the etiologies?

5. What are the treatment options?

Case ranking/difficulty:

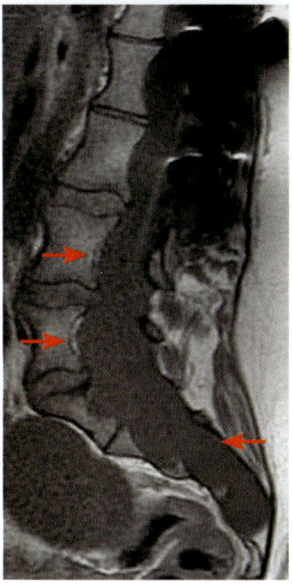

Sagittal proton density image demonstrates diffuse dural ectasia with dilation of the thecal sac and marked posterior vertebral body scalloping.

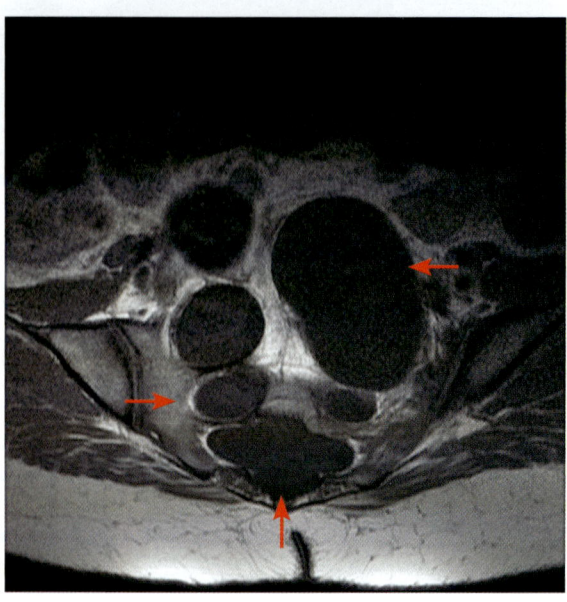

Axial T1 image demonstrates dilation of the thecal sac and multiple nerve root sleeves, as well as an anterior sacral meningocele.

Answers

1. The differential of a cystic mass includes dural ectasia, arachnoid cyst, epidermoid cyst, and schwannoma.

2. Dural ectasia can cause back pain and scoliosis from erosion of the vertebral bodies and pedicles, which can be complicated by pathologic fracture.

3. Scalloping of the posterior bodies as well as enlarged thecal sac and nerve root sleeve diameter can be used to diagnose dural ectasia.

4. Dural ectasia can be seen in ankylosing spondylitis, Ehlers-Danlos, neurofibromatosis type 1, and Marfan syndrome.

5. Conservative management is most appropriate unless complications such as fracture, spondylolisthesis, or scoliosis have occurred, which can necessitate surgical fixation.

Pearls

- Dural ectasia is common in patients with Marfan syndrome.
- It is diagnosed when the thecal sac diameter is greater at the S1 level than at the L4 level.
- It is one of the major criteria for the diagnosis of Marfan disease, which is an autosomal dominant connective tissue disorder.
- Dural ectasia can also be seen in Ehlers-Danlos syndrome, neurofibromatosis type 1, and ankylosing spondylitis.
- It is important to recognize as it can be associated with posterior vertebral body scalloping, which can lead to fracture, spondylolisthesis, or scoliosis.
- If there are associated complications, spinal fusion can be considered.

Suggested Readings

Habermann CR, Weiss F, Schoder V, et al. MR evaluation of dural ectasia in Marfan syndrome: reassessment of the established criteria in children, adolescents and young adults. *Radiology*. 2005;234:535-541.

Lundy R, Rand-Hendriksen S, Hald JK, et al. Dural ectasia in Marfan syndrome: a case control study. *AJNR*. 2009;30:1534-1540.

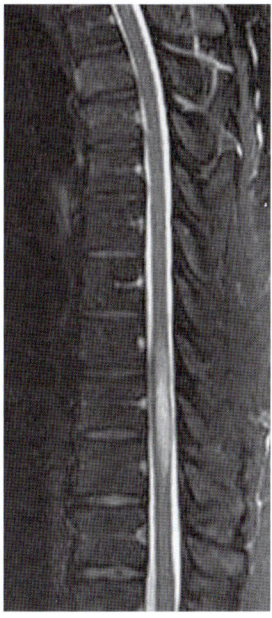 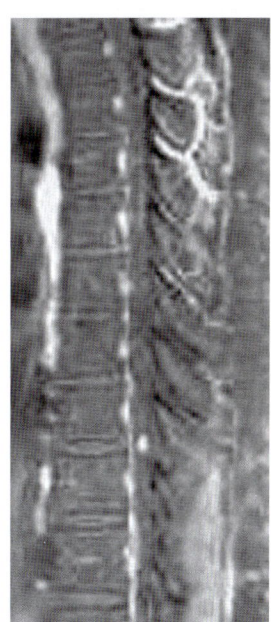

1. What should be included in the differential diagnosis?

2. What WHO grade are these lesions?

3. In patients with this lesion as part of a syndrome, what are other components?

4. What is the most common location within the cord?

5. What are the treatment options?

Case ranking/difficulty:

Category: Spinal cord

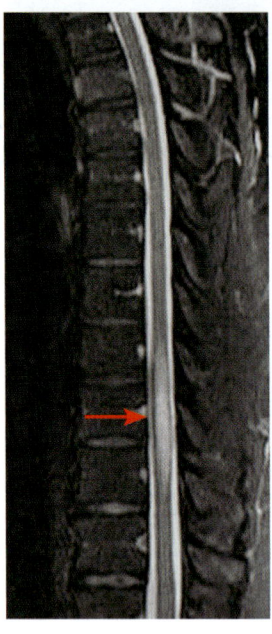

Sagittal T2 image demonstrates expansion and hyperintensity within the lower thoracic cord.

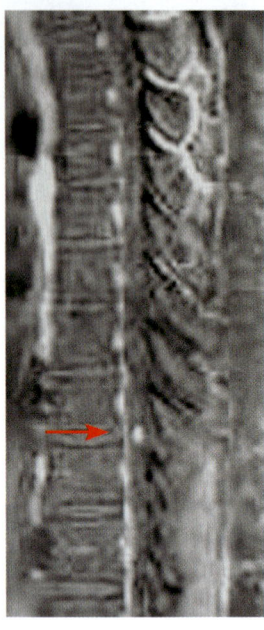

Sagittal T1 image after contrast administration demonstrates enhancing nodule at the T9-T10 level.

Answers

1. Hypervascular enhancing lesions in this location include astrocytoma, ependymoma, metastasis, vascular malformation, and hemangioblastoma.

2. Hemangioblastomas are WHO grade I and generally do not degenerate into higher grade tumors.

3. Von Hippel Lindau syndrome includes hemangioblastoma, endolymphatic sac tumors, retinal angiomas pheochromocytoma, hepatic/pancreatic and epididymal cysts, and renal cell carcinoma.

4. The thoracic spine is the most common location.

5. If patients are symptomatic, surgical resection can be considered, usually after embolization to decrease intraoperative complications. Stereotactic radiosurgery can be used in patients with multiple lesions.

- Most hemangioblastomas are sporadic (2/3).
- 1/3 occurring in conjunction with Von Hippel Lindau syndrome. These patients usually present at a younger age with multiple lesions.
- These are low-grade tumors and treatment may consist of serial imaging follow-up.
- If lesions are symptomatic, surgical resection or stereotactic radiosurgery may be performed with consideration of preoperative embolization to decrease complications.

Suggested Readings

Chamberlain MC, Tredway TL. Adult primary intradural spinal cord tumors: a review. *Curr Neurol Neurosci Rep.* 2011;11:320-328.

Rogers SR, Phalke VV, Anderson J, Riccelli LP, Gonda S, Pollock JM. HEALSME: differential diagnosis for intramedullary spinal cord lesions. *Neurographics.* 2012;2:13-226.

Pearls

- The classic imaging appearance of a hemangioblastoma is a dorsal-enhancing nodule with an intraspinal cyst.
- While flow voids may be seen, these are usually not present until the tumor is greater than 2 cm in dimension.

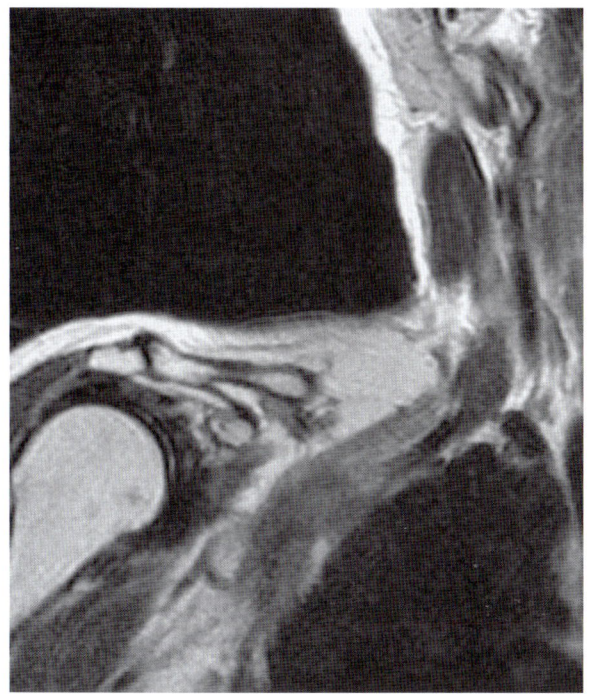 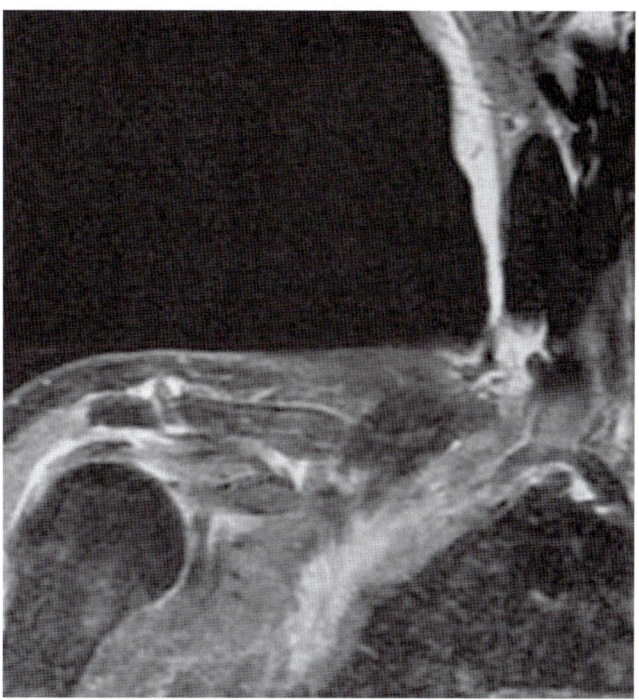

1. What should be included in the differential diagnosis?

2. What are the most common primary malignancies to metastasize to the brachial plexus?

3. What are the presenting symptoms?

4. What is one of the earliest imaging signs of brachial plexus involvement by a Pancoast tumor?

5. What are the treatment options?

Case ranking/difficulty:

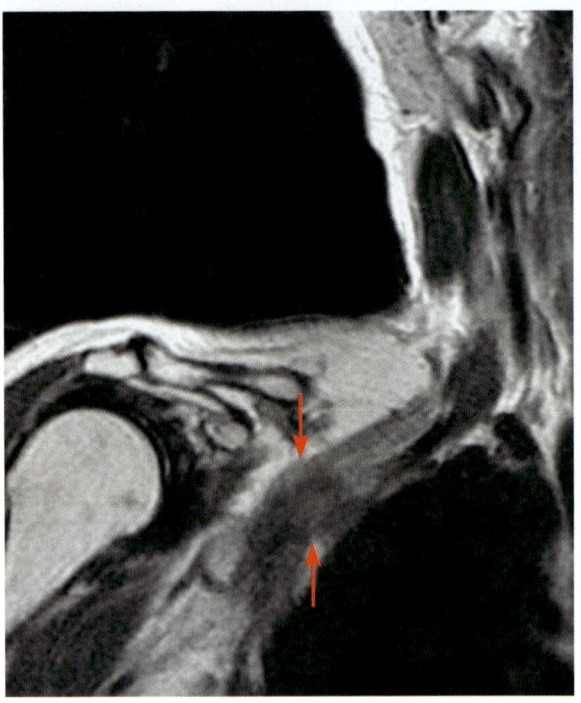

Coronal T2 image demonstrates hyperintensity and soft tissue along the right brachial plexus.

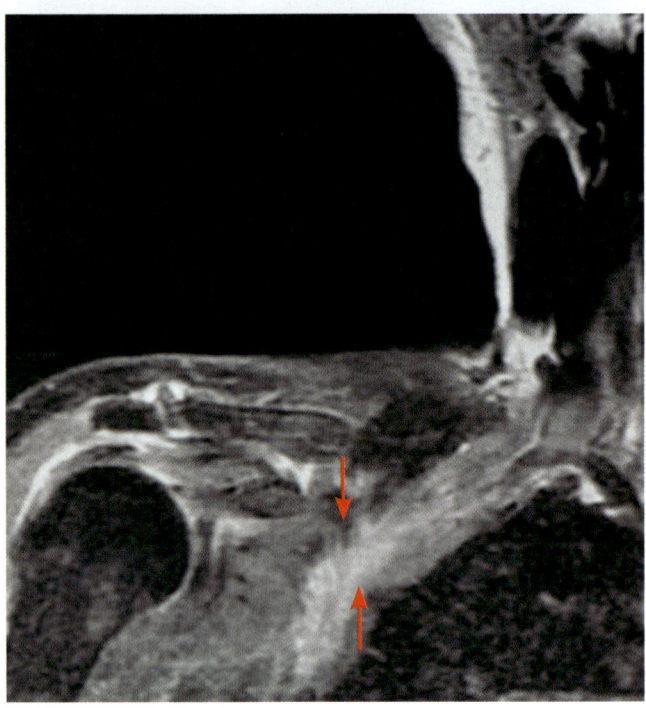

Coronal T1 postgadolinium image demonstrates enhancement of the right brachial plexus with nodular soft tissue.

Answers

1. The differential diagnosis includes radiation plexopathy, primary nerve tumor, metastasis, and inflammatory plexopathy. Metastasis to the brachial plexus often has a more nodular enhancement pattern than radiation or inflammatory plexopathy.

2. Breast and lung carcinoma, as well as lymphoma, leukemia, and multiple myeloma, are among the most common to involve the brachial plexus. Head and neck cancers may also involve the brachial plexus.

3. Pain, Horner syndrome, and hand weakness are all symptoms of metastatic infiltration of the brachial plexus. Lymphedema is more commonly seen in association with post-radiation plexopathy.

4. Effacement of the interscalene fat pad is one of the earliest signs of brachial plexus involvement by Pancoast tumor.

5. Radiation and chemotherapy are the primary modalities used to treat brachial plexus metastatic infiltration, depending on the primary malignancy. Surgical resection of adjacent masses is possible; however, resection or sclerosis of the brachial plexus can be potentially devastating with loss of function of the upper extremity.

Pearls

- Metastatic infiltration of the brachial plexus may occur via hematogenous, lymphatic, or direct spread.
- In patients who have undergone treatment, it is important to differentiate post-radiation and inflammatory enhancement from metastatic infiltration.
- When differentiating metastatic infiltration from post-radiation or inflammatory plexopathy, the pattern of enhancement is key.
- Generally, metastatic infiltration demonstrates a more nodular pattern of contrast enhancement.

Suggested Readings

Castillo M. Imaging the anatomy of the brachial plexus. *AJR*. 2005;185:S196-S204.

Sureka J, Cherian RA, Alexander M, Thomas BP. MRI of brachial plexopathies. *Clin Radiol*. 2009;64:208-218.

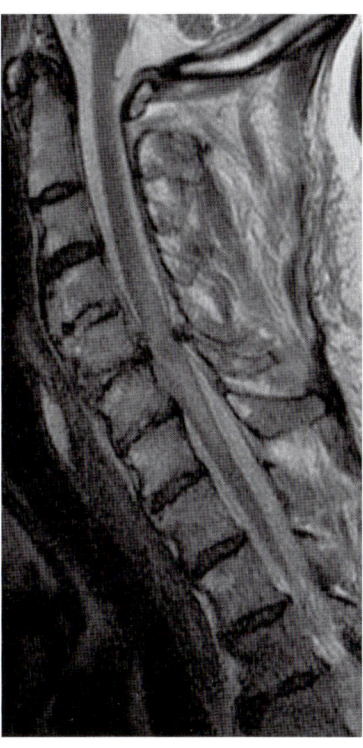

1. What is the differential diagnosis of focal T2 hyperintense signal within the spinal cord?

2. What are indications for obtaining MRI in the setting of cervical spine trauma?

3. What are the imaging findings of this abnormality?

4. What are the grades of the Frankel scale?

5. What are the treatment options?

Case ranking/difficulty:

Sagittal T2 image demonstrates cord expansion and T2 hyperintensity.

Answers

1. T2 hyperintensity within the cord is nonspecific and may represent any of the etiologies listed, making correlation with patient's history critical.

2. MRI should be considered in settings in which there is concern for ligamentous and/or cord injury.

3. The signal intensity within the cord in acute / subacute injury can vary depending on the amount of edema (T1 hypointensity, T2 hyperintensity) and hemorrhage (T1 hyperintensity, T2 hypointensity). In the acute to subacute phase, the cord is usually normal size to enlarged, but in the chronic phase, myelomalacia can develop.

4. Grade A—complete loss of function

   Grade B—intact sensation, loss of motor function

   Grade C—intact sensation, intermediate motor function (2-3/5)

   Grade D—intact sensation, near complete motor function (4/5)

   Grade E—normal function

   This Frankel classification model can be used in conjunction with imaging to help determine patient prognosis.

5. Treatment is directed at decreasing the cord edema, while treating associated injuries and/or instability. There is no known role of cord hematoma evacuation.

Pearls

- Multifactorial spinal canal stenosis is most common in the elderly.
- This leads to a higher incidence of spinal cord injuries in the setting of relatively minor trauma.
- A high index of suspicion is required to make the diagnosis, and advanced imaging with MRI is usually required.
- Focal T2 hyperintensity within the cord is nonspecific, but can be evaluated in the clinical context.

Suggested Readings

Goldberg A, Kershah SM. Advances in imaging of vertebral and spinal cord injury. *J Spinal Cord Med*. 2010;33:105-116.

ter Haar M, Naidoo SM, Govender S, Parag P, Esterhuizen TM. Acute traumatic cervical spinal cord injuries: correlating MRI findings with neurological outcome. *SA Orthop J*. 2011;10:35-41.

Neck mass

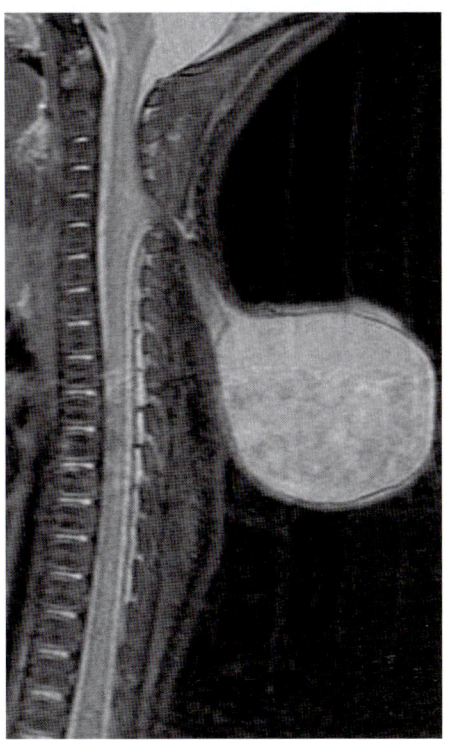

1. What is the etiology?

2. What are included in the classification scheme?

3. What are key differences between cervical and lumbosacral myelomeningoceles?

4. What should be included in the differential diagnosis of a cystic neck mass in a neonate?

5. What are the treatment options?

Case ranking/difficulty:

Category: Thecal sac

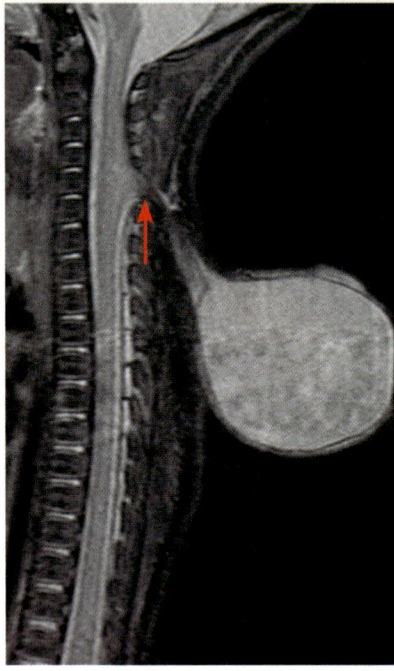

Sagittal STIR image demonstrates posterior exophytic mixed fluid intensity mass with connection to underlying thecal sac and distortion of the cord.

Answers

1. Cervical myelomeningoceles are secondary to abnormal neurulation with failure of the neural fold to fuse.

2. Cervical myelomeningoceles have been subdivided into meningoceles, meningocystoceles, and limited dorsal myeloschisis. Most recently, these have been further divided into three subgroups: cystic spinal dysraphism with a stalk, cystic spinal dysraphism without meningocele or stalk, and myelocystocele. There are few accepted universal classifications.

3. Cervical myelomeningoceles have a higher incidence of associated neurological deficits; however, there is a lower rate of association with Chiari II malformation or hydrocephalus. While preoperative imaging of the spine is usually not indicated in lumbosacral myelomeningoceles, it can be helpful in cervical lesions. While both myelomeningoceles can be associated with urological dysfunction, this can be evaluated following closure of the spinal dysraphic defect.

4. There are many etiologies for a cystic neck mass in a neonate, including cystic hygroma, cystic lymphadenopathy, myelomeningocele, branchial cleft malformation, and lymphangioma; however, myelomeningocele and hygroma are often more posteriorly distributed.

5. Initial treatment should consist of surgical resection with intradural exploration and cord untethering. There is no indication to spare the neural tissue within the defect as it has been shown to be nonfunctional. Syringosubarachnoid shunt placement may be indicated in cases of refractory syrinx; however, it is not a first-line treatment option.

Pearls

- Cervical myelomeningocele is a rare subtype of myelomeningoceles, representing less than 10% of all myelomeningoceles.
- Like classic lumbosacral myelomeningoceles, these may occur in conjunction with Chiari II malformation.
- However, they may be seen as an isolated anomaly or in association with hydrocephalus or syringomyelia.
- The pathogenesis is secondary to abnormal neurulation with incomplete fusion of the neural fold.
- Patients generally have distal, but variable, neurological deficits.
- Treatment consists of surgical resection of the meningeal sac; however, most patients achieve better neurological outcome with the addition of untethering of the cord.

Suggested Readings

Habibi Z, Nejat F, Tajik P, Kazmi SS, Kajbafzadeh AM. Cervical myelomeningocele. *Neurosurgery.* 2006;58:1168-1175.

Odebode TO, Udoffa SU, Nzeh AD. Cervical myelomeningocele and hydrocephalus without neurological deficit: a case report. *AEJSA.* 2007;2:60-62.

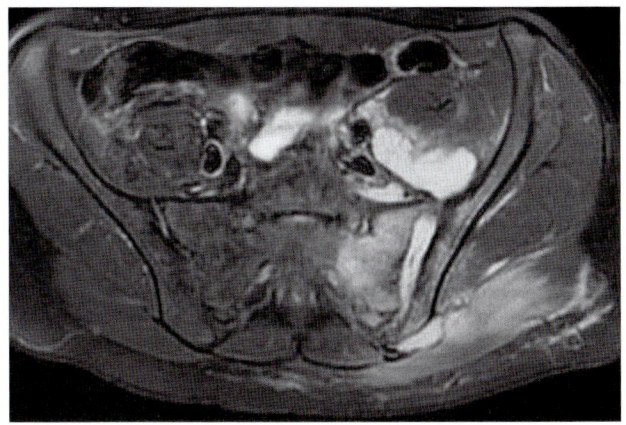 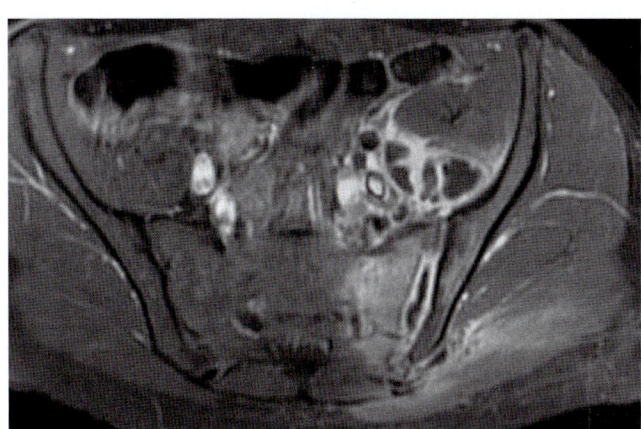

1. What should be included in the differential diagnosis?

2. What are common presenting symptoms?

3. What is the most sensitive finding on physical exam?

4. Which entities tend to have unilateral or asymmetric sacroiliac joint involvement?

5. What are the treatment options?

Case ranking/difficulty:

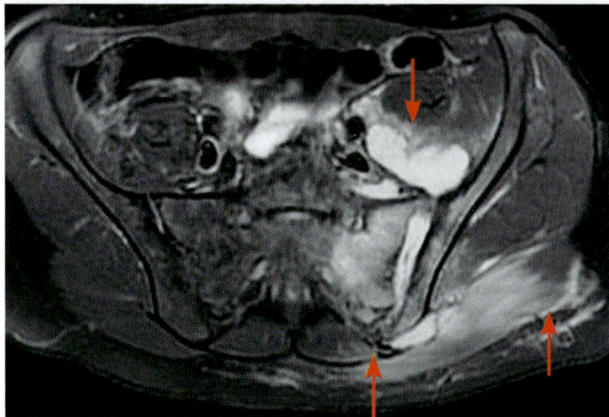

Axial T2 image demonstrates hyperintense fluid within the sacroiliac joint, extending into the pelvis, with associated marrow edema within the ilium and sacrum. There is extension into the gluteal musculature.

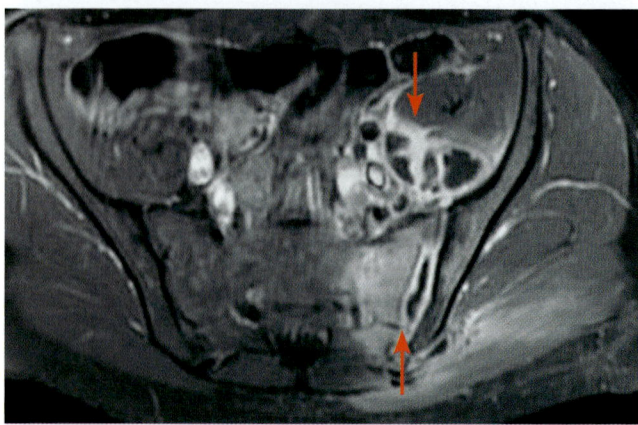

Axial T1 image following contrast administration demonstrates peripherally enhancing fluid collection within the sacroiliac joint, extending into the pelvis, with associated marrow edema within the ilium and sacrum.

Answers

1. Metastatic disease, primary bone tumor, ankylosing spondylitis, psoriatic arthritis, and infection may all involve the sacroiliac joints, either unilaterally or bilaterally.

2. Fever and limp are the predominant symptoms. Other symptoms may include back pain, lower quadrant pain, and radiculopathy.

3. The FABERE test (flexion-abduction-external rotation-extension) of the hip is usually positive for eliciting pain.

4. Unilateral or asymmetric sacroiliac involvement can be seen in Reiter syndrome, pyogenic sacroiliitis, and psoriatic arthritis. Ankylosing spondylitis is usually bilateral and symmetric with prominent ankylosis (fusion) across the sacroiliac joints.

5. Primary treatment is antibiotics with supplemental drainage of associated soft tissue abscesses and debridement. Surgical fixation is often necessary following debridement to avoid pelvic instability.

- The inferior one-third of the sacroiliac joint is lined by synovium and may have fluid; however, any fluid seen in the upper two-thirds is always abnormal.
- The most common pathogen is *Staphylococcus aureus* (up to 75% of patients) with additional isolates including *Streptococcus*, *Haemophilus influenzae*, *Escherichia coli*, and *Salmonella*.
- Imaging relies heavily on MRI for evaluation of soft tissue and osseous involvement.
- Initial treatment consists of appropriate antibiotic coverage with consideration of soft tissue abscess drainage.
- Debridement of the sacroiliac joint may be performed, if extensive bone involvement or intraspinal extension is visualized, but often leads to instability requiring surgical fusion.

Suggested Readings

Murphey MD, Wetzel LH, Bramble JM, Levine E, Simpson KM, Lindsley HB. Sacroiliitis: MR imaging findings. *Radiology*. 1991;180:239-244.

Quintana AM, Gutierrez BM, Lovillo MSC, Neth O, Santaella IO. Pyogenic sacroiliitis in children—a diagnostic challenge. *Clin Rheumatol*. 2011;30:107-113.

Pearls

- Pyogenic sacroiliitis is uncommon and often presents in patients with suppressed immune system.
- Up to 10% of patients report a prior history of trauma to the sacroiliac joint.
- It can be difficult to diagnose as the symptoms overlap with a variety of abdominal and pelvic pathologies.

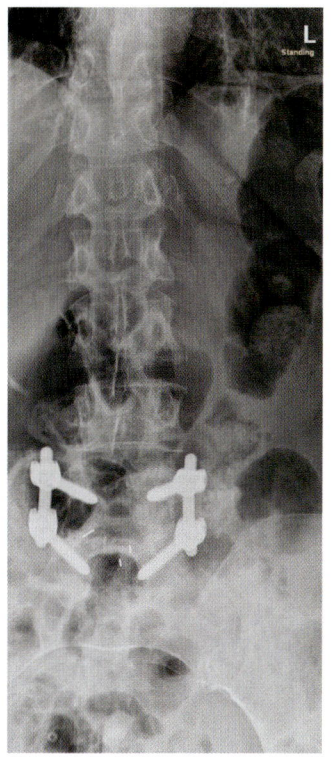 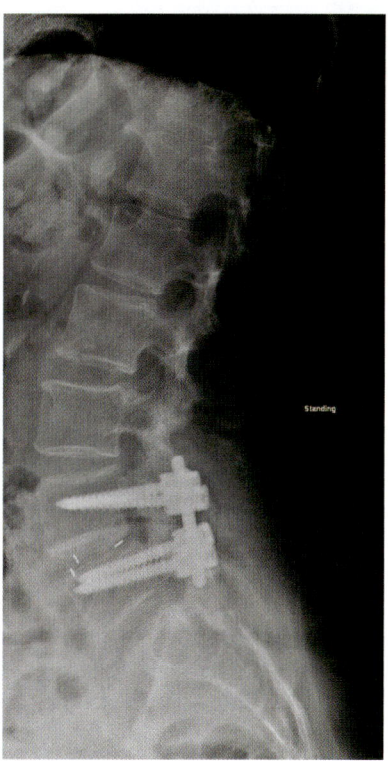

1. What is this procedure called?

2. Name some indications for this procedure?

3. Describe the major surgical steps of this procedure.

4. Which are the disadvantages of this procedure?

5. Name potential complications of this procedure.

Case ranking/difficulty: **Category:** Vertebral body

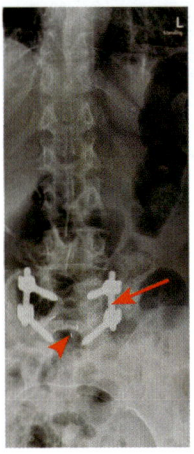
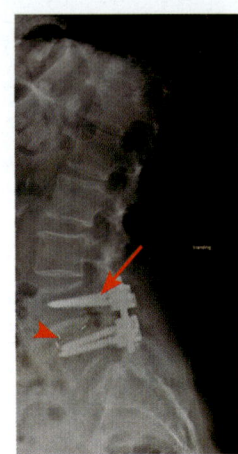

AP radiograph of the lumbar spine in a patient who was previously treated with PLIF. Note short rods (*arrow*) between cannulated pedicular screws at L4-L5 used for spinal stabilization. A synthetic cage was placed in the evacuated intervertebral disc space (*arrowhead*).

Lateral radiograph of the lumbar spine shows normal alignment of the lumbar vertebrae. L4-L5 disc has been evacuated and replaced with a synthetic cage (*arrowhead*) which restores the disc space height. Pedicular screws (*arrow*) and rods were used to stabilize the spine.

Answers

1. Posterior lumbar interbody fusion (PLIF) is a surgical procedure that involves a lumbar discectomy followed by placement of bone graft into the evacuated intervertebral disc space in order to achieve spinal fusion. It is often supplemented by simultaneous posterolateral spine fusion surgery.

2. PLIF is indicated in patients with symptomatic disc prolapse or foraminal stenosis in which previous spinal surgery has failed, in patients with significant discogenic or facet joint pain that has not responded to conservative measures, in spondylolisthesis, and in spinal instability.

3. The procedure is performed via a posterior midline incision. The erector spinae muscles are stripped off the laminae on both sides before a laminectomy is performed. The facet joints may also be undercut to provide more room for exiting nerve roots. A discectomy is then performed followed by insertion of a cage made of either allograft bone or synthetic material (PEEK or titanium) into the intervertebral disc space. Pedicle screws may be inserted in the levels above and below in order to stabilize the spine. The procedure is different from posterolateral fusion in which the bone graft is placed between the transverse processes to stimulate fusion between adjacent transverse processes.

4. PLIF has certain disadvantages. The posterior approach does not allow comprehensive evacuation of the intervertebral disc space, which decreases the surface area available for fusion. An anterior approach also allows the use of a larger spinal implant, which results in superior stabilization. The posterior approach may render surgery much more difficult in patients with spinal deformity and, rarely, the cage may retropulse into the spinal canal.

5. The main risk of the procedure is nonunion, which may require further surgery to attempt spinal fusion. Fusion rates of PLIF are, however, reported to be as high as 95%. The risk is increased in patients who have had previous spinal surgery, in multiple-level fusion surgery, in previous radiotherapy, and in obese patients. Other complications of the procedure include infection and hemorrhage. The patient's pain may not subside even when successful spine fusion has been achieved.

Pearls

- Posterior lumbar interbody fusion (PLIF) involves a lumbar discectomy followed by placement of bone graft into the evacuated intervertebral disc space in order to achieve spinal fusion.
- PLIF is indicated in patients with symptomatic disc prolapse or foraminal stenosis in which previous spinal surgery has failed, in patients with significant discogenic or facet joint pain that has not responded to conservative measures, in spondylolisthesis, and in spinal instability.
- The procedure is performed via a posterior midline incision.
- A discectomy is then performed followed by insertion of a cage made of either allograft bone or synthetic material into the intervertebral disc space.
- Pedicle screws may be inserted at the levels above and below in order to stabilize the spine.
- The main risk of the procedure is nonunion, which may require further surgery to attempt spinal fusion.
- The patient's pain may not subside even when successful spine fusion has been achieved.

Suggested Readings

Ahsan MK, Hossain MA, Sakeb N, Khan SI, Zaman N. Instrumented posterior lumbar interbody fusion (PLIF) with interbody fusion device (cage) in degenerative disc disease (DDD): 3 years outcome. *Mymensingh Med J.* 2013 Oct;22(4):798-806.

Pannell WC, Savin DD, Scott TP, Wang JC, Daubs MD. Trends in the surgical treatment of lumbar spine disease in the United States. *Spine J.* 2013 Oct 31.

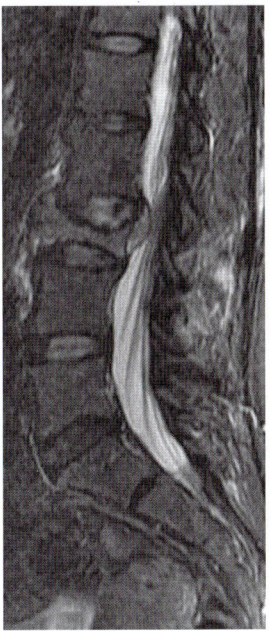 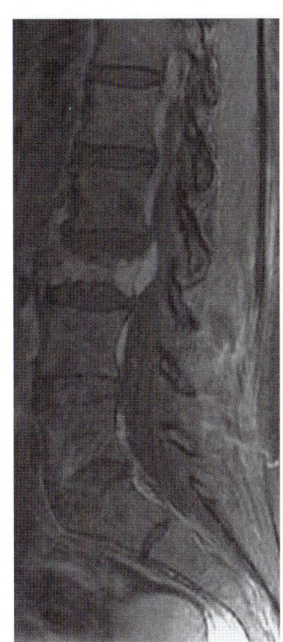

1. What should be included in the differential diagnosis?

2. What are common presenting symptoms?

3. Which location within the spine is most commonly affected?

4. What are common patterns of extension?

5. What are the treatment options?

Case ranking/difficulty:

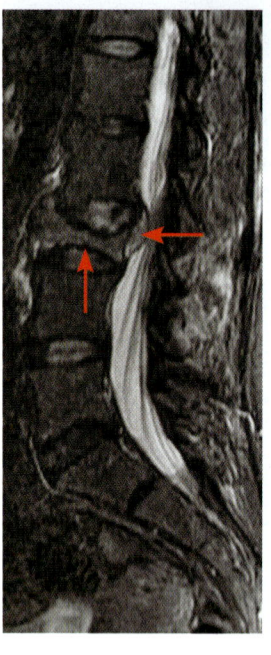

Sagittal STIR image demonstrates compression of L3 vertebral body with heterogeneous signal, and an epidural soft tissue mass.

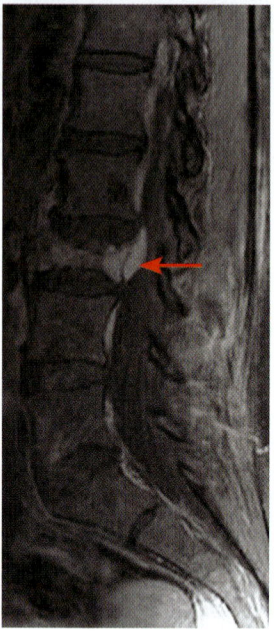

Sagittal T1 image following gadolinium administration demonstrates enhancement of the vertebral body with anterior epidural extension.

Answers

1. Potential causes of vertebral body lesions and pathologic fracture include chondrosarcoma, lymphoma, metastasis, multiple myeloma, and plasmacytoma.

2. Presenting symptoms depend on vertebral body and intraspinal extension and include pain, radiculopathy, myelopathy, and pathologic fracture.

3. 80% of spinal lesions arise in the posterior elements. Sacral lesions generally arise in the body and ala.

4. Potential patterns of extension include adjacent vertebral body, paravertebral soft tissue, epidural space, and neural foramina.

5. Surgical resection is the primary treatment, with stabilization as needed. Adjuvant radiation and chemotherapy may be used.

Pearls

- Osteosarcoma rarely occurs in the spine; however, it is the second most common primary osseous neoplasm in the spine after multiple myeloma.

- The risk factors include Paget disease and prior radiation therapy; however, these risk factors are more commonly seen in extremity osteosarcoma.
- Patients with primary spinal osteosarcoma tend to be slightly older than extremity osteosarcoma patients.
- Patients often present with pain or pathologic fracture.
- Evaluation for paravertebral soft tissue aids in making the diagnosis of pathologic fracture, rather than benign compression fracture.
- Primary treatment is surgical resection (with fixation as needed) with adjuvant radiation and chemotherapy.

Suggested Readings

Makhdoomi R, Nayil K, Ramzan A, Baba K, Bhat S, Sheikh S. Primary osteosarcoma of the cervical spine: a case report and literature review. *Neurosurg Q*. 2010;20:250-252.

Schwab J, Gasbarrini A, Bandiera S, et al. Osteosarcoma of the mobile spine. *Spine*. 2012;37:E381-E386.

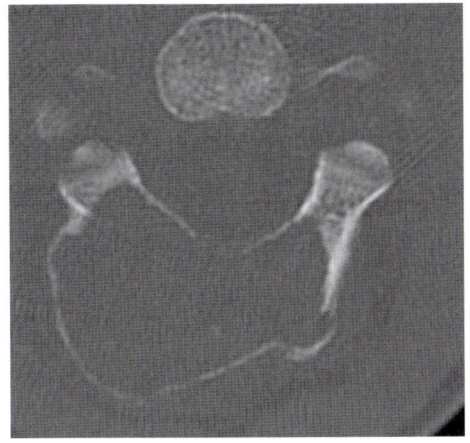 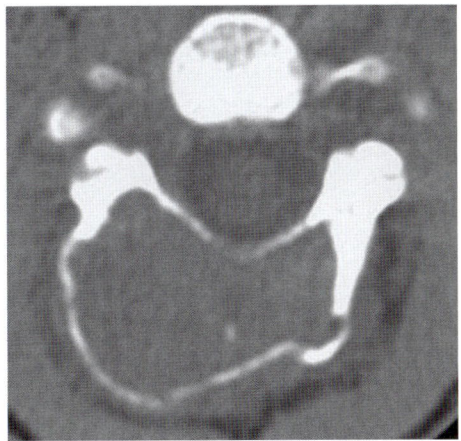 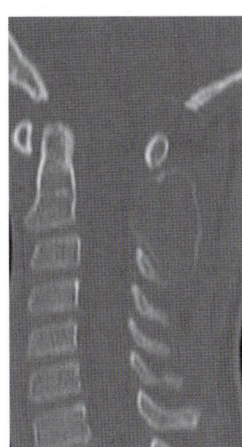

1. This abnormality can be associated with which other bone lesions?

2. What parts of the vertebral body can be involved?

3. What are common presenting symptoms?

4. What is the classic imaging appearance?

5. What are the treatment options?

Case ranking/difficulty:

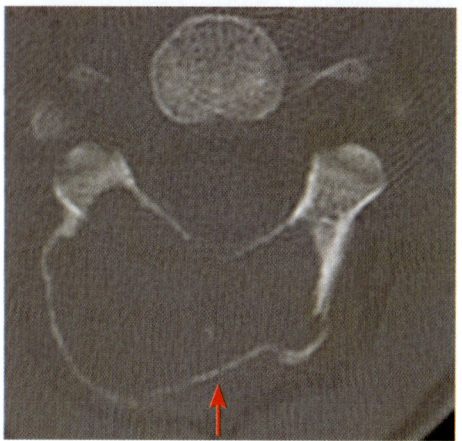

Axial CT image in bone windows demonstrates expansile and lucent lesion involving the bilateral laminae and spinous process.

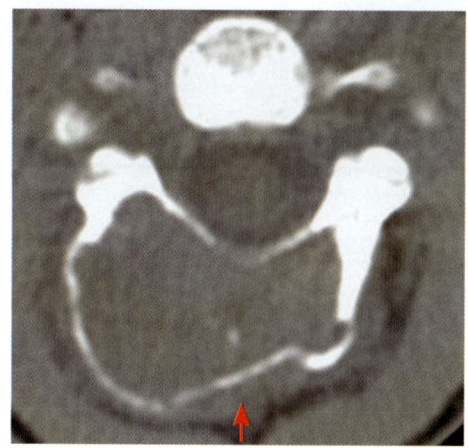

Axial CT image in soft tissue windows demonstrates expansile and lucent lesion involving the bilateral laminae and spinous process.

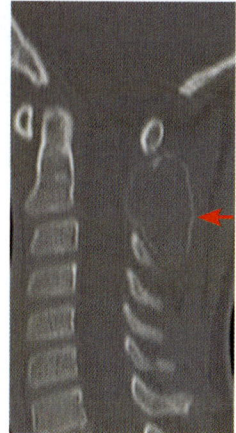

Sagittal CT image demonstrates expansile and lucent lesion involving the C2 spinous process.

Answers

1. Aneurysmal bone cyst is classified as primary if not associated with another lesion and secondary if associated with another lesion, such as osteoblastoma, telangiectatic osteosarcoma, giant cell tumor, or chondroblastoma.

2. Aneurysmal bone cyst can affect any part of the vertebral body.

3. The most common presenting symptom is pain; others include palpable mass, scoliosis/kyphosis, myelopathy, and radiculopathy. Depending on location and size, aneurysmal bone cyst can present with any of these symptoms.

4. Classically isolated aneurysmal bone cyst presents as a lucent expansile lesion without significant internal matrix. The lesion may be multiloculated with fluid-fluid levels depending on previous hemorrhage.

5. Surgical excision is the treatment of choice, but given the vascular nature of the lesions this is sometimes preceded by arterial embolization. In cases where complete surgical excision is not possible, curettage and/or radiotherapy may be employed.

Pearls

- Aneurysmal bone cysts (ABC) are benign osseous lesions of uncertain etiology.
- They represent approximately 1% of primary bone tumors, and up to 20% of ABC are found in the spine.
- ABC are classified as primary if they are isolated lesions, or secondary if another lesion is found in association with the ABC.
- ABC involve all spinal levels, as well as multiple parts of the vertebral column.
- They generally appear as expansile lucent lesions on radiographs or CT with complex signal on MRI and possible fluid-fluid levels, given the predilection for superimposed hemorrhage.

Suggested Readings

Boriani S, De Iure F, Campanacci L, et al. Aneurysmal bone cyst of the mobile spine: report on 41 cases. *Spine*. 2001;26:27-35.

Papagelopoulus PJ, Currier BL, Shaughnessy WJ, et al. Aneurysmal bone cyst of the spine: management and outcome. *Spine*. 1998;23:621-628.

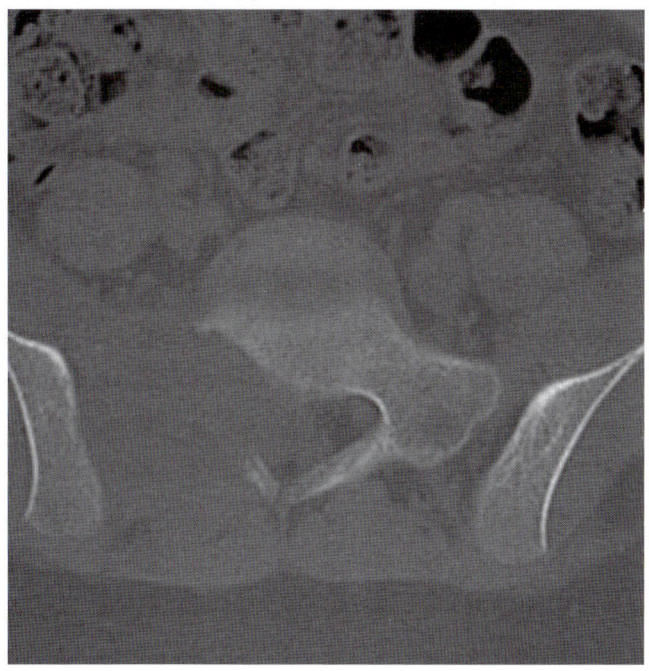 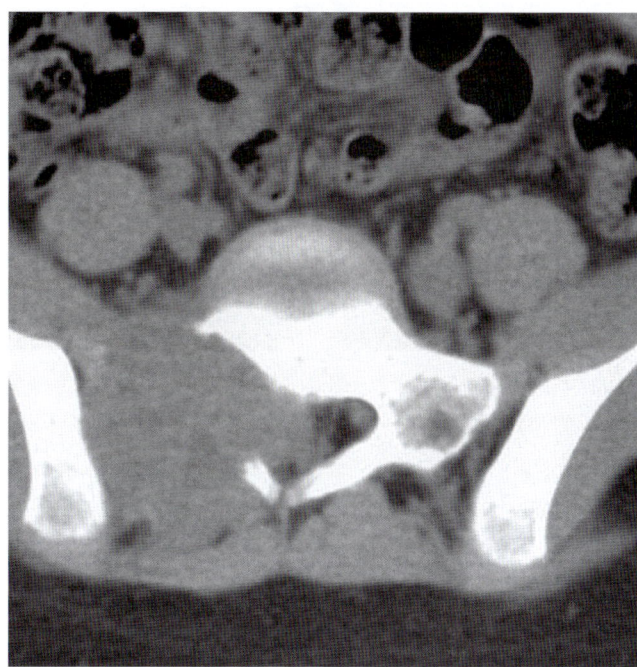

1. What should be included in the differential diagnosis?

2. What other lesions can be seen in conjunction with this abnormality?

3. What are common presenting symptoms?

4. What portion of the spine is most commonly affected?

5. What are the treatment options?

Case ranking/difficulty:

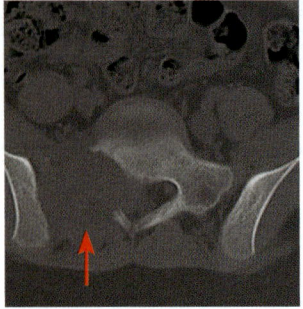

Axial CT image in bone windows demonstrates erosion of right S1 vertebral body and lamina with extension to the sacroiliac joint.

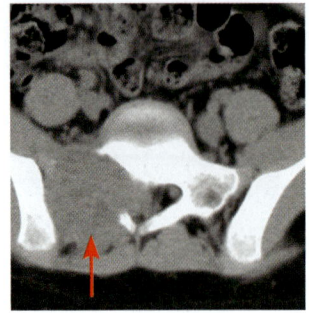

Axial CT image in soft tissue window demonstrates soft tissue mass without internal matrix or calcification. Mass extends into the spinal canal and displaces the thecal sac and traversing nerve root in the lateral recess.

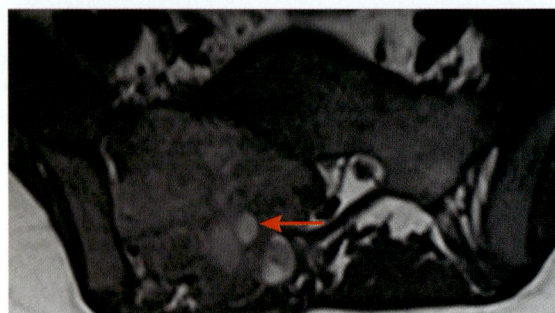

Axial T1 image demonstrates multiple loculations with focal areas of spontaneous T1 hyperintensity, consistent with blood products.

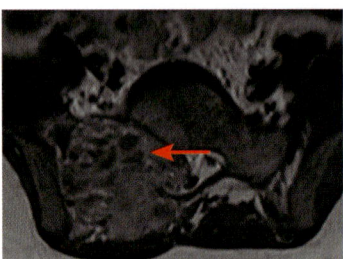
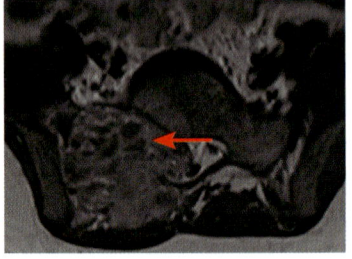

Axial T1 post-contrast image demonstrates enhancement of the solid septae within the mass.

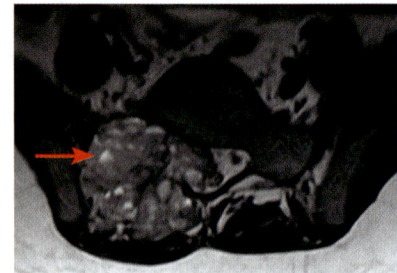

Axial T2 image demonstrates multiple areas of fluid intensity, consistent with cysts, interspersed between low T2 septae.

Answers

1. The differential of lytic expansile osseous lesions include aneurysmal bone cyst, lytic metastasis, telangiectatic osteosarcoma, and unicameral bone cyst. In skeletally mature patients, giant cell tumor and chondrosarcoma should also be considered. Chordoma should be included, but is classically more midline in location.

2. Secondary aneurysmal bone cyst can be seen in conjunction with chondroblastoma, giant cell tumor, osteoblastoma, and telangiectatic osteosarcoma.

3. Pain is the most common presenting symptoms; others include palpable mass, myelopathy, radiculopathy, and scoliosis.

4. Thoracic and lumbar spine account for approximately two-thirds of cases. The sacrum is the least likely location (approximately 10%).

5. Embolization and resection are the primary treatment options with fixation as needed to maintain stability. Curettage and packing may also be employed. Conservative management may be considered as the lesions generally stop growing after childhood and there is no risk of malignant degeneration.

Pearls

- Aneurysmal bone cysts only represent approximately 1% of all primary bone tumors; however, one-fifth of the lesions are found within the spine.
- Classification of lesions is dependent on the absence/presence of an associated lesion (primary/secondary).
- The classic imaging appearance is an expansile lytic lesion that demonstrates lobulation and internal fluid-fluid levels.
- Within the spine, any portion of the spinal column may be involved.
- Treatment is geared at resection with fusion as needed for stability.

Suggested Readings

Boriani S, De Iure F, Campanacci L, et al. Aneurysmal bone cyst of the mobile spine: report on 41 cases. *Spine*. 2001;26:27-35.

Papagelopoulus PJ, Currier BL, Shaughnessy WJ, et al. Aneurysmal bone cyst of the spine: management and outcome. *Spine*. 1998;23:621-628.

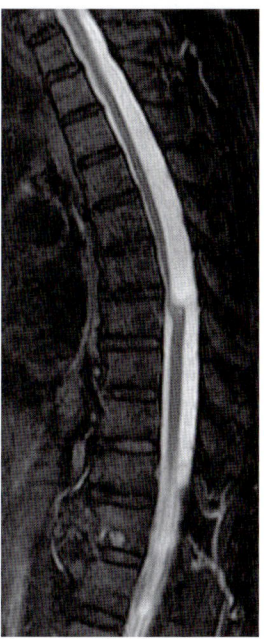 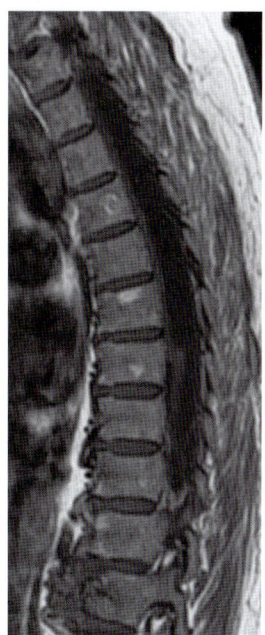

1. In which location may these lesions occur?

2. What should be included in the differential diagnosis?

3. What are the etiologies?

4. What is included in the classification scheme?

5. What are the treatment options?

Case ranking/difficulty:

Category: Spinal canal

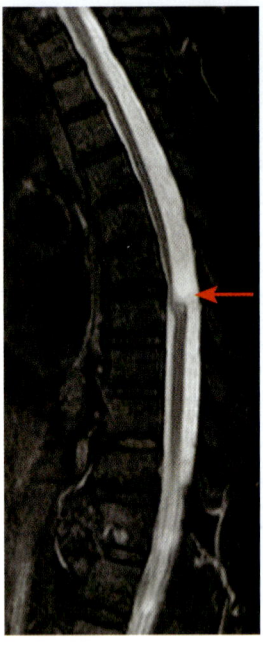

Sagittal T2 image demonstrates fluid intensity mass in the dorsal spinal canal with mass effect on and deformity of the cord.

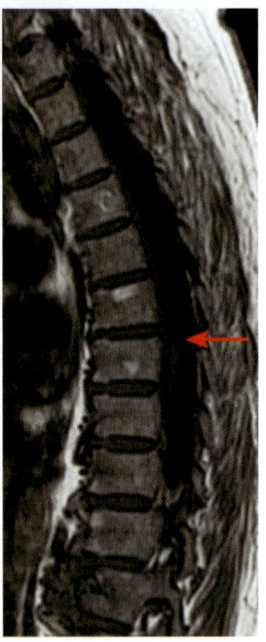

Sagittal T1 image demonstrates fluid intensity mass in the dorsal spinal canal with mass effect on and deformity of the cord.

Answers

1. Intracranial arachnoid cysts are far more common than spinal arachnoid cysts. Within the spine, arachnoid cysts may occur within the intradural extramedullary or extradural compartments. Fluid collections within the foramina are nerve sheath cysts; however, an intraspinal lesion may extend through a foramen.

2. Transdural spinal cord herniation occurs secondary to a dural tear, usually at the level of a disc herniation. Facet synovial cyst tends to be more localized at the level of the facet joint. Dural ectasia also presents with vertebral body remodeling; however, this fluid space freely communicates with the thecal sac.

3. Arachnoid cyst is divided into primary and secondary. Primary arachnoid cyst is felt to arise from a congenital diverticulum or dural defect. Secondary arachnoid cysts are secondary to inflammatory changes or dural tear.

4. The Nabors classification system:

   Type 1A: Extradural arachnoid cyst

   Type 1B: Sacral meningocele

   Type 2: Tarlov cyst

   Type 2: Spinal nerve root diverticulum

   Type 3: Intradural arachnoid cyst

5. Complete resection is the preferred treatment; however, if this is not feasible, cyst fenestration or marsupialization or shunt placement can be performed.

Pearls

- Arachnoid cysts are uncommon lesions that may occur within the extradural or intradural extramedullary spaces.
- They are usually located dorsal to the cord and often extend over two to four vertebral segments.
- They are most common within the thoracic spine and generally follow cerebrospinal fluid signal on all MRI sequences. Heavily T2-weighted sequences can be helpful in evaluation.
- Filling of arachnoid cysts with contrast following myelography is variable but usually delayed.

Suggested Readings

Hoy RJ, Faulder KC. Spinal arachnoid cysts. *Aust Radiol.* 1968;12:344-354.

Kendall BE, Valentine AR, Keis B. Spinal arachnoid cysts: clinical and radiological correlation with prognosis. *Neuroradiology.* 1982;22:225-234.

Kumar A, Sakia R, Singh K, Sharma V. Spinal arachnoid cyst. *J Clin Neuroscience.* 2011;18:1189-1192.

Nakagawa A, Kusaka Y, Jokura H, Shirane R, Tominaga T. Usefulness of constructive interference in steady state (CISS) imaging for the diagnosis and treatment of a large extradural spinal arachnoid cyst. *Minim Invasive Neurosurg.* 2004;47:369-372.

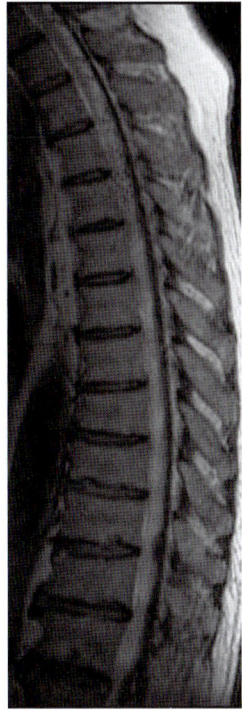 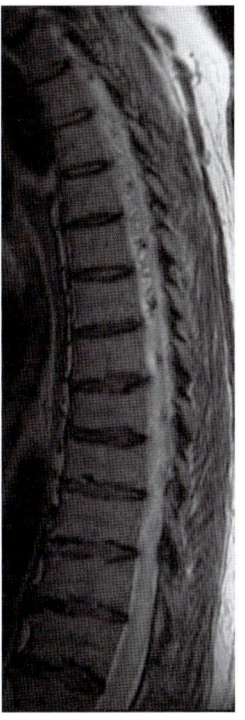 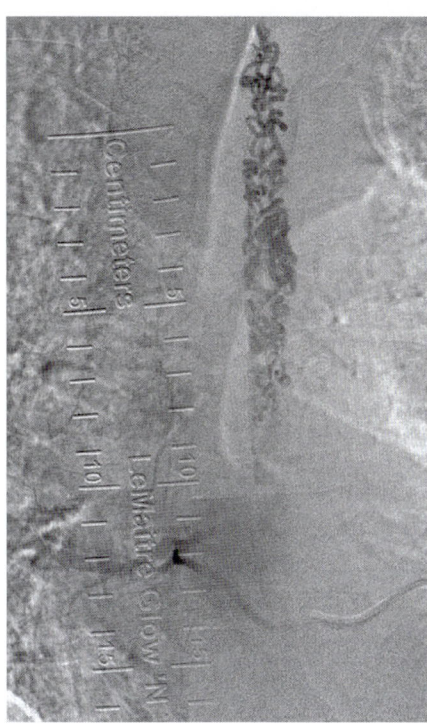

1. What should be included in the differential diagnosis?

2. What are common presenting symptoms?

3. What are the most helpful findings for differentiating this abnormality from cord infarction?

4. What is the classification system?

5. What are the treatment options?

Case ranking/difficulty: 🐛🐛

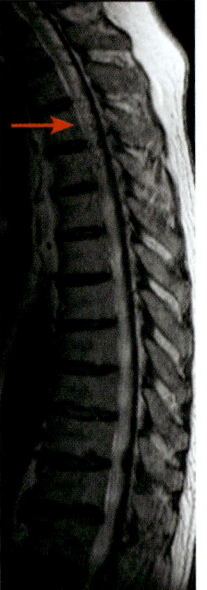

Sagittal T2 image demonstrates multiple flow voids in the thecal sac.

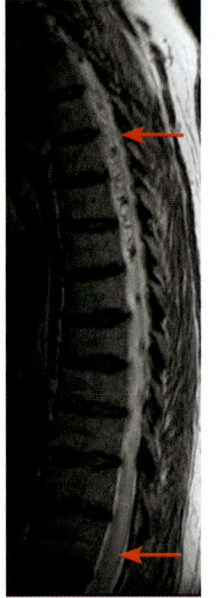

Parasagittal T2 image demonstrates multiple flow voids surrounding the thoracic cord and hyperintensity and enlargement of the distal cord.

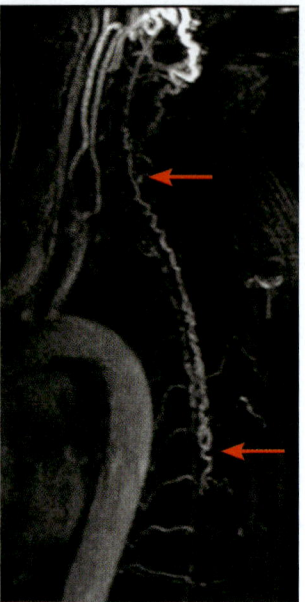

Sagittal oblique contrast enhanced MRA image demonstrates tangle of abnormal vessels overlying the thecal sac.

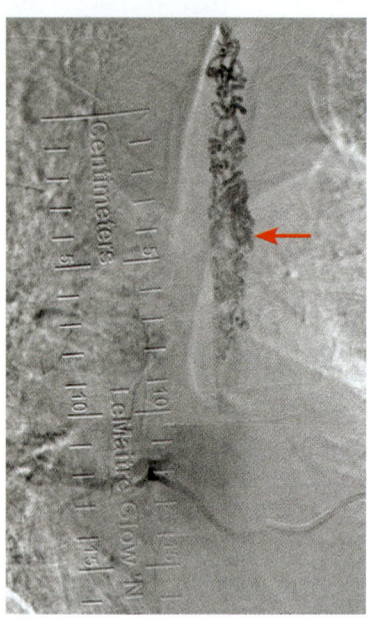

AP image from a selective right T6 intercostal artery injection demonstrates a tangle of vessels.

Answers

1. Linear areas of signal heterogeneity within the cerebrospinal fluid could be caused by dural arteriovenous fistula, arteriovenous malformation, cerebrospinal fluid pulsation artifact, nerve roots, and nerve sheath tumors.

2. The most common presentation is slowly progressive lower extremity weakness; other symptoms include back pain, impotence, bowel and bladder incontinence, and subarachnoid hemorrhage. Hemorrhage is unusual.

3. Both dural arteriovenous fistula and cord infarction can present with cord T2 hyperintensity and enhancement. Spinal cord infarction should have an acute presentation and is less likely to have associated dilated pial veins.

4. Type 1: Dural arteriovenous malformation

   Type 2: Intramedullary glomus type arteriovenous malformation

   Type 3: Juvenile type arteriovenous malformation

   Type 4: Intradural extramedullary/perimedullary arteriovenous fistula

5. Treatment options consist of onyx embolization and surgical resection. Polyvinyl alcohol and Gelfoam embolization are contraindicated given the high rate of recanalization.

Pearls

- Dural arteriovenous fistulas are the most common spinal vascular malformation and are classified as Type 1.
- Patients are generally middle aged to elderly males who present with progressive lower extremity weakness, though to originate from myelopathic changes from venous hypertension.
- These lesions most often occur between the T5 and L3 levels.
- Imaging workup usually consists of MRI, including dynamic angiography if possible.
- Digital subtraction angiography can be used to refine delineation of feeding vessels, as well as perform embolization of lesions.
- Surgical resection or obliteration may also be required.

Suggested Readings

Da Costa L, Dehdashti AR, TerBrugge KG. Spinal cord vascular shunts: spinal cord vascular malformations and dural arteriovenous fistulas. *Neurosurg Focus*. 2009;26:E6.

Muralidharan R, Saladino A, Lanzino G, Atkinson JL, Rabinstein AA. The clinical and radiological presentation of spinal dural arteriovenous fistula. *Spine*. 2011;36:E1641-1647.

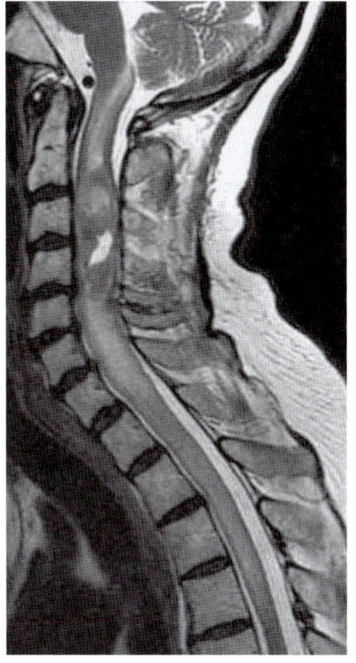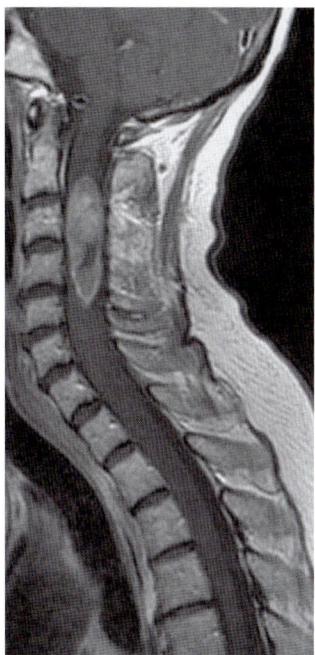

1. What should be included in the differential diagnosis?

2. What are common presenting symptoms?

3. What location within the spinal cord is most commonly affected?

4. What are common imaging appearances?

5. What are the treatment options?

Case ranking/difficulty:

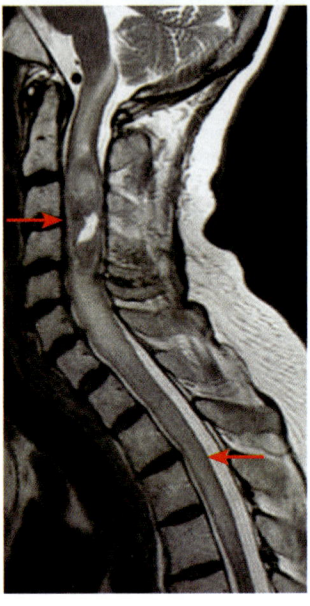

Sagittal T2 image demonstrates heterogeneous, centrally necrotic intramedullary mass extending from C2 to C5 with surrounding T2 hyperintensity, consistent with edema.

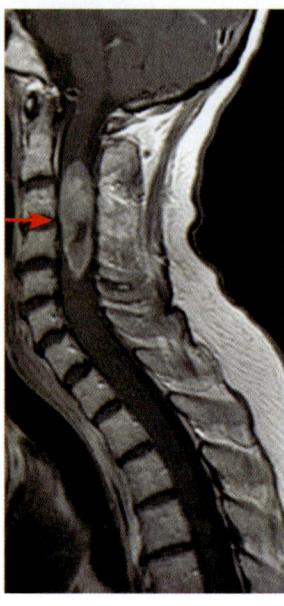

Sagittal T1 image following gadolinium administration demonstrates peripheral and nodular enhancement of the intramedullary lesion.

Answers

1. An enhancing intramedullary lesion with surrounding vasogenic edema can represent astrocytoma, ependymoma, metastasis, demyelinating disease, and hemangioblastoma. As in the brain, metastases often have edema out of proportion to lesion size.

2. Potential presenting symptoms include pain, myelopathy, bowel and bladder dysfunction, paraparesis, and Brown-Sequard syndrome.

3. The cervical cord is most commonly affected, followed by thoracic cord and then conus.

4. Spinal cord metastases are generally solitary lesions that have edema greater than would be expected for lesion size. These lesions tend to be rapidly progressive and are usually seen in patients with diffuse metastatic disease.

5. Treatment options can include conservative management, analgesia, radiation, chemotherapy, and surgical resection, depending on patient symptomatology and overall prognosis.

Pearls

- While spinal cord metastases are rare, they should be considered in the differential of a cord lesion in a patient with a primary malignancy.

- The most common malignancies to metastasize to the spinal cord are lung and breast, but any primary may.
- Patients usually present with pain and weakness, which may be insidious or rapid in onset.
- There are no imaging features that clearly define a metastatic lesion, and biopsy is often required for diagnosis.
- Metastases generally enhance and often have edema out of proportion to lesion size.
- Spinal cord metastases affect the cervical spine most commonly and are usually solitary, although they can be seen in conjunction with other sites of metastatic disease.
- Treatment is geared at the primary malignancy with adjunct steroids to reduce cord edema.
- Surgical resection and radiotherapy may be considered in some patients to alleviate symptoms.
- Overall survival following diagnosis is poor, generally less than 1 year.

Suggested Readings

Do-Dai DD, Brooks MK, Goldkamp A, Erbay S, Bhadelia RA. Magnetic resonance imaging of intramedullary spinal cord lesions: a pictorial review. *Curr Probl Diagn Radiol.* 2010;39:160-185.

Rogers SR, Phalke VV, Anderson J, Riccelli LP, Gonda S, Pollock JM. HEALSME: Differential diagnosis for intramedullary spinal cord lesions. *Neurographics.* 2012;2:13-26.

Motor cycle collision with left arm paralysis

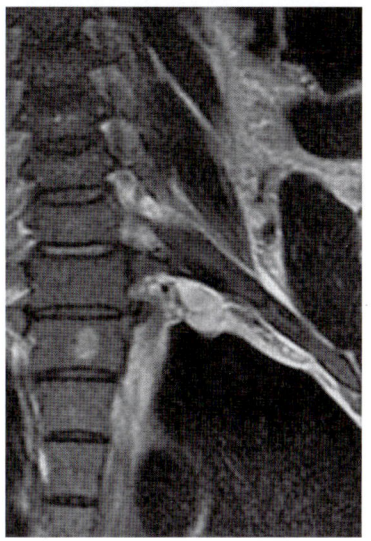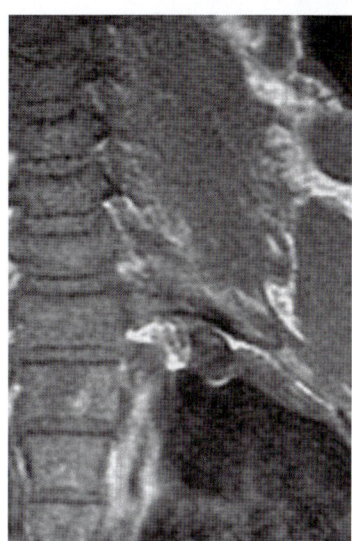

1. What are common presenting symptoms?

2. What are etiologies of this abnormality?

3. What forms the brachial plexus?

4. What are associated abnormalities?

5. What are the treatment options?

Case ranking/difficulty: **Category:** Nerve roots/Nerve plexus/Peripheral nerves

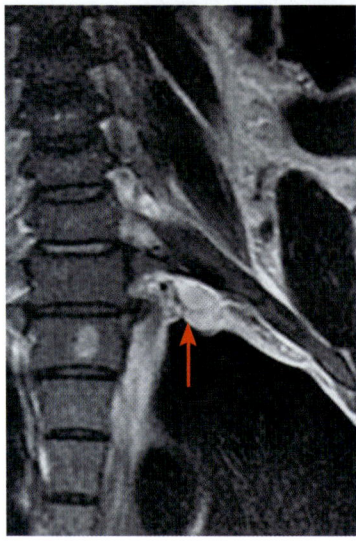

Coronal T2 image demonstrates fluid intensity collections arising from the left T1 nerve root.

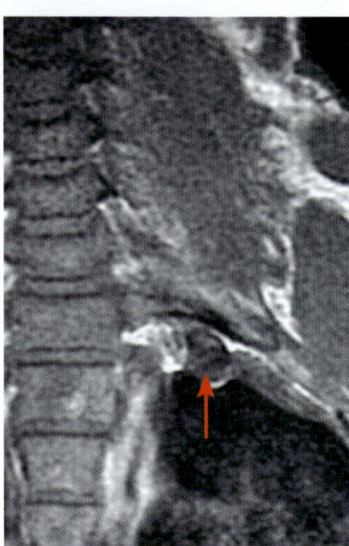

Coronal T1 image demonstrates fluid intensity collections arising from the left T1 nerve root.

Answers

1. The brachial plexus has both motor and sensory components and both can be affected by injury. Diaphragmatic paralysis can occur from injuries involving the C3, C4, and C5 nerve roots.

2. Potential mechanisms of brachial plexus abnormalities include neuropraxia, avulsion, infiltration, and compression.

3. During the fifth to sixth week of gestation, the ventral rami of C5 to T1 form the brachial plexus.

4. Associated injuries can include spinal cord injury. Diaphragmatic paralysis results from injury to the C3-C5 nerve roots. Scapular winging results from injury to C5 to C7. Horner syndrome results from injury to infraclavicular plexus.

5. For neuropraxic injuries, treatment consists of physical therapy. If there is a brachial plexus avulsion, this can be treated with either primary reanastomosis and/or nerve grafting depending on the gap distance. Prolonged immobilization should be avoided because it can lead to a frozen joint.

Pearls

- Brachial plexopathy symptoms tend to be vague and nonspecific.
- Cases of neuropraxic (stretching) injuries and avulsions tend to present with motor symptoms.
- Pseudomeningoceles develop in approximately 80% of traumatic avulsions and result from a tear in the meningeal sheath with extravasation of cerebrospinal fluid.
- A radiologist should attempt to define the gap distance between the avulsed nerve segments, which can be important information for a surgeon planning potential reanastomosis.
- In the neonatal population, consider brachial plexus injuries related to delivery, which can result in Erb palsy (injury to C5 and C6) or Klumpke palsy (injury to C8 and T1).

Suggested Readings

Castillo M. Imaging the anatomy of the brachial plexus: review and self-assessment module. *AJR.* 2005;185:S196-S204.

Sureka J, Cherian RA, Alexander M, Thomas BP. MRI of brachial plexopathies. *Clin Radiol.* 2009;64:208-218.

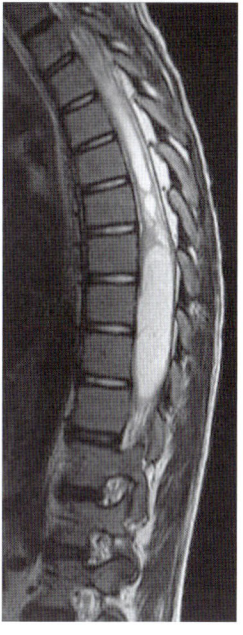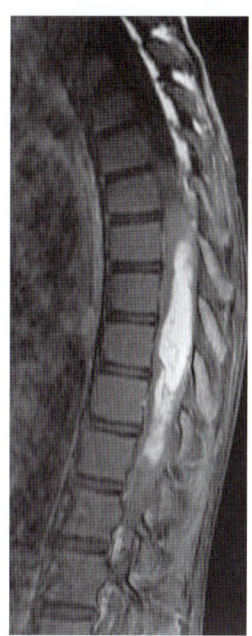

1. What should be included in the differential diagnosis?

2. What are common presenting symptoms?

3. What are associated complications?

4. What are 5-year survival rates?

5. What are the treatment options?

Case ranking/difficulty: 🦠🦠   **Category:** Spinal cord

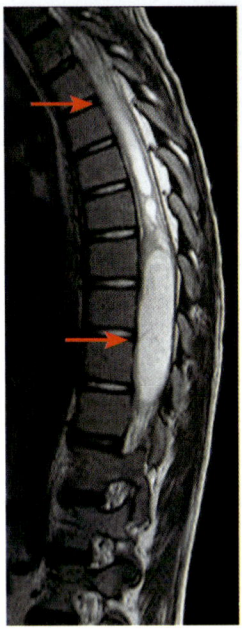

Sagittal T2 image demonstrates irregular fluid collection within the thoracic cord, which is expanded.

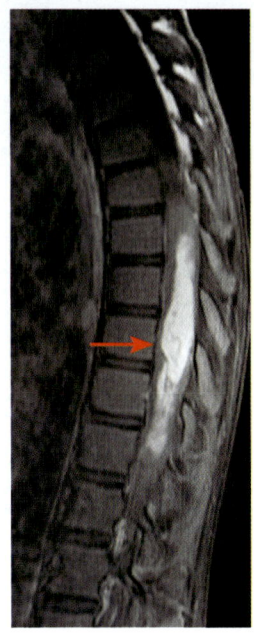

Sagittal T1 image following gadolinium administration demonstrates intramedullary enhancing mass.

Answers

1. The differential for multisegment T2 hyperintensity within the cord includes astrocytoma, ependymoma, and syringomyelia. Differentiating syrinx from underlying tumor is an important role for contrast administration in spinal imaging.

2. The symptoms of holocord astrocytoma are nonspecific and include pain, progressive scoliosis, myelopathy, radiculopathy, and dysesthesia.

3. Potential complications of holocord astrocytoma include permanent neurological deficit, disseminated metastatic disease, osseous remodeling of the spinal canal, and scoliosis.

4. For WHO grade I astrocytoma, the 5-year survival is approximately 80%, in contrast to the higher-grade tumors, which average 30%.

5. Microsurgical resection is often employed for debulking followed by chemotherapy. However, radiation therapy may be used in refractory cases. Given their slow-growing nature, conservative management might be appropriate.

Pearls

- Astrocytoma is the most common spinal cord tumor in children with the majority being low grade (WHO grade I and II).
- Holocord astrocytomas are less common and usually demonstrate large cystic components.
- Presenting symptoms are usually nonspecific and include progressive scoliosis, pain, and myelopathy.
- Once the diagnosis is confirmed, treatment can consist of chemotherapy with consideration of surgical resection and radiotherapy.
- Large cysts associated with holocord astrocytoma can mimic syrinx; this is the reason to give contrast to identify enhancing tumor.

Suggested Readings

Merchant TE, Kiehna EN, Thompson SJ, Heideman RL, Sanford RA, Kun LE. Pediatric low-grade and ependymal spinal cord tumors. *Pediatr Neurosurg*. 2000;32:30-36.

Schittenhelm J, Ebner FH, Tatagiba M, et al. Holocord pilocytic astrocytoma—case report and review of the literature. *Clin Neurol and Neurosurg*. 2009;111:203-207.

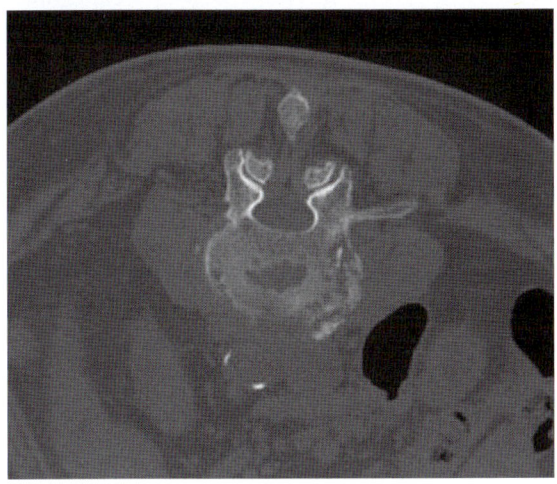 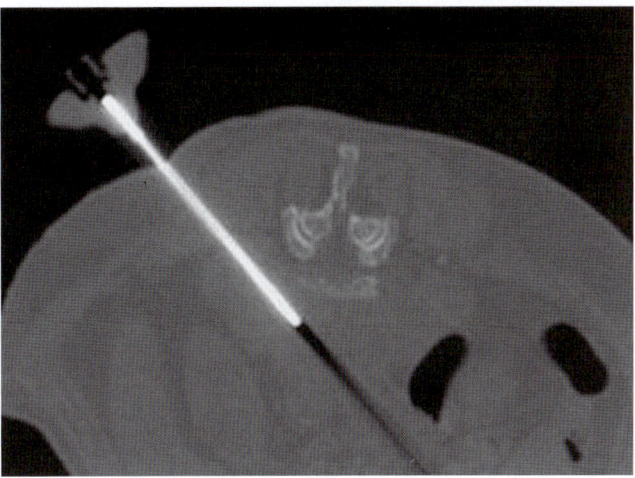

1. What is this procedure called?

2. Which approaches are commonly used?

3. Why is this procedure performed?

4. What is the diagnostic yield of this procedure?

5. How can the diagnostic yield of this procedure be improved?

Case ranking/difficulty:

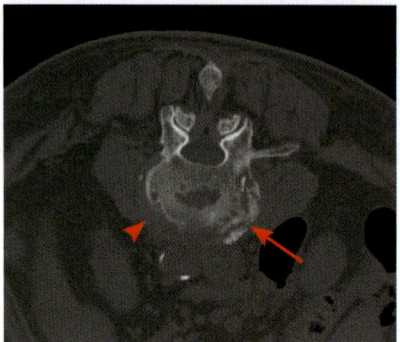

Axial CT image at the level of L3-L4 intervertebral disc. There are erosive endplate changes (*arrow*) and a small paravertebral collection (*arrow*). Previous MRI of the lumbar spine showed probable spondylodiscitis at L3-L4.

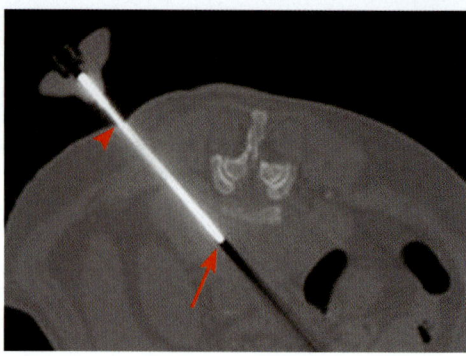

CT-guided biopsy of L3-L4 intervertebral disc using a posterolateral approach (*arrowhead*). The tip of the needle was advanced into the intervertebral disc (*arrow*) before three core samples were obtained.

Answers

1. Spondylodiscitis commonly affects elderly and immunocompromised patients and the clinical manifestations are nonspecific often leading to a delay in the diagnosis.

2. Two approaches, namely the transpedicular and posterolateral approaches, are commonly used and one should aim to include both subchondral bone and disc material in the biopsy track. The procedure is performed under either fluoroscopic or CT guidance. CT shows the needle position better and is generally considered to be a safer option. In some institutions, percutaneous disc aspiration and biopsy for suspected spondylodiscitis has become a routine procedure.

3. Although MR imaging is quite sensitive and specific to diagnose spondylodiscitis, it has certain limitations. Early stages of spondylodiscitis are notoriously difficult to differentiate from Modic type 1 changes. Other differential diagnoses, particularly in early stages, include dialysis-related disc changes, seronegative spondyloarthropathy, amyloidosis, and crystal deposition disease.

4. Microorganism are, however, only cultivated in about 57% of cases. Reasons for a negative culture include the initiation of antibiotic treatment prior to biopsy, insufficient number of microorganisms in the specimen, and the absence of living infectious agents within the sampled tissue.

5. When the biopsy tract includes the subchondral bone, the diagnostic yield is increased substantially. This may be explained by the fact that discitis secondary to hematogenous spread starts in the subchondral part of

the vertebra before spreading to the disc. Sampling of paravertebral abscesses is often negative as the fluid aspirated is usually sterile. Even when the diagnosis of spondylodiscitis is made on imaging, a microbiologic diagnosis is desirable as this helps target antibiotic therapy according to drug sensitivities. Biopsy also provides a sample for histopathological assessment. Histology may confirm spondylodiscitis even when no specific infectious agent is isolated on microbiology and a combination of the two is therefore the optimum.

Pearls

- Spondylodiscitis commonly affects elderly and immunocompromised patients.
- Biopsy should be performed before initializing antibiotic treatment.
- Two approaches namely the transpedicular and posterolateral approaches are commonly used and one should aim to include both subchondral bone and disc material in the biopsy track.

Suggested Readings

Michel SC, Pfirrmann CW, Boos N, Hodler J. CT-guided core biopsy of subchondral bone and intervertebral space in suspected spondylodiskitis. *AJR Am J Roentgenol.* 2006 Apr;186(4):977-980.

Phadke DM, Lucas DR, Madan S. Fine-needle aspiration biopsy of vertebral and intervertebral disc lesions: specimen adequacy, diagnostic utility, and pitfalls. *Arch Pathol Lab Med.* 2001 Nov;125(11):1463-1468.

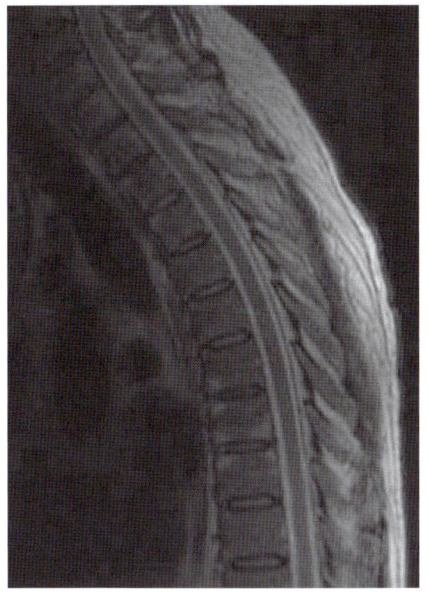 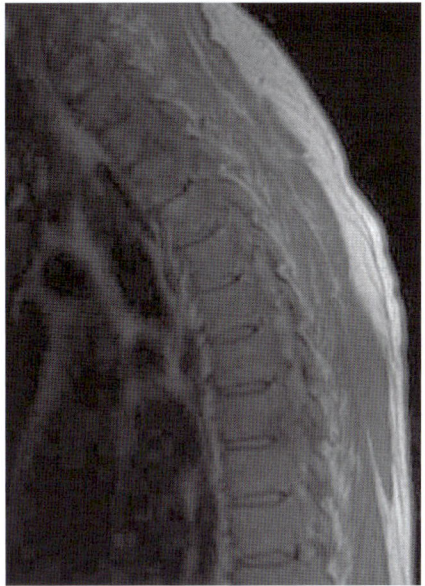 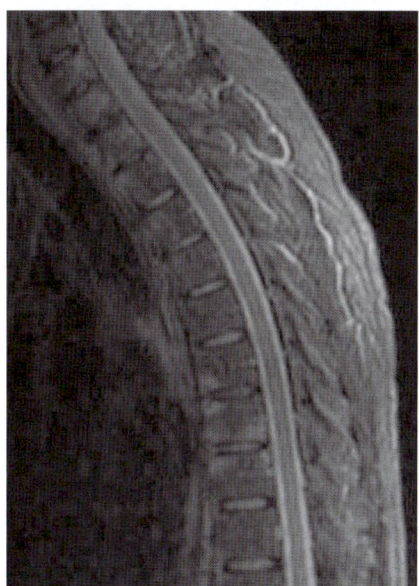

1. What is the most likely diagnosis?

2. Which site is typically affected?

3. Which part of the spinal column is typically affected?

4. Which imaging modality best images this condition?

5. Why should these lesions not be overlooked?

Case ranking/difficulty: **Category:** Vertebral body

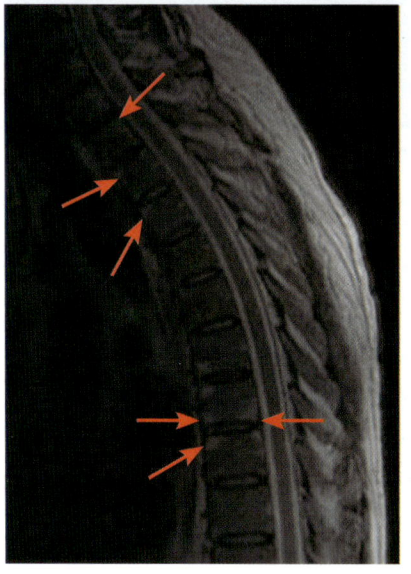

Sagittal T2-weighted sequence of the thoracic spine. There are multiple sharply margined triangular T2 hyperintense "corner" abnormalities (*arrows*). No associated osteophyte formation or Schmorl nodes are seen.

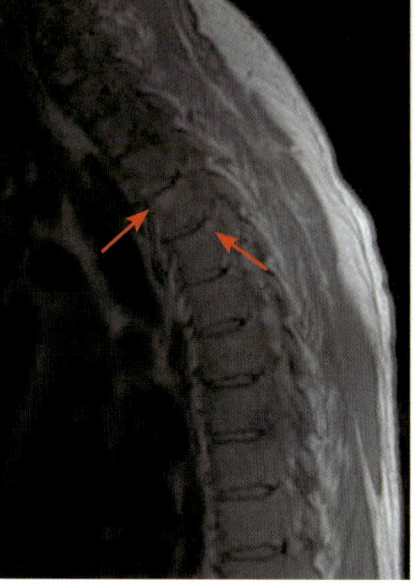

Sagittal T1-weighted sequence of the thoracic spine shows focal areas of T1 hyperintensities (*arrows*), which correspond to the abnormalities seen on the T2 sequence. This represents focal fatty marrow due to chronic inflammation.

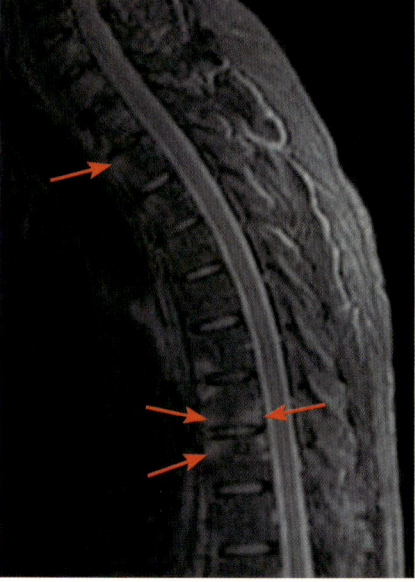

Sagittal STIR sequence demonstrates hyperintense vertebral corners (*arrows*) affecting multiple thoracic vertebrae.

Answers

1. Romanus lesions are early spinal imaging findings in ankylosing spondylitis. The specificity and positive predictive value (PPV) of Romanus lesions are 96% and 92%, respectively.

2. They characteristically affect the site of attachment of the annulus fibrosus fibers to the vertebral endplate. As the discovertebral junction is an enthesis, anterior and posterior spondylitis are effectively a form of enthesitis.

3. The "corner sign" in ankylosing spondylitis is frequently seen at the thoracolumbar junction as opposed to degenerative corner lesions, which are more common in the lumbar spine.

4. MRI is more sensitive compared to radiography and can detect changes in ankylosing spondylitis much earlier. The *MR corner sign* refers to a sharply margined triangular or less frequently quadrant-shaped nonerosive corner abnormality, which is not associated with osteophyte formation or Schmorl nodes. The most frequent pattern of signal intensity in these lesions corresponds to Modic type 2 changes. Romanus lesions are often seen as focal T1 hyperintensities secondary to focal fatty marrow due to chronic inflammation. The "corners" appear hyperintense on both STIR and T2-weighted sequences.

5. The sign should not be overlooked as it raises the possibility of ankylosing spondylitis, which should therefore be further evaluated.

Pearls

- Romanus lesions are early spinal imaging findings in ankylosing spondylitis.
- The *MR corner sign* refers to a sharply margined triangular nonerosive corner abnormality, which is not associated with osteophyte formation or Schmorl nodes.
- The most frequent pattern of signal intensity in these lesions corresponds to Modic type 2 changes.

Suggested Readings

Hermann KG, Althoff CE, Schneider U, et al. Spinal changes in patients with spondyloarthritis: comparison of MR imaging and radiographic appearances. *Radiographics*. 2005;25(3):559-569.

Kim NR, Choi JY, Hong SH, et al. "MR corner sign": value for predicting presence of ankylosing spondylitis. *AJR Am J Roentgenol*. 2008;191(1):124-128.

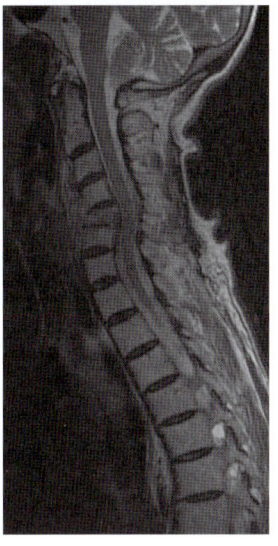 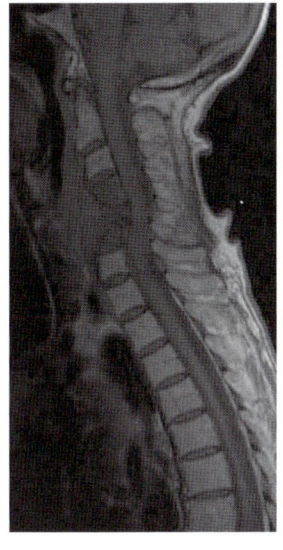 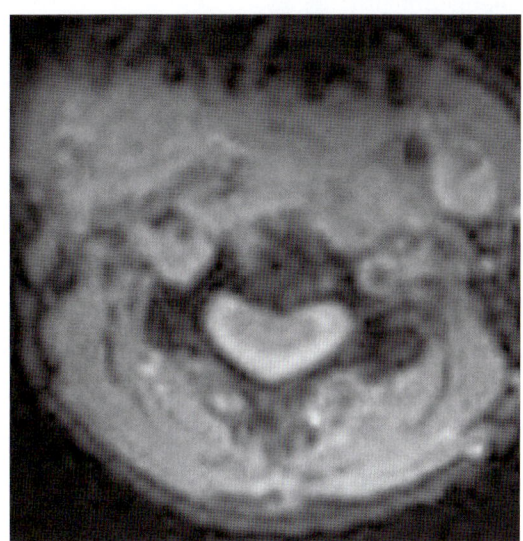

1. What is the most likely diagnosis?

2. Which symptoms are encountered in this condition?

3. Which CNS manifestations are seen in this condition?

4. Which imaging modality best images the condition?

5. Name some risk factors for CNS involvement in this disease.

Case ranking/difficulty:

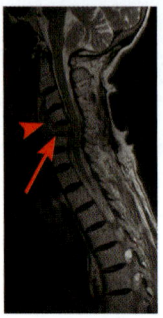

Sagittal T2-weighted sequence of the cervical and upper thoracic spine shows a pre-vertebral soft tissue mass in the cervical region (*arrowhead*) consistent with a conglomerate of lymph nodes. There is obvious involvement of the vertebral marrow (*arrow*). Note the reversal of the cervical lordosis.

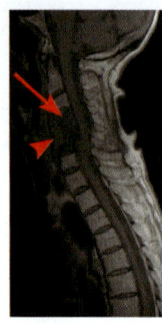

Sagittal T1-weighted sequence of the cervical and upper thoracic spine demonstrates a pre-vertebral soft tissue mass in the cervical region (*arrowhead*). The extent of vertebral marrow involvement (*arrow*) is better appreciated on this sequence.

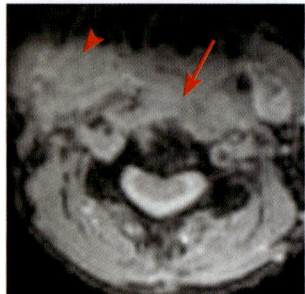

Axial T2 sequence confirms the large pre-vertebral soft tissue mass (*arrow*). Also note the conglomerate of lymph nodes along the right carotid sheath (*arrowhead*).

Answers

1. Lymphoma is a relatively common heterogeneous group of malignancies that usually originates from lymph nodes and is subdivided into Hodgkin disease and non-Hodgkin lymphoma (NHL) on the basis of pathology. Hodgkin disease is primarily a nodal disease but extranodal involvement has been described. Non-Hodgkin lymphoma is eight times more common than Hodgkin disease.

2. Lymphadenopathy is the primary presentation in lymphoma.

   Lymphoma may present with certain nonspecific symptoms. These include a variety of systemic symptoms (the so-called B symptoms), which include fever, weight loss, and night sweats.

   Fatigue, dyspnea, itching, and anorexia are also encountered.

3. CNS lesions may include intracranial masses, leptomeningeal involvement, spinal cord compression, and peripheral neuropathies. The latter may also complicate chemotherapy.

4. MRI is the imaging modality of choice in CNS lymphoma and it is exquisitely sensitive to detect intra- or extramedullary spinal involvement. Vertebral and paravertebral involvement, invasion of the epidural space, and leptomeningeal disease may all be assessed. 18F-FDG PET has been reported to be more sensitive than bone scintigraphy in patients with lymphoma and was shown to detect early bone marrow involvement before cortical changes could be seen by bone scintigraphy.

   Lymphoma is a known radiological "imitator" and should be included in the differential diagnosis of almost any mass lesion seen anywhere in the body.

5. CNS involvement is estimated to happen in up to 10% of lymphoma patients. Immunodeficiency is the major risk factor for developing CNS lymphoma.

Pearls

- Lymphoma is a heterogeneous group of malignancies that usually originates from lymph nodes.
- It is subdivided into Hodgkin disease and non-Hodgkin lymphoma (NHL) on the basis of pathology.
- Extranodal involvement may occur in the absence of significant lymphadenopathy when it is regarded as primary extranodal lymphoma of the affected organ.
- CNS involvement happens in up to 10% of lymphoma patients.
- Lymphoma is a known radiological "imitator" and should be included in the differential diagnosis of almost any mass lesion.

Suggested Readings

Metser U, Lerman H, Blank A, Lievshitz G, Bokstein F, Even-Sapir E. Malignant involvement of the spine: assessment by 18F-FDG PET/CT. *J Nucl Med*. 2004 Feb;45(2):279284.

Thomas AG, Vaidhyanath R, Kirke R, Rajesh A. Extranodal lymphoma from head to toe: part 1, the head and spine. *AJR Am J Roentgenol*. 2011 Aug;197(2):350-356.

Vanneuville B, Janssens A, Lemmerling M, de Vlam K, Mielants H, Veys EM. Non-Hodgkin's lymphoma presenting with spinal involvement. *Ann Rheum Dis*. 2000 Jan;59(1):12-14.

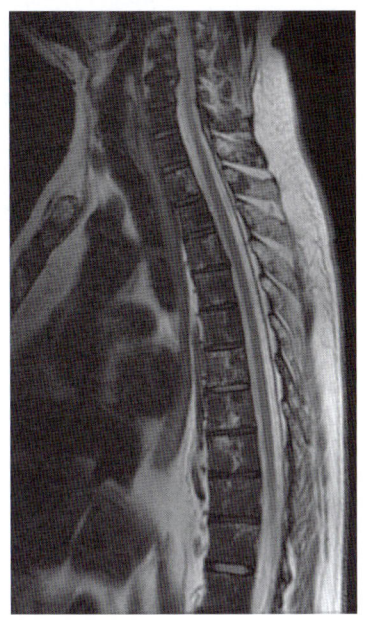
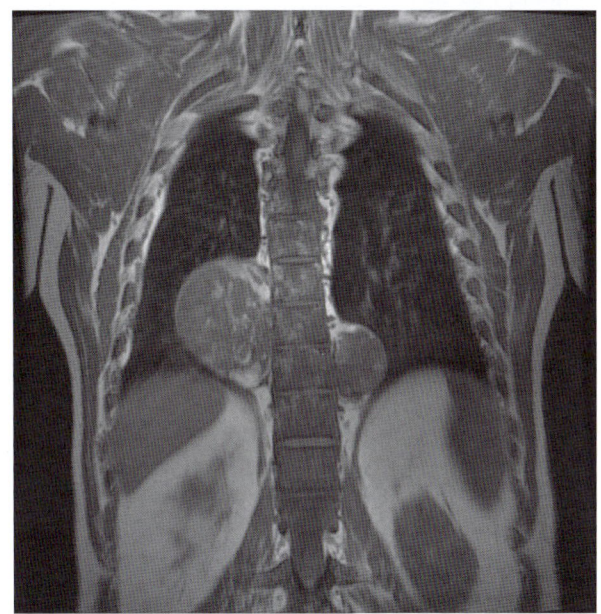

1. What is the most likely diagnosis?

2. What should be included in the differential diagnosis?

3. In which conditions may EMH occur?

4. In which hematological disorders may EMH occur?

5. In which organs does EMH occur?

Case ranking/difficulty:

Category: Paraspinal soft tissue

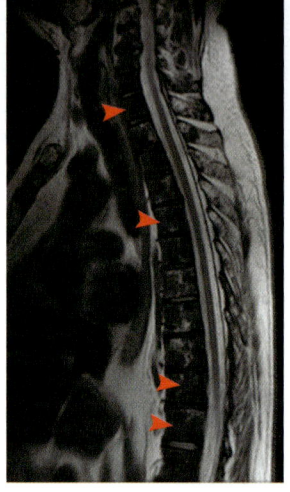

Note the diffusely abnormal signal intensity of the vertebral bone marrow (*arrowheads*), which appears hypointense and heterogenous.

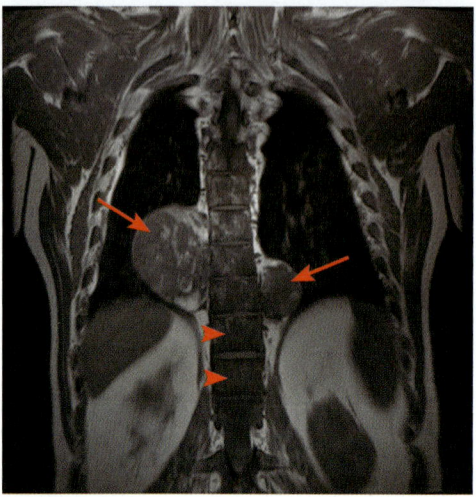

Coronal T1-weighted image showing two large paraspinal masses (*arrows*) in the lower thoracic region. Note again the abnormal vertebral bone marrow signal, which appears hypointense compared to the intervertebral discs.

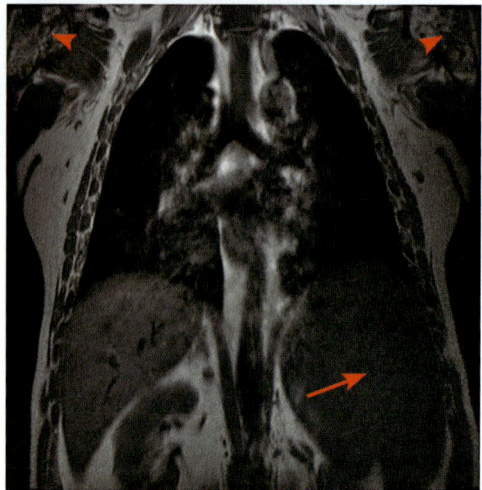

Coronal T1-weighted image demonstrates splenomegaly (*arrow*) and abnormal bone marrow in the humeral heads (*arrowheads*).

Answers

1. Extramedullary hematopoiesis (EMH) is a rare myeloproliferative disorder of clonal origin seen in patients with prolonged anemias. It is a physiological compensatory mechanism that leads to the formation of normal blood cells outside the bone marrow when the latter is unable to meet the circulatory demands.

2. Differential diagnoses of a paraspinal lesion include neurogenic tumors, lymphoma, metastasis, paravertebral abscess, and lateral meningocele.

3. EMH occurs with prolonged anemias including hemolytic anemias, myeloproliferative disorders, and neoplasia.

4. Extramedullary hematopoiesis (EMH) is seen in patients with prolonged anemias, myeloproliferative disorders, neoplasia, and following marrow irradiation.

5. EMH may occur in various sites including the spleen, liver, kidneys, heart, lymph nodes, skin, thymus, breast, prostate, adrenal glands, ovaries, intestines, and the CNS. During fetal life, hematopoiesis occurs in these sites but stops just before birth. The extramedullary hematopoietic tissues, however, retain their ability to produce red blood cells.

Pearls

- Extramedullary hematopoiesis is a myeloproliferative disorder seen in prolonged anemias.
- EMH may occur at various sites where hematopoiesis occurred during fetal life.
- Extramedullary hematopoiesis is a rare cause of a paraspinal mass.
- The MR signal intensity of extramedullary hematopoiesis varies depending on the activity of the hematopoietic tissue.

Suggested Readings

Georgiades CS, Neyman EG, Francis IR, Sneider MB, Fishman EK. Typical and atypical presentations of extramedullary hemopoiesis. *AJR Am J Roentgenol*. 2002 Nov;179(5):1239-1243.

Ginzel AW, Kransdorf MJ, Peterson JJ, Garner HW, Murphey MD. Mass-like extramedullary hematopoiesis: imaging features. *Skeletal Radiol*. 2012 Aug;41(8):911-916.

Kaleem A, Ansari S, Koirala R, Agarwal M, Chaudhary S. Paraspinal and presacral extramedullary hematopoiesis: a rare manifestation of polycythemia vera. *Iran J Radiol*. 2013 September;10(3):164-168.

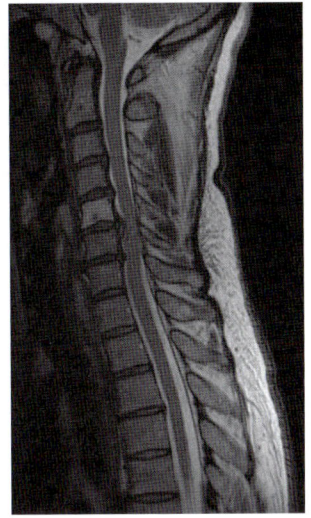 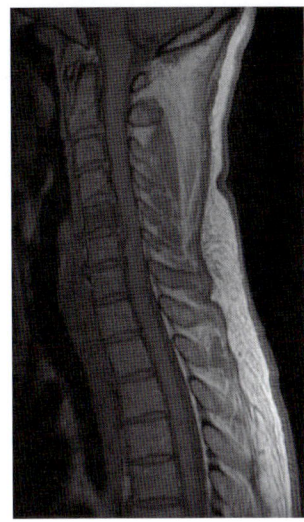 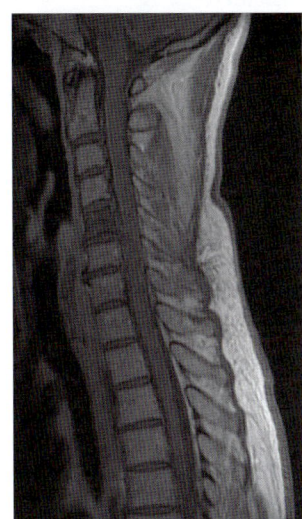

1. What is the most likely diagnosis?

2. What should be included in the differential diagnosis?

3. Which conditions form part of the spectrum of notochordal lesions?

4. Which imaging modality best images this condition?

5. How does the condition usually present?

Case ranking/difficulty: **Category:** Vertebral body

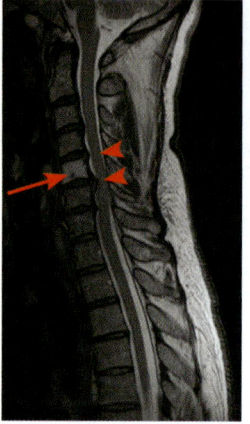

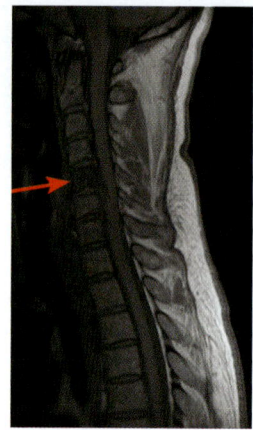

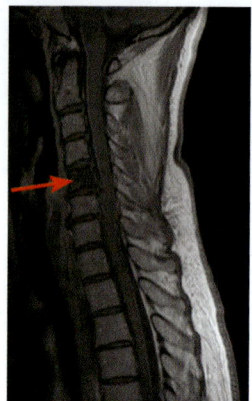

Sagittal T2-weighted sequence of the cervical spine showing replacement of C5 vertebral marrow with a homogenously hyperintense signal (*arrow*). Note that the affected vertebra is not expanded. There are multilevel disc bulges in the mid to lower cervical spine (*arrowheads*) with cord impingement at C5-C6. The latter was likely responsible for the presenting symptoms.

Sagittal T1-weighted sequence of the cervical spine showing replacement of C5 vertebral marrow with a homogenously hypointense signal (*arrow*). Note that the vertebral marrow should be brighter than the intervertebral disc on T1.

Contrast-enhanced sagittal T1-weighted sequence of the cervical spine showing replacement of C5 vertebral marrow with a homogenously hypointense signal (*arrow*). The intravertebral lesion does not enhance following contrast administration.

Answers

1. Benign notochordal cell tumour (BNCT) is a benign intravertebral lesion of notochord origin. BNCTs are found in the clivus or vertebral bodies in up to 20% of autopsy series and are detected with increasing frequency in vivo on cross-sectional imaging studies.

2. The main differential diagnoses include chordoma, hemangioma, plasmacytoma, Paget disease, atypical infections, lymphoma, and metastatic disease.

3. The spectrum of notochordal lesions includes chordoma, notochordal vestiges of the intervertebral disc, and ecchordosis physaliphora.

4. Small BNCTs may be radiologically occult. Larger lesions, on the other hand, may demonstrate nonspecific radiographic findings. Bone scintigraphy is typically negative. BNCTs often appear as sclerotic lesions on CT. MRI demonstrates a homogenous T2 hyperintense and T1 hypointense lesion replacing the vertebral marrow. They appear as well-circumscribed lesions that do not extend beyond or destroy the affected vertebra.

   Chordomas can often be distinguished radiologically by their aggressive growth as they cause extensive bone destruction and soft tissue invasion. Unlike BNCTs, chordomas enhance following contrast administration.

5. BNCTs are often found as incidental findings on imaging. Less commonly larger lesions may become symptomatic due to canal/exiting foraminal compromise. Clinical symptoms depend on the lesion location and

include back pain, limitation of movement, and sensory (paresthesia and anesthesia) and motor disturbances.

Pearls

- Benign notochordal cell tumor (BNCT) is a benign intravertebral lesion of notochord origin.
- The spectrum of notochordal lesions includes chordoma, notochordal vestiges of the intervertebral disc, and ecchordosis physaliphora.
- BNCTs are often found as incidental findings on imaging.
- MRI demonstrates a well-defined homogenous T2 hyperintense and T1 hypointense lesion that does not extend beyond or destroy the affected vertebra.
- Differential diagnoses include chordoma, vertebral hemangioma, plasmacytoma, Paget disease, atypical infections, lymphoma, and metastatic disease.

Suggested Readings

Amer H, Hameed M. Intraosseous benign notochordal cell tumor. *Arch Pathol Lab Med*. 2010 Feb;134(2):283-288.

Yamaguchi T, Iwata J, Sugihara S, et al. Distinguishing benign notochordal cell tumors from vertebral chordoma. *Skeletal Radiol*. 2008 Apr;37(4):291-299.

Yamaguchi T, Suzuki S, Ishiiwa H, Shimizu K, Ueda Y. Benign notochordal cell tumors—a comparative histological study of benign notochordal cell tumors, classic chordomas, and notochordal vestiges of fetal intervertebral discs. *Am J Surg Pathol*. 2004;28(6):756-761.

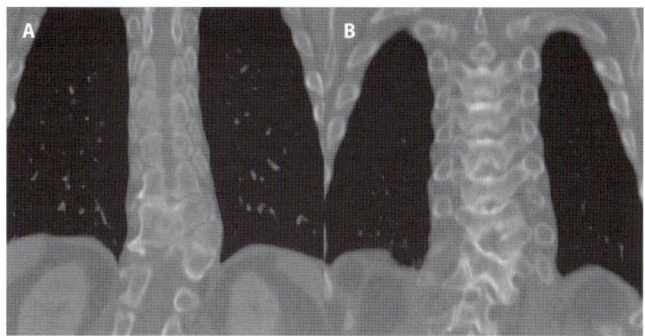 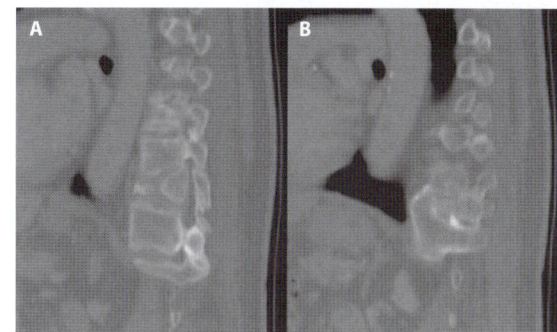

1. What is the most likely diagnosis?

2. Which syndromes are associated with this condition?

3. How can the condition manifest clinically?

4. Describe clinical and pathological characteristics of this condition.

5. Which treatments may be beneficial in this condition?

Case ranking/difficulty:

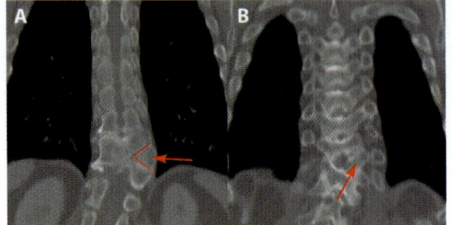

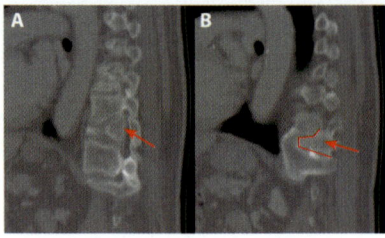

Coronal CT reconstructions show a wedge-shaped hemivertebra in the lower thoracic spine (*arrow*, panel A) with a unilateral transverse process (*arrow*, panel B). The hemivertebra causes a scoliotic curvature, convex to the left.

Answers

1. Hemivertebrae form part of the spectrum of segmentational anomalies and result from failure of development of one half of the vertebral body. Two lateral chondrification centers appear in developing vertebrae during the sixth week of gestation. By the seventh to eighth week of gestation the two centers unite to form the primary ossification center of the vertebral body. Failure of one of the chondrification centers to develop results in a hemivertebra.

2. There are several recognized associations that include cleidocranial dysostosis, Gorlin syndrome, VACTERL, gastroschisis, Aicardi syndrome, and OEIS complex.

3. Affected individuals are often asymptomatic. Neurologic problems are secondary to severe angulation of the spine, instability of the spinal column, spinal canal stenosis, and subluxation or fracture of the adjacent vertebrae. Symptomatic patients may present with motor (limb weakness or paralysis), sensory or autonomic dysfunction (urinary or fecal incontinence), and back/neck pain.

4. Hemivertebrae may involve single or multiple spinal levels and are a common cause of congenital scoliosis and kyphosis. The hemivertebra acts as a wedge within the spinal column, resulting in a curvature away from the side where it is present. The most common location of a hemivertebra is within the midthoracic spine.

   Hemivertebrae are classified according to their orientation (ie, dorsal, ventral, or lateral) and attachment to adjacent vertebrae. The orientation of the hemivertebra determines whether the anomalous curvature results in kyphosis, scoliosis, or lordosis.

   The attachment is described in terms of segmentation as follows:

   1) Fully segmental when the hemivertebra is not attached to either the vertebra above or below.
   2) Semisegmental when the hemivertebra is fused with one of the adjacent vertebrae with no intervening disc.

Sagittal CT reconstructions again demonstrate a wedge-shaped hemivertebra (*arrow*, panel A). A unilateral pedicle (*arrow*, panel B) and articulation with adjacent vertebrae is seen.

   3) Nonsegmental if the hemivertebra is connected to both vertebrae above and below.
   4) Incarcerated when the hemivertebra is joined to the adjacent levels by their pedicles.

   Antenatal ultrasonography reveals an asymmetrical vertebral body and distortion in the shape of the spine on coronal and sagittal scanning.

5. Treatment is conservative in asymptomatic cases. Spinal cord decompression and vertebral stabilization are offered if the deformity is progressive and for symptom relief.

Pearls

- Hemivertebrae form part of the spectrum of segmentational anomalies and result from failure of development of one half of the vertebral body.
- Hemivertebrae may involve single or multiple spinal levels and are a common cause of congenital scoliosis and kyphosis.
- The most common location of a hemivertebra is within the midthoracic spine.
- Affected individuals are often asymptomatic.
- Hemivertebrae are classified according to their orientation and attachment to adjacent vertebrae.
- Antenatal ultrasonography reveals an asymmetrical vertebral body and distortion in the shape of the spine.
- Treatment is conservative in asymptomatic cases.
- Spinal cord decompression and vertebral stabilization are offered if the deformity is progressive and for symptom relief.

Suggested Readings

Humbert L, Steffen JS, Vialle R, Dubousset J, Vital JM, Skalli W. 3D analysis of congenital scoliosis due to hemivertebra using biplanar radiography. *Eur Spine J.* 2013 Feb;22(2):379-386.

McMaster MJ, David CV. Hemivertebra as a cause of scoliosis. A study of 104 patients. *J Bone Joint Surg Br.* 1986 Aug;68(4):588-595.

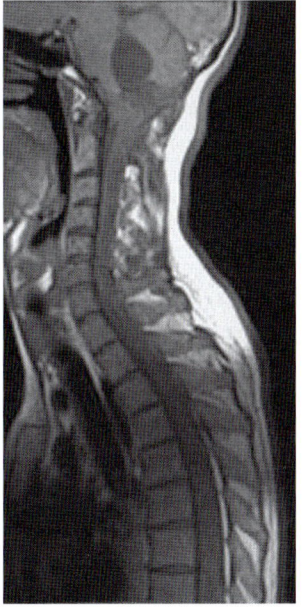 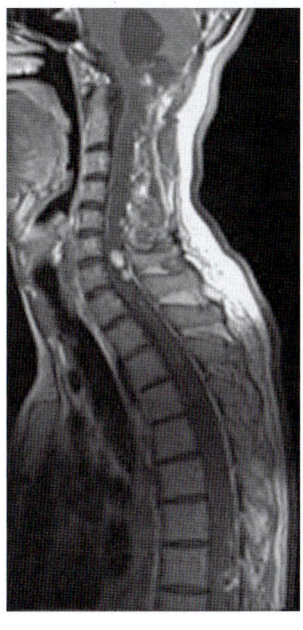 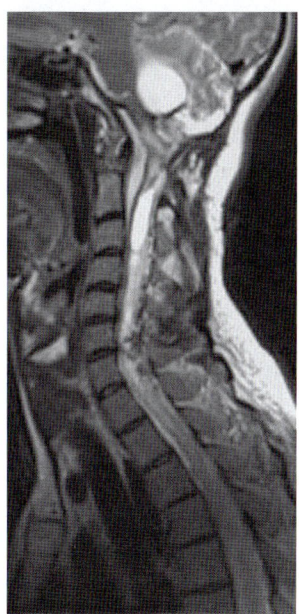 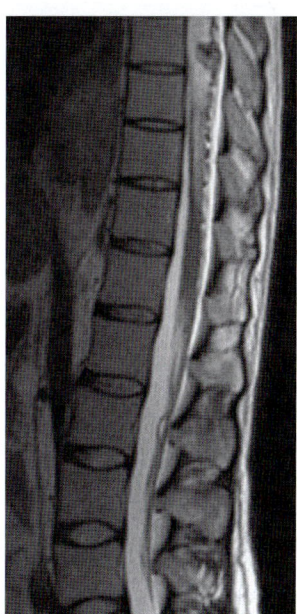

1. What is the most likely diagnosis?

2. What is the pattern of inheritance of this disease?

3. Which tumors are encountered in this disease?

4. Visceral cysts in this disease may affect:

5. Which of the following are diagnostic of this condition?

Case ranking/difficulty:

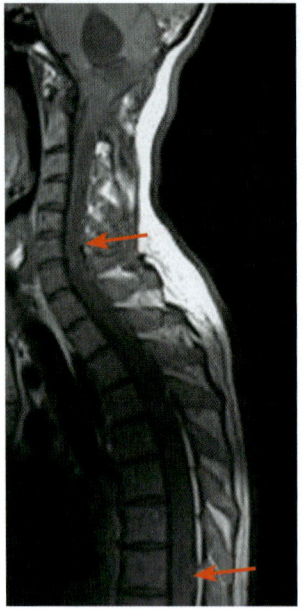

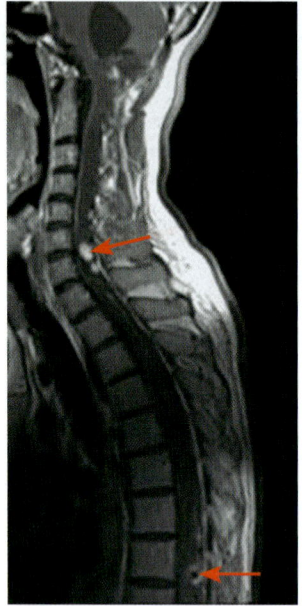

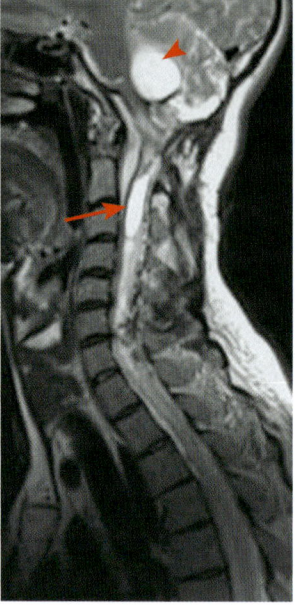

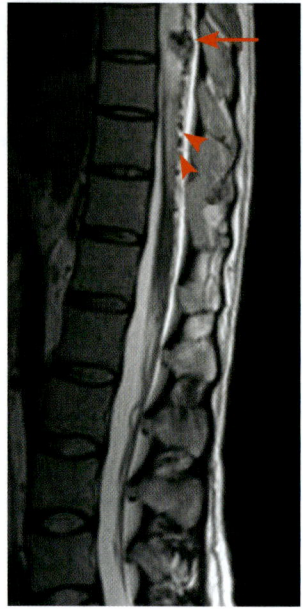

Non contrast T1-weighted sequence of the cervical and upper thoracic spine. It is difficult to identify the intradural lesions (*arrows*) on this sequence, but one can make out the abnormal adjacent flow voids.

Contrast-enhanced T1-weighted sequence of the cervical and upper thoracic spine shows multiple avidly enhancing intradural but extramedullary lesions (*arrows*) compatible with multiple hemangioblastomas.

T2-weighted sequence of the cervical and upper thoracic spine shows evidence of previous posterior fossa surgery (*arrowhead*) for a hemangioblastoma and a cervical cord syrinx (*arrow*).

T2-weighted sequence of the lower thoracic and lumbar spine shows a hypointense extramedullary lesion on the dorsal aspect of the cord (*arrow*) with adjacent abnormal flow voids (*arrowheads*), which correspond to abnormal draining/feeding vessels.

Answers

1. von Hippel-Lindau (vHL) disease is an autosomal dominant disorder caused by germline mutations in the vHL tumor suppressor gene located on chromosome 3p25-26.

2. vHL is an autosomal dominant disease. It demonstrates marked phenotypic variability and age-dependent penetrance.

3. The most frequent tumors in vHL are retinal and CNS hemangioblastomas and renal cell carcinomas.

   Pheochromocytomas, pancreatic islet tumors, endolymphatic sac tumors, and head and neck paragangliomas are less frequently encountered tumors.

4. Visceral cysts in vHL are found in bone, kidneys, liver, pancreas, and epididymis. The spleen, omentum, mesentery, adrenal glands, and lungs may also be affected.

5. The diagnostic criteria of vHL disease are:

   a) More than one CNS hemangioblastoma

   b) One hemangioblastoma *plus* a visceral manifestation of vHL

   c) One visceral manifestation *plus* a known family history

Pearls

- vHL is an autosomal dominant disorder.
- CNS hemangioblastomas are a cardinal feature of vHL.
- Frequent tumors in vHL are CNS hemangioblastomas and renal cell carcinomas.
- Less frequent tumors include pheochromocytomas, pancreatic islet tumors, endolymphatic sac tumors, and head and neck paragangliomas.
- Visceral cysts are very common and may affect multiple body systems.
- vHL may be further subclassified into Type 1, Type 2A, and Type 2B.

Suggested Readings

Maher E, Neumann H, Richard S. von Hippel-Lindau disease: a clinical and scientific review. *Eur J Hum Genet.* June 2011;19(6):617-623.

Zhang Q, Ma L, Li W, Chen J, Ju Y, Hui X. Von Hippel-Lindau disease manifesting disseminated leptomeningeal hemangioblastomatosis: surgery or medication? *Acta Neurochirurgica.* 2011 Jan;153(1):48-52.

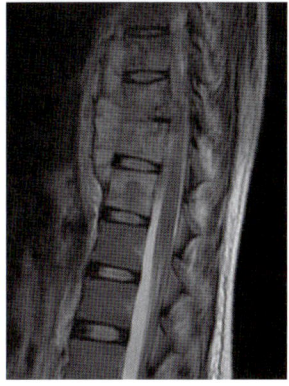 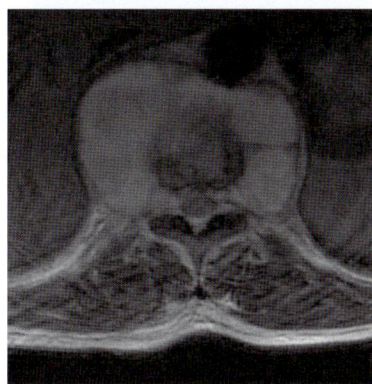 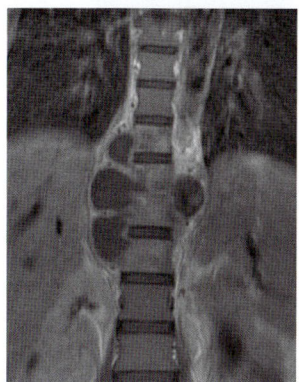

1. What is the most likely diagnosis?

2. Which features are typical of this condition?

3. Pulmonary involvement can be demonstrated in:

4. Which imaging modality best images this condition?

5. Which site is preferentially affected?

Case ranking/difficulty:

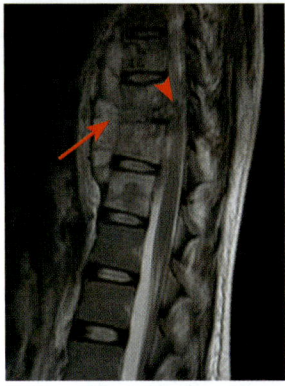

Sagittal T2-weighted sequence of the lower thoracic and lumbar spine showing edematous changes in T9-T12 vertebral bodies in keeping with spondylitis. Note the large abscess in the anterior paraspinal space (*arrow*), and a smaller epidural collection posteriorly (*arrowhead*).

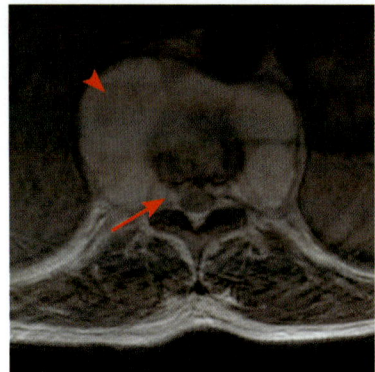

Axial T2-weighted sequence at the level of T11 vertebral body shows a large paraspinal abscess (*arrowhead*), which extends through the intervertebral foramina into the lateral recesses (*arrow*) causing narrowing of the spinal canal.

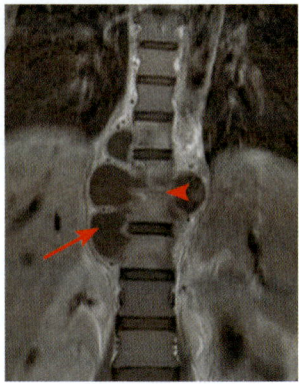

Coronal T1-weighted sequence of the thoracic spine shows large bilateral paraspinal collections with ring enhancement in keeping with abscess formation (*arrow*). Note the loss of disc space at T10-T11 (*arrowhead*) and the marrow edema in the adjacent vertebral bodies.

Answers

1. Tuberculosis is one of the commoner infections of the spine and its incidence is on the increase due to the development of multiple drug-resistant strains.

2. The infection usually spreads beneath the longitudinal ligaments to affect multiple (often contiguous) vertebrae. This is referred to as "subligamentous" spread and preferentially occurs beneath the anterior longitudinal ligament. The posterior vertebral elements are hence often spared. Slow collapse of the affected vertebrae results in an acute kyphotic angulation or "gibbus" deformity. Cord compression may result from this angulation coupled with the formation of large epidural collections and bone fragments. Tuberculous spondylitis may result in large paraspinal abscesses, sometimes being completely painless and without frank pus, when they are referred to as "cold abscesses." Infection limited to a single vertebra is less common and results in vertebral collapse and development of a vertebra plana deformity.

3. Pulmonary tuberculous involvement can only be demonstrated in up to 50% of cases.

4. MRI is the imaging modality of choice as it delineates the extent of infectious involvement, the presence and size of epidural collections, and canal compromise. CT can demonstrate anterior vertebral body destruction or collapse, narrowing of the intervertebral disc, and the presence of paraspinal collections.

The earliest sign is involvement of the anterosuperior vertebral endplate or subtle irregularity of the anterior vertebral body. Focal areas of erosion and osseous destruction can be seen on plain radiography at these sites.

5. Spinal involvement results from hematogenous seeding to the vertebral bodies. There is preferential involvement of the thoracolumbar region, with the cervical spine and sacrum being rarely involved.

Pearls

- The incidence of tuberculous spondylitis is on the increase worldwide due to the development of multiple drug-resistant strains.
- Spinal involvement results from hematogenous seeding to the vertebral bodies.
- MRI is the imaging modality of choice as it delineates the extent of infectious involvement, the presence and size of epidural collections, and canal compromise.

Suggested Readings

Dagirmanjian A, Schils J, McHenry M, Modic MT. MR imaging of vertebral osteomyelitis revisited. *AJR Am J Roentgenol.* 1996 Dec;167(6):1539-1543.

Gouliamos AD, Kehagias DT, Lahanis S, et al. MR imaging of tuberculous vertebral osteomyelitis: pictorial review. *Eur Radiol.* 2001;11(4):575-579.

Recurrent meningitis

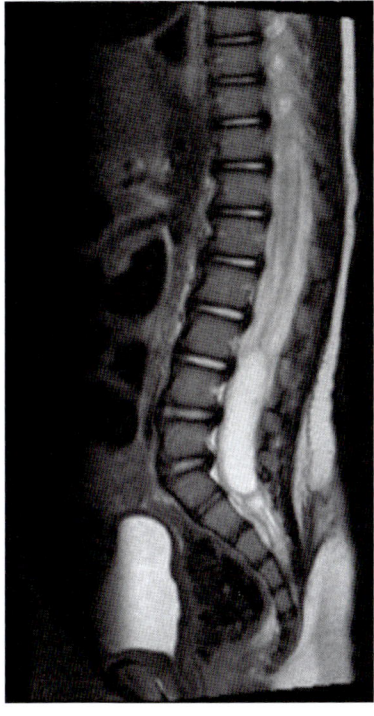 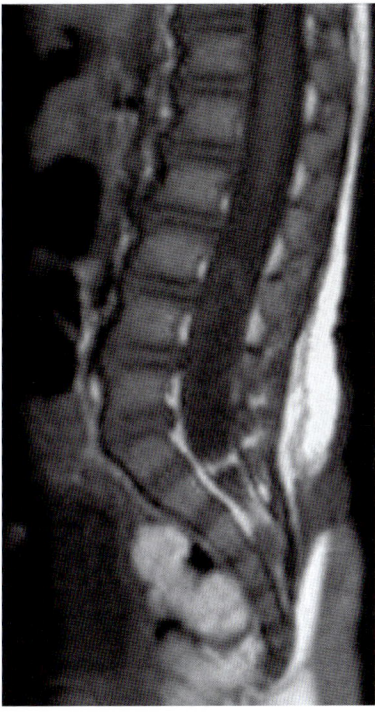 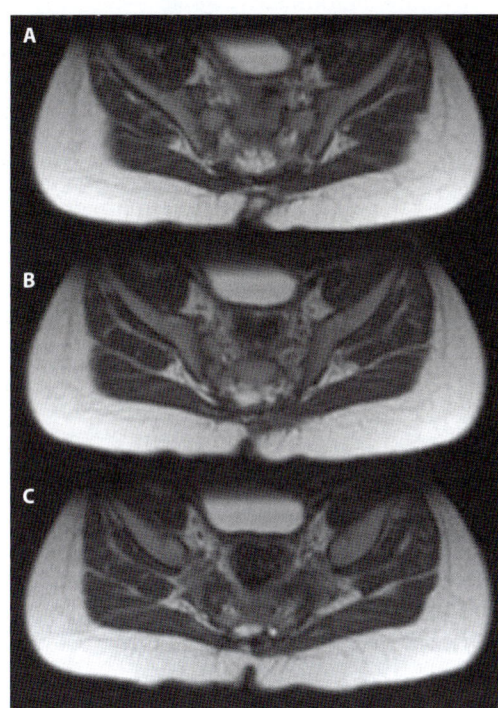

1. What is the most likely diagnosis?

2. Where is the anomaly frequently seen?

3. Which clinical findings may be seen in this condition?

4. Which vertebral anomalies are associated with this condition?

5. Name potential complications of this condition.

Case ranking/difficulty:

Category: More than one category

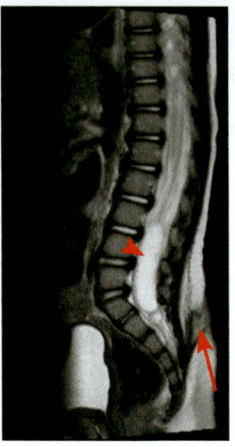

Sagittal T2-weighted sequence shows a linear hypointense tract extending from the skin to the sacral canal (*arrow*) compatible with a dorsal dermal sinus. There is an associated hyperintense "sausage-shaped" T2 hyperintense lesion in the lower lumbar canal (*arrowhead*).

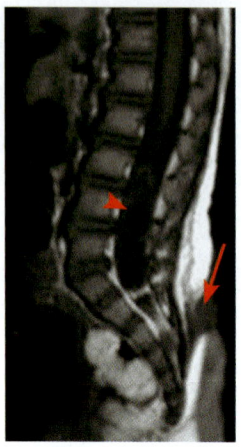

Sagittal T1-weighted sequence again demonstrates a linear tract (*arrow*) crossing the subcutaneous tissues of the back to reach the spinal canal. The oval-shaped lesion in the lumbar canal also follows the CSF signal on T1 and represents an epidermoid (*arrowhead*).

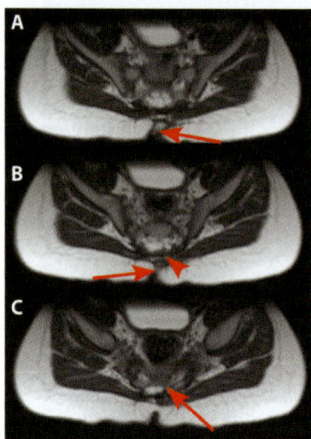

Consecutive axial T1-weighted images at the level of the sacral bone demonstrates a hypointense tract extending from the skin surface (*arrow*, panel A), across the subcutaneous fat (*arrow*, panel B) to reach the sacral canal (*arrowhead*, panel B and *arrow*, panel C).

Answers

1. A dorsal dermal sinus is a rare form of spinal dysraphism in which an anomalous epithelial-lined tract extends from the skin to the spinal cord, cauda equina, or arachnoid. It results from failure of the cutaneous and neural ectoderm to separate during neurulation resulting in a focal segmental adhesion.

2. Dorsal dermal sinuses are commonly encountered in the lumbosacral region. Less often they are seen in the occipital region. The sinus is lined by stratified squamous epithelium and extends from the skin surface to either terminate superficially within the subcutaneous layers or else extends deeply through the fascia and vertebrae to communicate directly with the thecal sac or intradural compartment.

3. A small dimple along the back may be found on clinical examination and they are often associated with hyperpigmentation of the overlying skin, a hairy nevus, and capillary angioma. The sinus ostium is seen in a midline location or more rarely in a paramedian location.

4. Up to 50% of dorsal dermal sinuses end in an associated spinal dermoid, epidermoid, or lipoma. The latter may compress the adjacent neural structures resulting in neurologic symptoms. Apart from inclusion tumors, the condition is also associated with spinal teratoma, split-cord malformations, and tethered spinal cord.

5. Complications include CSF leaks and recurrent infections leading to meningitis, epidural or subdural abscess formation, or less commonly a cord abscess.

   Meningitis can be either pyogenic due to bacterial ascent from the skin along the tract, or less frequently chemical meningitis secondary to the release of cholesterol crystals from spinal inclusion tumors.

Pearls

- A dorsal dermal sinus is a rare form of spinal dysraphism.
- Up to 50% end in an associated spinal dermoid, epidermoid, or lipoma.

Suggested Readings

Cox EM, Knudson KE, Manjila S, Cohen AR. Unusual presentation of congenital dermal sinus: tethered spinal cord with intradural epidermoid and dual paramedian cutaneous ostia. *Neurosurg Focus*. 2012 Oct;33(4):E5.

Unsinn KM, Geley T, Freund MC, Gassner I. US of the spinal cord in newborns: spectrum of normal findings, variants, congenital anomalies, and acquired diseases. *Radiographics*. 2000 Jul-Aug;20(4):923-938.

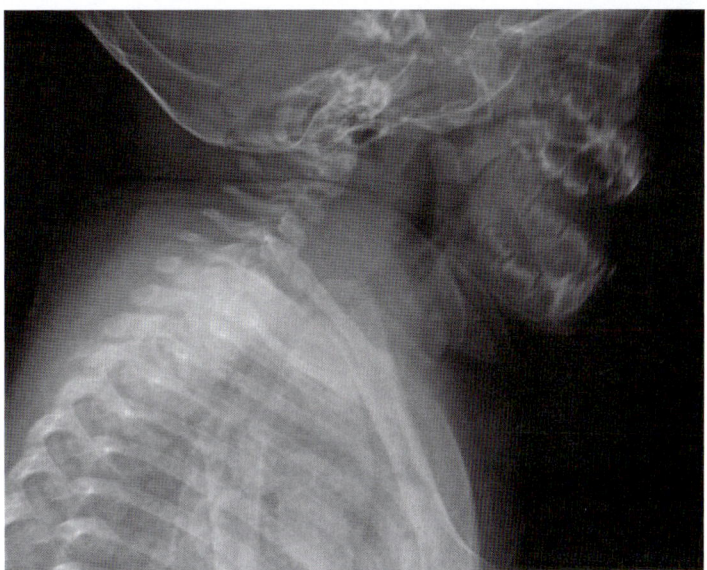

1. What is the prevertebral soft tissue space?

2. What should be included in the differential diagnosis?

3. Describe the normal measurements of the prevertebral space.

4. How should the radiograph be acquired?

5. Describe other soft tissue signs on the lateral cervical radiograph.

Case ranking/difficulty:

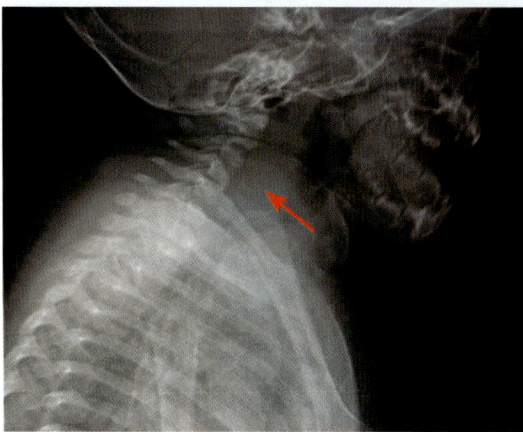

Lateral radiograph of the cervical spine in an 18-month-old girl. There is abnormal widening of the prevertebral soft tissue space (*arrow*) with anterior displacement of the pharynx and trachea at the level of C3-C4 vertebral bodies.

Answers

1. The prevertebral soft tissue space should always be assessed carefully on a lateral radiograph of the cervical spine, particularly in the setting of trauma where abnormal widening of the space may point to serious spinal injury.

   The retropharyngeal space and the prevertebral soft tissue space are two distinct spaces. The former extends from the skull base to the level of the carina. It is located between the prevertebral fascia and the buccopharyngeal mucosa. The prevertebral soft tissue space is a potential space between the anterior aspect of the cervical spine and the prevertebral fascia.

2. Assessment of the thickness and contours of the prevertebral soft tissues is also important in the evaluation of infectious conditions of the retropharyngeal space. The prevertebral soft tissue space may also be widened in the presence of a neoplastic or inflammatory mass.

3. The prevertebral space is usually measured at C2 and C6 levels. At the former level the space should measure less than 7 mm or <50% of the width of C2 body. At C6, the prevertebral space should not be wider than 22 mm or the width of C6 vertebral body. Various studies have, however, demonstrated that these measurements should only be used as a guide and soft tissue abnormalities should always be interpreted in light of other clinical signs, osseous findings, and the mechanism of injury. It was also shown using these measurements in isolation results in a large proportion of cervical spine fractures being missed.

4. The patient's neck should be in the extended position and the radiograph should be obtained in end inspiration. The prevertebral soft tissues may appear falsely widened if the patient is swallowing at the time of exposure or if the neck is flexed resulting in a "pseudomass."

5. Other soft tissue signs should be assessed when evaluating the lateral cervical spine radiograph.

   1) There is normally a "step-off" between the posterior wall of the trachea and the posterior pharyngeal wall at the level of the larynx, which usually corresponds to C4 level. This may be lost in the presence of retropharyngeal cellulitis or abscess formation.

   2) The air–soft tissue interface between the posterior pharynx and the prevertebral soft tissues should also be assessed. The interface is normally very sharp but may become indistinct in the presence of an inflammatory process in the retropharyngeal space.

   3) The contour of the prevertebral soft tissue space should follow the contour of the anterior aspect of the cervical spine.

Pearls

- The prevertebral soft tissue space should always be assessed carefully on a lateral radiograph of the cervical spine, particularly in the setting of trauma.
- The patient's neck should be in the extended position and the radiograph should be obtained in end inspiration.
- The retropharyngeal space and the prevertebral soft tissue space are two distinct spaces.
- The prevertebral space at C2 should measure less than 7 mm or <50% of the width of C2 body.
- At C6, the prevertebral space should not be wider than 22 mm or the width of C6 vertebral body.
- Assessment of the thickness and contours of the prevertebral soft tissues is also important in the evaluation of infectious conditions of the retropharyngeal space.
- The prevertebral soft tissue space may also be widened in the presence of a neoplastic or inflammatory mass.
- Other soft tissue signs should be assessed when evaluating a lateral cervical spine radiograph.

Suggested Readings

DeBehnke DJ, Havel CJ. Utility of prevertebral soft tissue measurements in identifying patients with cervical spine fractures. *Ann Emerg Med*.1994 Dec;24(6):1119-1124.

Matar LD, Doyle AJ. Prevertebral soft-tissue measurements in cervical spine injury. *Australas Radiol*. 1997 Aug;41(3):229-237.

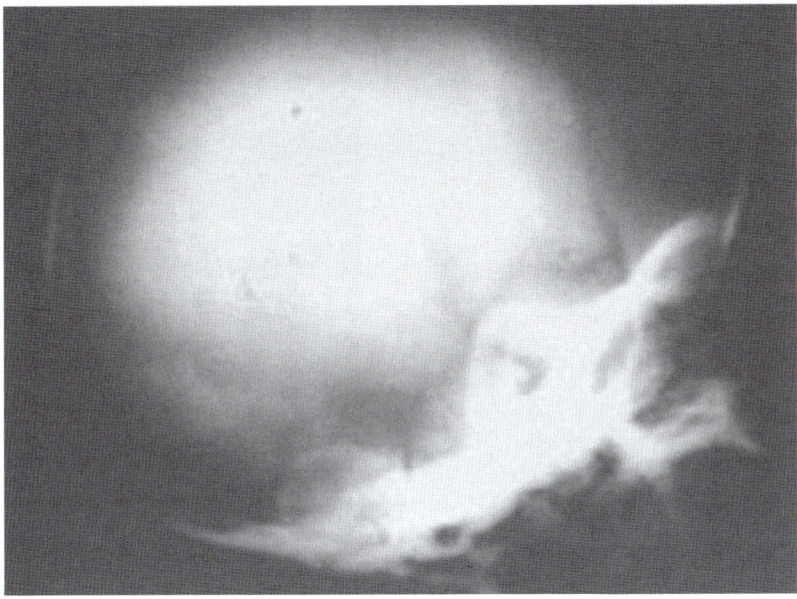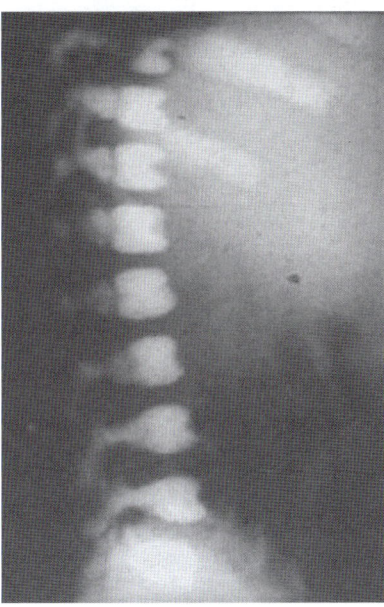

1. What are the pertinent radiologic findings?

2. What conditions are included in the differential, and what is the most likely diagnosis?

3. What is the pathogenesis for this entity?

4. Which form of the disease is most severe?

5. What are some of the complications of this entity?

Category: Vertebral body

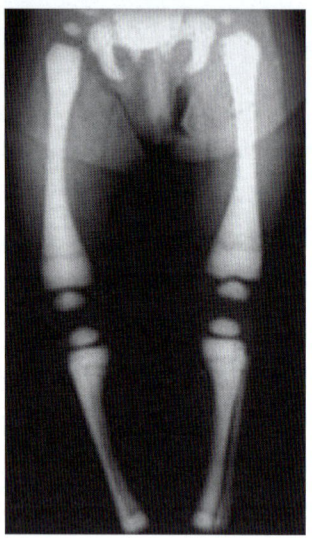

Another patient. Generalized increase in bone density with Erlenmeyer flask deformity.

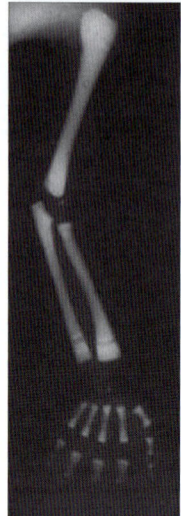

Another patient. Generalized increase in bone density. All images courtesy of Dr. Akbar Bonakdarpour.

Answers

1. There is a generalized increase in bone density with sclerosis in the base of skull and "sandwich" vertebrae. Although fractures are frequent, none are demonstrated here.

   Medullary sclerosis with relative sparing of the cortices, and Erlenmeyer flask deformities, is typically seen in the extremities.

2. Lead toxicity, pyknodysostosis, Paget disease, osteoblastic metastasis, and osteopetrosis are all in the differential for osteosclerosis. Given the age of the patient, the most likely diagnosis is osteopetrosis.

3. Osteopetrosis is a result of a failure of osteoclasts to resorb bone.

4. The infantile autosomal recessive variant of osteopetrosis has a much higher morbidity and mortality.

5. The bones are dense in osteopetrosis, but weak. Therefore, fractures and fracture complications such as delayed/nonunion as well as osteomyelitis may occur. Encroachment on the medullary space may result in anemia. Other complications include nerve compression and abnormal dentition.

Pearls

- Osteopetrosis is a disease resulting from a failure of osteoclastic activity.
- There is an increase in bone density; however, the bones are weaker and prone to fractures and complications of fractures.
- Two main forms exist: the more severe infantile autosomal recessive form and the milder adult autosomal dominant form.
- Adult forms may be diagnosed incidentally, or with mild anemia.
- The bones are dense with medullary sclerosis and relative sparing of the cortices. Erlenmeyer flask deformity can be seen.
- Adult Type 1 form shows uniform increase in bone density of the long bones, spine, and skull.
- Adult Type 2 form shows the classic "bone in bone" appearance, with "sandwich vertebrae." The pelvis, spine, and skull base are often affected.

Suggested Readings

Ihde LL, Forrester DM, Gottsegen CJ, et al. Sclerosing bone dysplasias: review and differentiation from other causes of osteosclerosis. *Radiographics.* 2011;31(7):1865-1882.

Vanhoenacker FM, De Beuckeleer LH, Van Hul W, et al. Sclerosing bone dysplasias: genetic and radioclinical features. *Eur Radiol.* 2000 Nov;10(9):1423-1433.

Quadriplegia of an acute onset

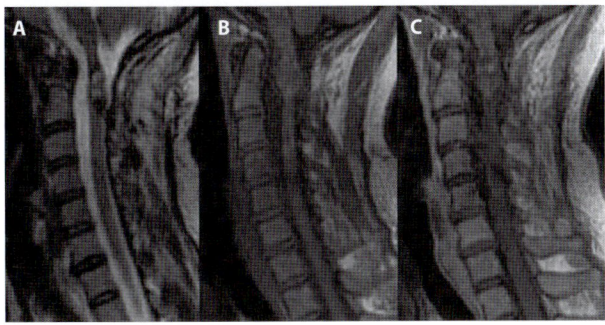 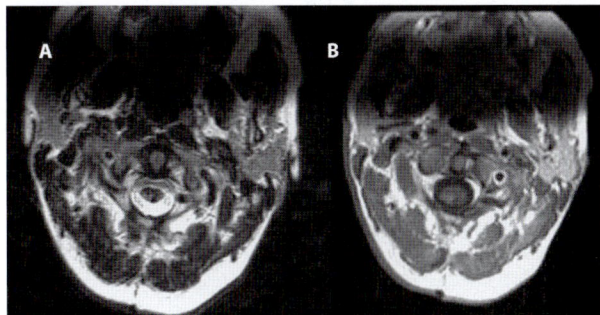

1. What is the most likely diagnosis?

2. What should be included in the differential diagnosis?

3. Which MR features are typical of this condition?

4. Which imaging modality best images this condition?

5. Describe clinical and pathological characteristics of this condition.

Case ranking/difficulty:

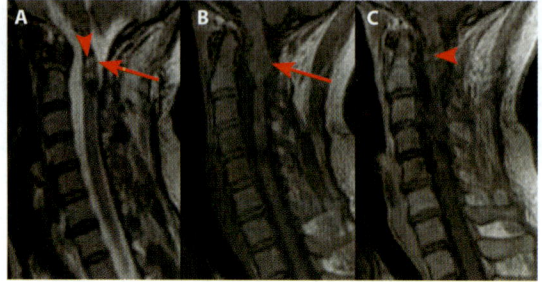

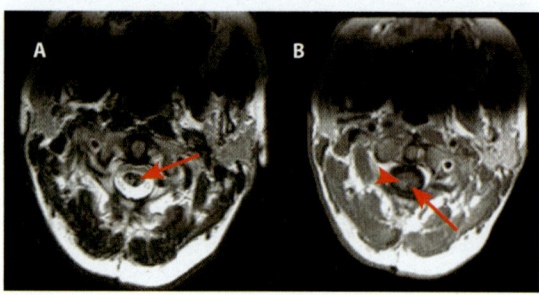

There is an oval-shaped intramedullary lesion in the cervical cord (*arrow*, panel A), which expands the cord. The lesion is surrounded by a hypointense hemosiderin rim (*arrowhead*, panel A). The lesion (*arrow*, panel B) demonstrates subtle contrast enhancement (*arrowhead*, panel C).

Axial MRI sequences (panel A = T2; panel B = T1) of the cervical spine at the level of the odontoid peg confirms the intramedullary location of the lesion, which is surrounded by a hypointense hemosiderin rim (*arrows*, panels A and B). Hyperintense T1 signal is noted within the lesion (*arrowhead*, panel B).

Answers

1. Spinal cavernomas are well-circumscribed vascular malformations composed of closely packed capillary-like vessels with no intervening spinal tissue.

2. Intramedullary lesions including primary spinal tumors (eg, astrocytoma, ependymoma, and hemangioblastoma), metastatic lesions, and inflammatory lesions (demyelination and transverse myelitis) should be included in the differential diagnosis.

3. Cavernomas do not have prominent vascular supply or venous drainage and are angiographically occult lesions. Magnetic resonance imaging is virtually diagnostic for spinal cavernomas. They are seen as having mixed signal intensity on T1-weighted sequences and are surrounded by a prominent hemosiderin ring on both T1- and T2-weighted images. A pathognomonic "popcorn" appearance of mixed hyperintensity and hypointense blood-containing locules may also be demonstrated.

4. Magnetic resonance imaging is virtually diagnostic of spinal cavernomas. The lesion is occult angiographically and can be easily overlooked on CT.

5. Spinal cavernomas account for about 5% of all cavernomas and are clinically more aggressive than their cranial counterparts. Their location is often precarious and they are therefore more likely to be symptomatic compared to cranial cavernomas.

Sporadic and familial forms have been described. The former often presents with a single lesion, whereas multiple lesions characterize the inherited form.

Presentation may be acute secondary to intramedullary hemorrhage or chronic when it manifests as slowly progressive neurological decline. This progressive myelopathy is the result of repetitive microhemorrhages with formation of perifocal hemosiderosis and reactive gliosis. Clinical presentation also varies according to the location of the cavernoma.

Pearls

- Cavernomas are vascular malformations composed of closely packed capillary-like vessels.
- Spinal cavernomas account for about 5% of all CNS cavernomas.
- Presentation may be acute secondary to intramedullary hemorrhage or chronic when it manifests as slowly progressive neurological decline.
- Magnetic resonance imaging is virtually diagnostic for spinal cavernomas—a "popcorn" appearance is pathognomonic.

Suggested Readings

Hegde A, Mohan S, Tan KK, Lim CC. Spinal cavernous malformations: magnetic resonance imaging and associated findings. *Singapore Med J.* 2012 Sep;53(9):582-586.

Kivelev J, Niemelä M, Hernesniemi J. Characteristics of cavernomas of the brain and spine. *J Clin Neurosci.* 2012 May;19(5):643-648.

See-Sebastian EH, Marks ER. Spinal cord intramedullary cavernoma: a case report. *W V Med J.* 2013 May-Jun;109(3):28-30.

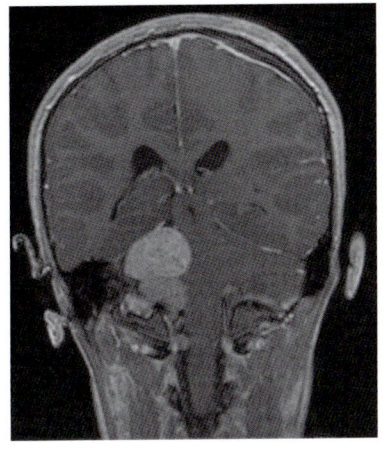 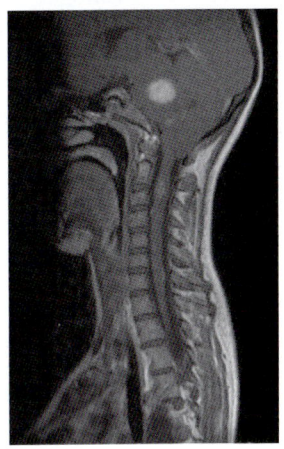 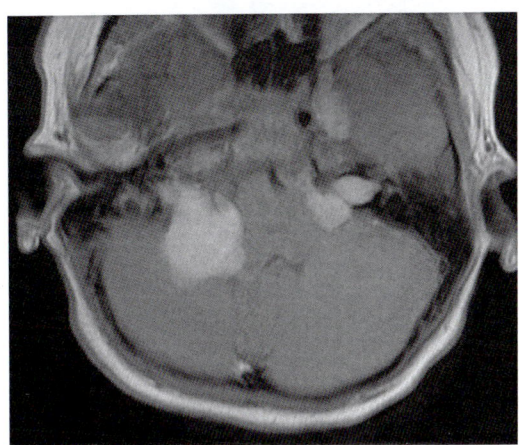

1. What is the most likely diagnosis?

2. Name the diagnostic criteria of this syndrome?

3. Which conditions are considered "neurocutaneous syndromes?"

4. Which pattern of inheritance does this condition have?

5. Which symptoms may occur in this condition?

Case ranking/difficulty:

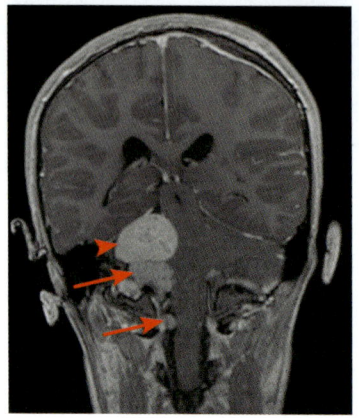

Contrast-enhanced scan at the level of the posterior fossa shows multiple enhancing extraaxial lesions including a vestibular schwannoma (*arrowhead*) and lower cranial nerve schwannomas (*arrows*).

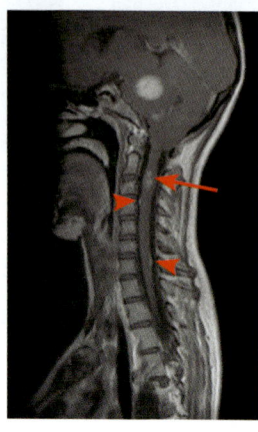

Post-contrast T1-weighted sequence demonstrates an intramedullary enhancing lesion, likely an ependymoma (*arrow*) and multiple intradural but extramedullary lesions (*arrowheads*).

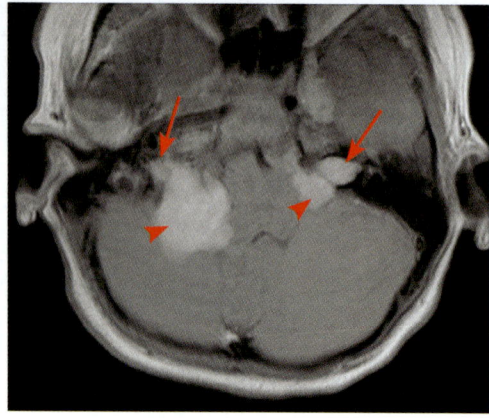

Bilateral enhancing cerebellopontine angle masses (*arrowheads*). The lesions extend through the porus acusticus into the internal auditory canals (*arrows*). Bilateral acoustic schwannomas are diagnostic of NF-2.

Answers

1. Multiple schwannomas, meningiomas, and ependymomas are diagnostic of neurofibromatosis type 2. The condition is sometimes referred to as "MISME syndrome."

2. Ferner et al described three sets of diagnostic criteria for neurofibromatosis type 2:

   1) Bilateral vestibular schwannomas or family history of NF-2 plus unilateral vestibular schwannoma or any two of meningioma, glioma, neurofibroma, schwannoma, and posterior subcapsular lenticular opacities.
   2) Unilateral vestibular schwannoma plus any two of meningioma, glioma, neurofibroma, schwannoma, and posterior subcapsular lenticular opacities.
   3) Two or more meningioma plus unilateral vestibular schwannoma or any two of glioma, schwannoma, and cataract.

3. Neurocutaneous syndromes include neurofibromatosis, tuberous sclerosis, Sturge-Weber syndrome, von Hippel-Lindau disease, ataxia telangiectasia, Wyburn-Mason syndrome, incontinentia pigmenti, and nevoid basal cell carcinoma syndrome.

4. The incidence of NF-2 is about 1 in 50,000. Half of the cases are secondary to de novo mutations. The affected gene is located on chromosome 22.

5. Vestibular schwannomas often present with neurosensory hearing loss, tinnitus, and headaches. Mass effect in the cerebellopontine angles may also result in facial nerve symptoms.

Pearls

- NF-2 is an autosomal dominant multiple neoplasia syndrome that results from mutations of the NF-2 tumor suppression gene located on chromosome 22.
- Affected individuals are at a propensity of developing multiple CNS tumors, ophthalmological lesions, cutaneous lesions, and peripheral neuropathy.

Suggested Readings

Asthagiri AR, Parry DM, Butman JA, et al. Neurofibromatosis type 2. *Lancet*. 2009 Jun 6;373(9679):1974-1986. Review.

Evans DG. Neurofibromatosis type 2 (NF2): a clinical and molecular review. *Orphanet J Rare Dis*. 2009 Jun 19;4:16. Review.

Ferner, Rosalie E, Susan M, Huson D. Gareth R. Evans. Neurofibromatoses in clinical practice. Springer, 2011.

Acute paraparesis and sphincter dysfunction

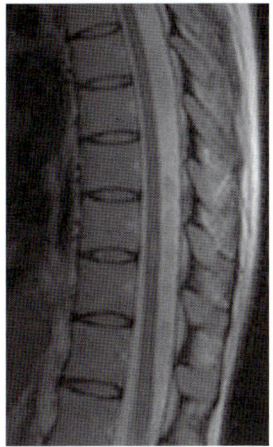 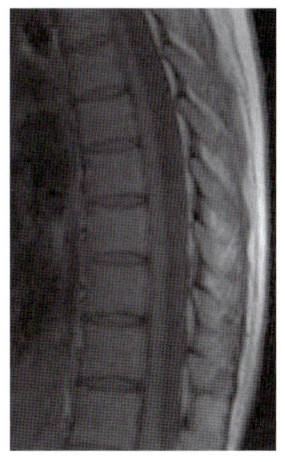 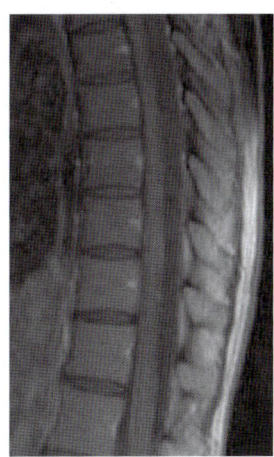 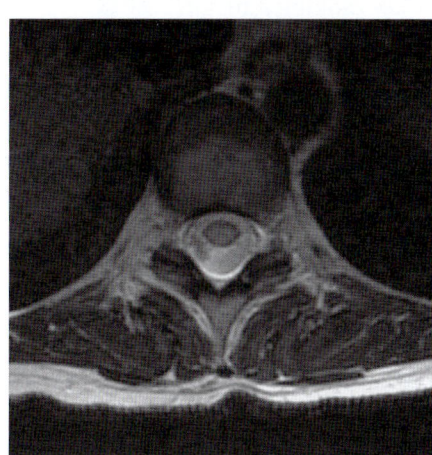

1. What is the most likely diagnosis?

2. Which underlying causes have been implicated in this condition?

3. What is a variant of this condition that affects three or more vertebral segments called?

4. Which imaging modality best images this condition?

5. Name some inclusion criteria proposed by the Transverse Myelitis Consortium Working Group.

Case ranking/difficulty:

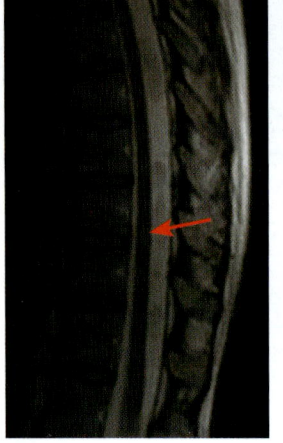

Sagittal T2-weighted sequence of the thoracic spine demonstrates an intramedullary hyperintense lesion (*arrow*) at T9-T10, which causes slight cord expansion.

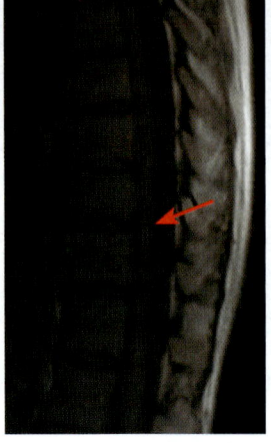

Sagittal T1-weighted sequence of the thoracic spine. Note that the intramedullary lesion (*arrow*) at T9-T10 is barely seen.

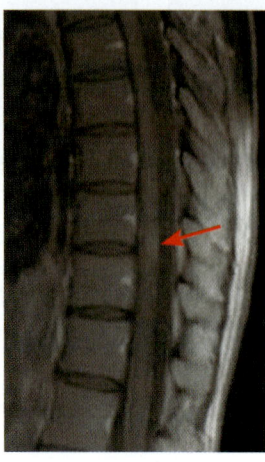

Contrast-enhanced sagittal T1-weighted sequence of the thoracic spine showing subtle enhancement of the intramedullary lesion (*arrow*).

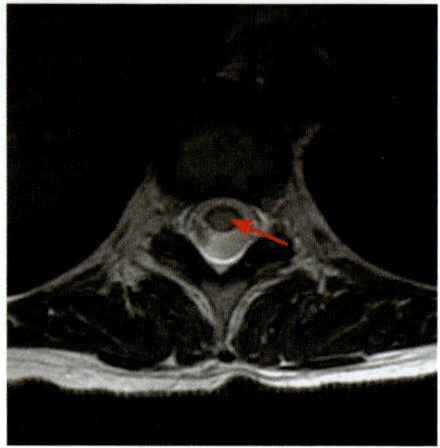

Axial T2-weighted sequence at the level of T10 confirms the intramedullary location of the lesion (*arrow*). Note that the lesion affects more than 2/3 of the cross-sectional area of the cord.

Answers

1. Transverse myelitis is a rare inflammatory disorder of the spinal cord that results in rapidly progressive weakness, sensory alterations, and autonomic dysfunction.

2. The etiology of transverse myelitis is protean and includes viral infections (eg, CMV), spinal cord injury, immune reactions, schistosomiasis, and spinal blood flow alterations.

3. The lesions may affect anywhere along the spinal cord and are usually restricted to a small cord portion. A variant of the condition is termed longitudinally extensive transverse myelitis (LETM), which extends over three or more vertebral segments.

4. MRI is the imaging investigation of choice and is essential to rule out differential diagnosis. The lesion is often seen as an ill-defined T2 hyperintense focus with variable enhancement post-contrast administration. The affected cord segment is expanded and the lesion typically affects more than two-thirds of the cross section of the cord.

5. Diagnostic criteria have been proposed by the Transverse Myelitis Consortium Working Group and include inclusion and exclusion criteria as follows:

   a) Inclusion criteria:
      - Development of sensory, motor, or autonomic spinal dysfunction
      - Bilateral signs and/or symptoms

   - A clearly defined sensory level
   - Exclusion of extraaxial compressive causes by neuroimaging
   - Inflammation within the spinal cord as demonstrated by CSF pleocytosis, increased IgG index, or gadolinium enhancement

   b) Exclusion criteria:
      - Previous radiation to the spine in the last 10 years
      - Arterial distribution clinical deficit consistent with thrombosis of the anterior spinal artery
      - Demonstration of a spinal AVM

Pearls

- Transverse myelitis results in rapidly progressive weakness, sensory alterations, and autonomic dysfunction.
- Diagnostic criteria have been proposed by the Transverse Myelitis Consortium Working Group and include inclusion and exclusion criteria.

Suggested Readings

Desanto J, Ross JS. Spine infection/inflammation. *Radiol Clin North Am.* 2011;49(1):105-27.

Transverse Myelitis Consortium Working Group. Proposed diagnostic criteria and nosology of acute transverse myelitis. *Neurology.* 2002;59 (4):499-505.

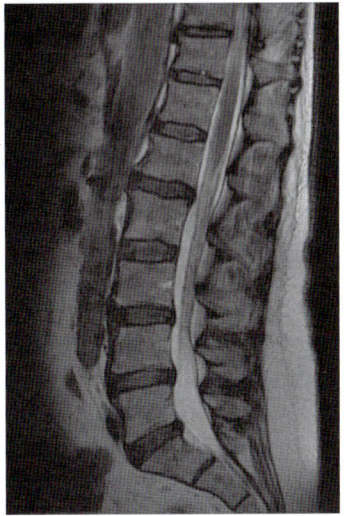
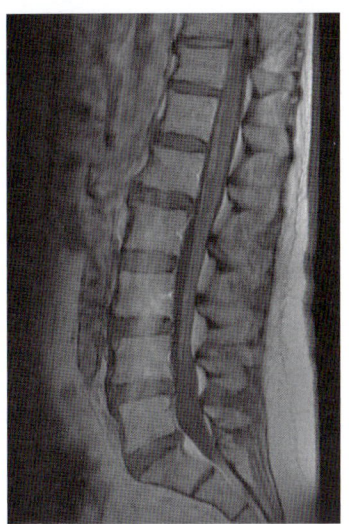

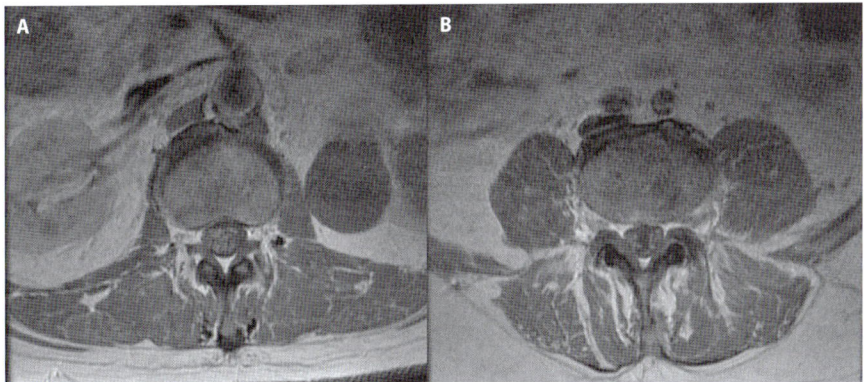

1. What is the most likely diagnosis?

2. What should be included in the differential diagnosis?

3. How can the condition manifest clinically?

4. Which imaging modality best images this condition?

5. Which imaging findings may be seen in this condition?

Case ranking/difficulty:

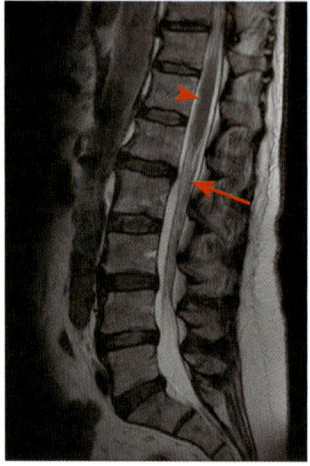

Sagittal T2-weighted sequence of the lumbar spine. The conus terminates at L1 level. Note abnormal thickening ventral to the conus medullaris (*arrowhead*) and along the cauda equina roots (*arrow*). The vertebrae are normal in height with preserved marrow signal.

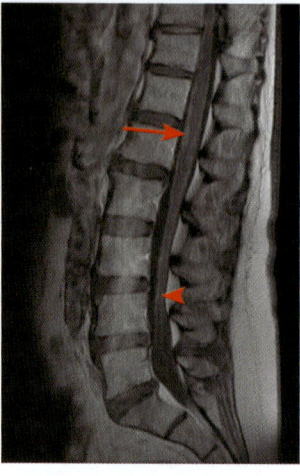

Contrast-enhanced sagittal T1-weighted sequence of the lumbar spine. There is abnormal thick leptomeningeal enhancement at the level of the conus (*arrow*) and along the cauda equina roots (*arrowhead*).

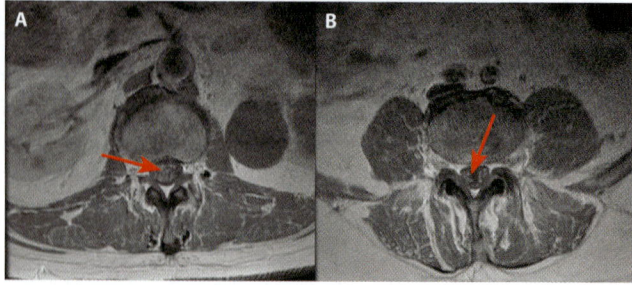

Post-contrast axial T1 images of the lumbar spine. Note diffuse nodular (*arrows*) leptomeningeal enhancement of the cauda equina roots.

Answers

1. Sarcoidosis is a multisystem granulomatous disease characterized by the formation of noncaseating granulomas. Neurosarcoidosis refers to the involvement of the central nervous system by sarcoidosis. Although the CNS may be involved in up to 25% of patients suffering from systemic sarcoidosis, only 5% of those affected are symptomatic.

2. The diagnosis of neurosarcoidosis is challenging as both the clinical symptoms and radiological findings are nonspecific and may mimic other conditions. Differential diagnoses include infectious, granulomatous, demyelinating, neoplastic, and connective tissue disorders. Definitive diagnosis of neurosarcoidosis can only be made by biopsy, which demonstrates epithelioid granulomas without caseation or staining for infectious agents.

3. Clinical manifestations of neurosarcoidosis depend on which site is affected. Cranial nerve palsies, symptoms of increased intracranial pressure, pituitary hormone deficiency, seizures, motor and sensory dysfunctions may be seen. Spinal cord involvement presents with lower extremity weakness and other signs of myelopathy.

4. MRI is the imaging modality of choice. Contrast-enhanced T1-weighted sequences are essential as subtle findings may be otherwise overlooked. Leptomeningeal enhancement can be focal or diffuse.

5. Spinal involvement may be further subclassified into
   1) Intradural extramedullary findings including leptomeningeal enhancement, isointense-enhancing root nodules, and clumping of cauda equina roots.
   2) Extradural findings include spondylodiskitis and paraspinal masses.
   3) Intramedullary sarcoidosis occurs in less than 1% of cases and causes severe neurologic sequelae.

Pearls

- Neurosarcoidosis refers to the involvement of the central nervous system by sarcoidosis—a multisystem granulomatous disease characterized by the formation of noncaseating granulomas.
- MRI is the imaging modality of choice.
- Early treatment with corticosteroids reduces the neurologic complications and disease morbidity.

Suggested Readings

Nozaki K, Judson MA. Neurosarcoidosis. *Curr Treat Options Neurol.* 2013 Aug;15(4):492-504.

Smith JK, Matheus MG, Castillo M. Imaging manifestations of neurosarcoidosis. *AJR Am J Roentgenol.* 2004 Feb;182(2):289-295.

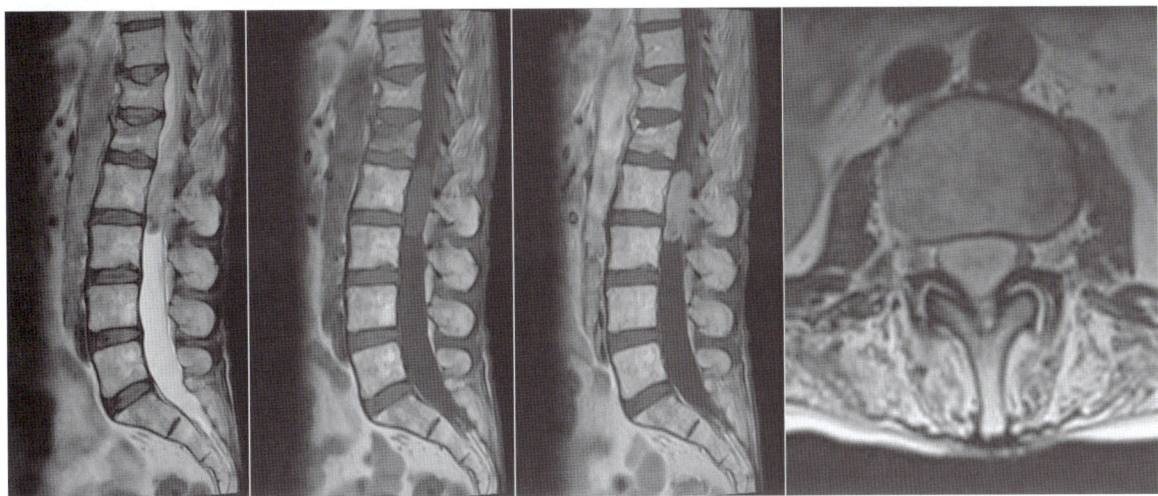

1. What should be included in the differential diagnosis?

2. What is the most likely diagnosis?

3. What is the classic imaging appearance of this condition?

4. Where do these lesions tend to occur?

5. What is the WHO classification of these lesions?

Case ranking/difficulty: **Category:** Filum

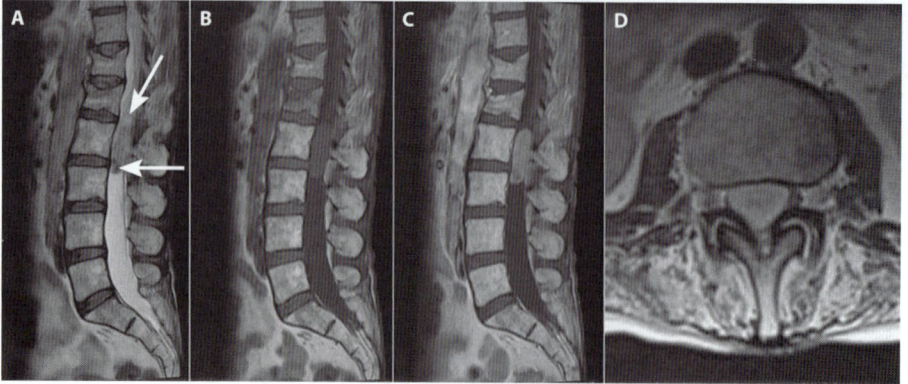

Sagittal T2-weighted image shows an oval-shaped heterogeneous mass at the level of L2 vertebral body. The mass is intradural and arises from the filum terminale. A subtle hypointense rim along the caudal aspect of the lesion and coarse hypointense foci at the inferior tumoral pole (*arrows*, Image A) represent blood products and are frequent findings in spinal ependymomas. The lesion enhances homogenously after contrast administration (Image B = precontrast T1; Image C = post-contrast T1) and reflects the hypervascular nature of the tumor. Image D clearly shows the intradural location of the tumor.

Answers

1. Schwannomas, paragangliomas, and metastases are often intradural extramedullary lesions that may be found in the region of the filum terminale. Disc prolapse is extradural, whereas cavernomas are usually intramedullary.

2. Myxopapillary ependymoma is a slow-growing tumor (WHO grade I) that arises predominantly in the region of the filum terminale.

3. Myxopapillary ependymomas typically appear as a hyperintense sausage-shaped mass in the region of the filum terminale. Intratumoral hemorrhage is common, which may result in characteristic hemosiderin caps. Enhancement postcontrast is typical.

4. Myxopapillary ependymomas typically occur in the region of the filum terminale.

5. Myxopapillary ependymomas are slow-growing tumors and are regarded as tumors of low-grade malignancy (WHO grade I).

Pearls

- Myxopapillary ependymomas are WHO grade I tumors that arise from the filum terminale and account for 13% of all ependymomas.
- They affect a younger population with a mean presentation age of 36 years.
- Myxopapillary ependymomas are intradural extramedullary masses that enhance post-contrast administration.
- Differential diagnoses include other subtypes of ependymoma, astrocytoma, hemangioblastoma, and nerve sheath tumors.
- Surgical resection may be possible and is associated with a more favorable outcome.

Suggested Readings

Schittenhelm J, Becker R, Capper D, et al. The clinico-surgico-pathological spectrum of myxopapillary ependymomas--report of four unusal cases and review of the literature. *Clin Neuropathol.* 2008 Jan-Feb;27(1):21-28.

Wippold FJ 2nd, Smirniotopoulos JG, Moran CJ, Suojanen JN, Vollmer DG. MR imaging of myxopapillary ependymoma: findings and value to determine extent of tumor and its relation to intraspinal structures. *AJR Am J Roentgenol.* 1995 Nov;165(5):1263-1267.

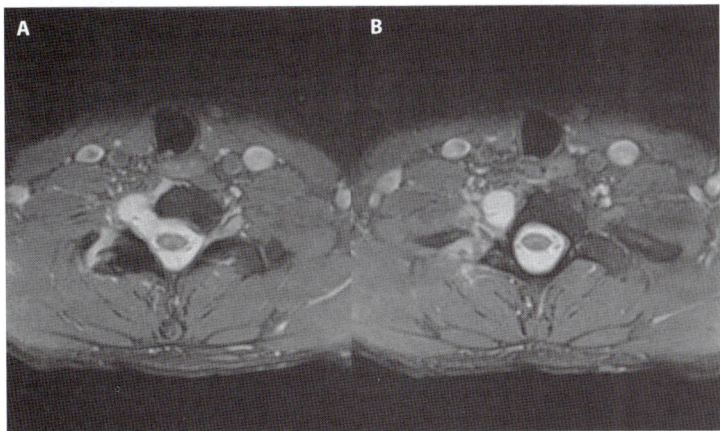
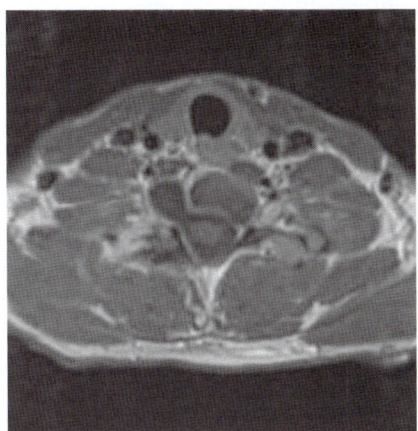

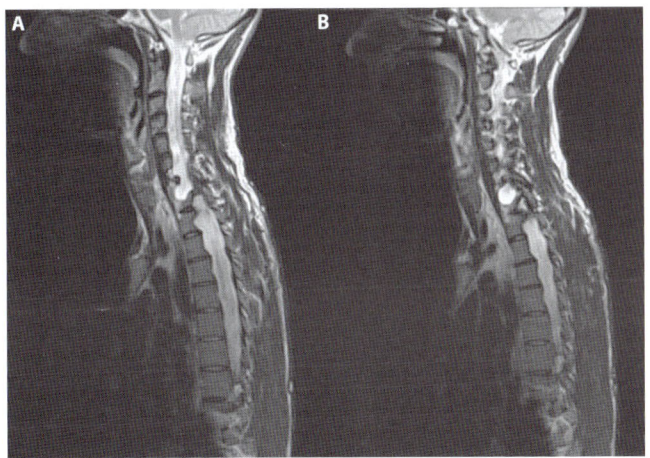

1. What is the most likely diagnosis?

2. What should be included in the differential diagnosis?

3. Which conditions are associated with this finding?

4. What is this finding called in the absence of an underlying condition?

5. What are the typical MR findings in this condition?

Case ranking/difficulty:

Category: Thecal sac

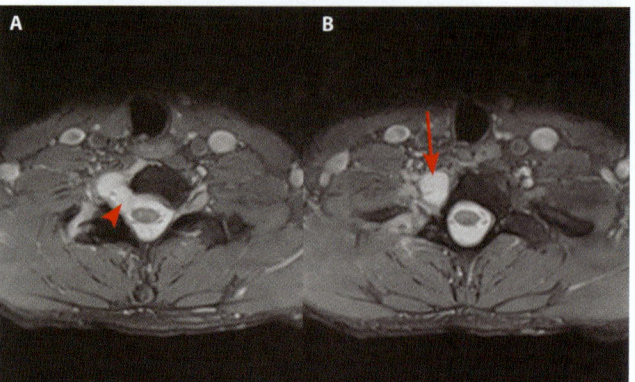

Axial T2-weighted sequence of the thoracic spine. Panel B is at a slightly more caudal level than panel A. A right lateral meningocele is seen (*arrow*) exiting through a widened right intervertebral foramen (*arrowhead*).

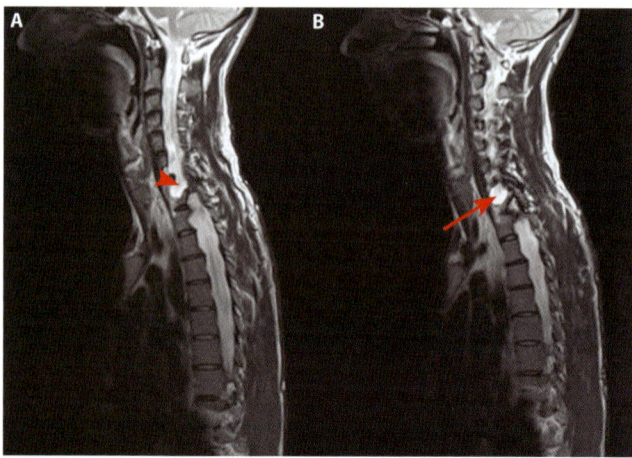

Sagittal T2-weighted sequence of the thoracic spine. Panel B is at a slightly more lateral plane than A. A lateral meningocele is seen (*arrow*) exiting through a widened right intervertebral foramen (*arrowhead*).

Answers

1. Lateral meningocele is a rare anomaly where protrusion of the dura mater and arachnoid extend laterally through an enlarged intervertebral foramen.

2. Extramedullary hematopoiesis, neurofibromatosis, and neurenteric cyst should also be included in the differential diagnoses.

3. Lateral meningocele may be associated with underlying syndromes including Marfan syndrome, Ehlers-Danlos syndrome, and neurofibromatosis type 1.

4. When multiple meningoceles are seen in the absence of an underlying condition, it is called Lehman syndrome or lateral meningocele syndrome.

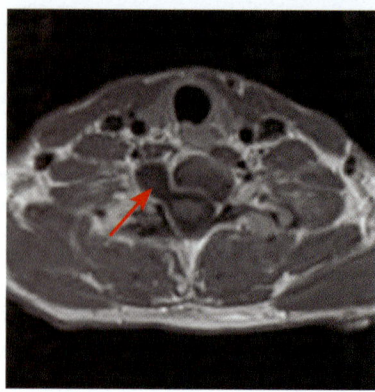

Contrast-enhanced axial T1-weighted sequence of the thoracic spine shows a right lateral meningocele (*arrow*). Note the widened intervertebral foramen.

5. Meningoceles appear as well-defined round, smooth, or lobulated paraspinal masses. The lesions follow CSF signal and appear hypointense on T1-weighted images and hyperintense on T2-weighted images. Enlarged neural foramina and vertebral scalloping may also be seen.

Pearls

- Lateral meningocele is a protrusion of the dura mater and arachnoid through an enlarged intervertebral foramen.
- Lateral meningocele may be associated with underlying syndromes including Marfan syndrome, Ehlers-Danlos syndrome, and neurofibromatosis type 1.
- Occasionally multiple lateral meningoceles may occur in the absence of an underlying condition when it is called Lehman syndrome.
- The lesions follow CSF signal on MRI.
- Surgical excision is only recommended in symptomatic lesions.

Suggested Readings

Alves D, Sampaio M, Figueiredo R, Leão M. Lateral meningocele syndrome: additional report and further evidence supporting a connective tissue basis. *Am J Med Genet A*. 2013 Jul;161A(7):1768-1772.

Gripp KW, Scott CI Jr, Hughes HE, et al. Lateral meningocele syndrome: three new patients and review of the literature. *Am J Med Genet*. 1997 Jun 13;70(3):229-239.

Kumar BE, Hegde KV, Kumari GL, Agrawal A. Bilateral multiple level lateral meningocoele. *J Clin Imaging Sci*. 2013 Jan 30;3:1.

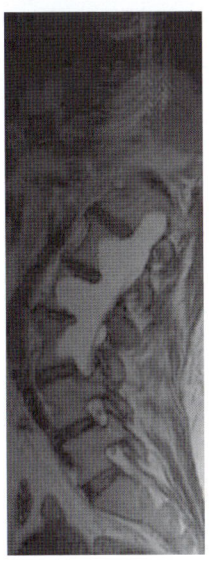 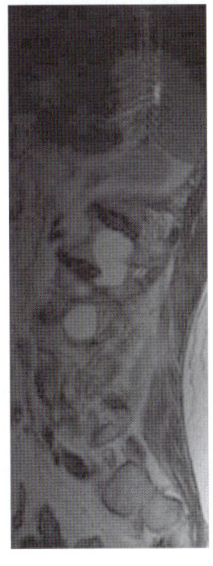 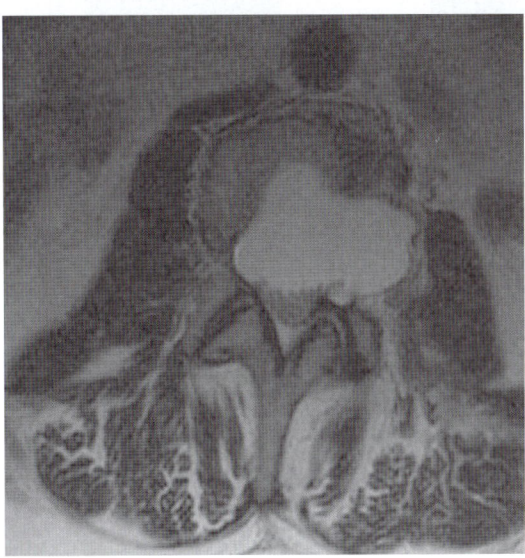

1. Name some "cardinal clinical features" of this condition.

2. Which conditions form part of the "neurocutaneous syndromes?"

3. Which conditions may cause posterior vertebral scalloping?

4. Which pattern of inheritance does this condition have?

5. Which CNS manifestations are seen in this condition?

Case ranking/difficulty:

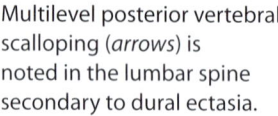

Multilevel posterior vertebral scalloping (*arrows*) is noted in the lumbar spine secondary to dural ectasia.

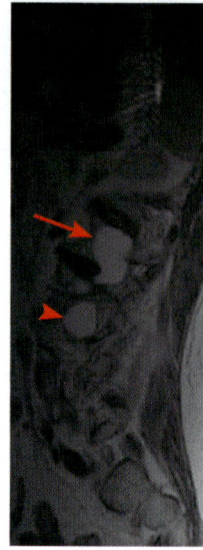

There is multilevel posterior vertebral scalloping (*arrow*) in the lumbar spine. Also note the enlargement of the intervertebral foramen (*arrowhead*).

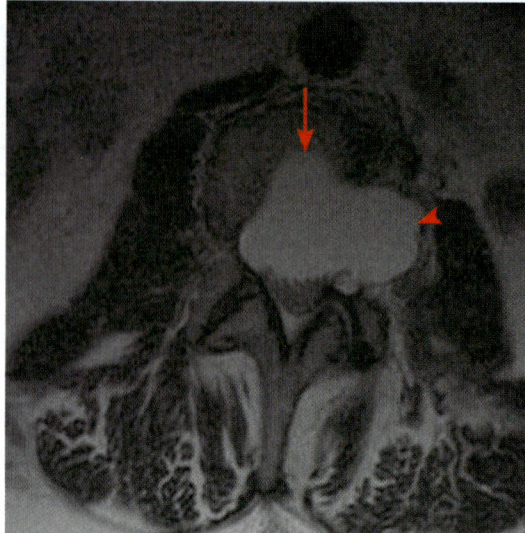

Axial image demonstrates posterior vertebral scalloping (*arrow*) and widening of the left intervertebral foramen (*arrowhead*).

Answers

1. Two out of seven "cardinal clinical features" need to be present for a diagnosis of Neurofibromatosis type 1 to be made. These include
   1) Six or more café-au-lait spots
   2) Two or more neurofibromas or 1 plexiform neurofibroma
   3) Axillary freckling
   4) Optic glioma
   5) Two or more Lisch nodules
   6) A distinctive osseous lesion
   7) A first-degree relative with NF-1

2. Neurocutaneous syndromes include neurofibromatosis, tuberous sclerosis, Sturge-Weber syndrome, von Hippel-Lindau disease, ataxia telangiectasia, Wyburn-Mason syndrome, incontinentia pigmenti, and nevoid basal cell carcinoma syndrome.

3. Posterior vertebral scalloping is seen in achondroplasia, acromegaly, neurofibromatosis type 1, mucopolysaccharidoses, and osteogenesis imperfecta tarda.

   Connective tissue disorders including Marfan disease and Ehlers-Danlos syndrome may also cause posterior vertebral scalloping secondary to dural ectasia.

4. NF-1 has an autosomal dominant inheritance with almost a 100% penetrance. However, 50% of cases are sporadic. The affected NF-1 gene is located on chromosome 17.

5. CNS findings in NF-1 include hydrocephalus, lateral and anterior meningoceles, cranial and spinal nerve neurofibromas, CNS hamartomas, cerebral gliomas, Moyamoya phenomenon, and spongiotic myelinopathy.

Pearls

- Neurofibromatosis type 1 is an autosomal dominant disorder.
- The NF-1 gene was mapped to chromosome 17q11•2.
- The diagnosis of neurofibromatosis type 1 requires two of the seven "cardinal" clinical criteria to be present.
- NF-1 patients have a higher incidence of tumors including pheochromocytomas, intestinal tumors and malignant nerve sheath tumors.
- Skeletal abnormalities occur in 25%-40% of NF-1 patients.
- Multiple spinal manifestations (including posterior vertebral scalloping, lateral meningoceles, and scoliosis) are seen in NF-1.

Suggested Readings

Hillier J, Moskovic E. The soft-tissue manifestations of neurofibromatosis type 1. *Clin Radiol.* 2005;(9):960.

Reynolds R, Browning G, Nawroz I, Campbell I. Von Recklinghausen's neurofibromatosis: neurofibromatosis type 1. *Lancet.* 2003 May 3;361(9368):1552.

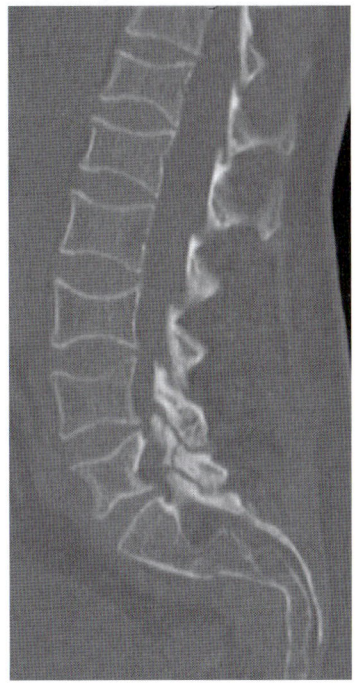 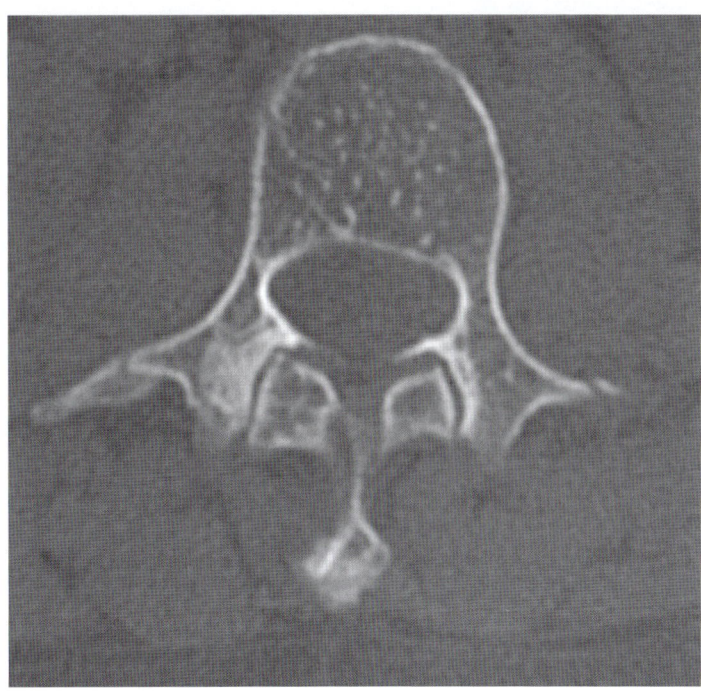

1. What features are demonstrated on the CT images?

2. What is the most likely diagnosis?

3. What is the underlying abnormality in all types of this condition?

4. Which type of the disease is usually the most severe?

5. Histologically, this entity may resemble what condition?

Case ranking/difficulty:

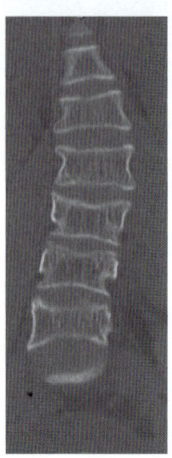

Pars interarticularis fracture (*arrowhead*), displaced S2 fracture (*arrow*), and diffuse osteoporosis with biconcave vertebral bodies.

Numerous biconcave vertebral bodies.

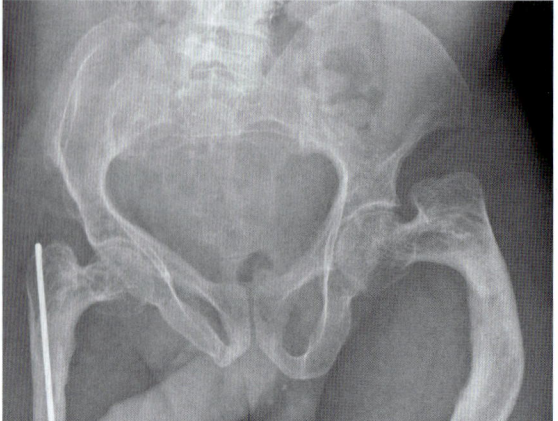

Marked pelvic bone and femoral deformity, osteoporosis, and treated right femoral fracture.

Answers

1. The bones are osteopenic with multiple fractures and deformity.

2. Type 1 osteogenesis imperfecta usually has mild disease and usually presents later in life. Severe disease but with survival beyond the first year suggests osteogenesis imperfecta (OI) type 3.

3. A defect in the quantity and/or quality of collagen is the underlying problem in osteogenesis imperfecta, with a defect in the quality being more problematic. In the Type 2 variant both the quality and quantity of collagen are affected, accounting for the severity of disease.

4. Type 2 osteogenesis imperfecta is the most severe type of osteogenesis imperfecta, with death in the first few weeks of life. Types 5 and 6 are variants of Type 4, and Types 7 and 8 are rare recessive forms.

5. Histologically, osteoporosis and osteogenesis imperfecta are almost identical in appearance.

Pearls

- Osteogenesis imperfecta is a disorder of either the quantity or quality of collagen, or both. Disorders of the collagen quality lead to more severe disease.
- The bones are osteopenic, and are prone to fractures.
- Type 1 disease is mild, with propensity for fracture but no deformity. These patients have blue sclera and deafness.
- Type 2 is most severe and is incompatible with life.
- Type 3 is more severe than Type 1, with multiple fractures and deformity.
- Type 4 is more severe than Type 1. This form is the type most often confused with nonaccidental injury.
- Prenatal ultrasound may be diagnostic, with thin calvaria that are easily compressible or fractured. Increased acoustic through transmission occurs.

Suggested Readings

Ablin DS, Greenspan A, Reinhart M, Grix A. Differentiation of child abuse from osteogenesis imperfecta. *AJR Am J Roentgenol*. 1990 May;154(5):1035-1046.

Ablin DS. Osteogenesis imperfecta: a review. *Can Assoc Radiol J*. 1998 Apr;49(2):110-123.

Neck pain and stiffness

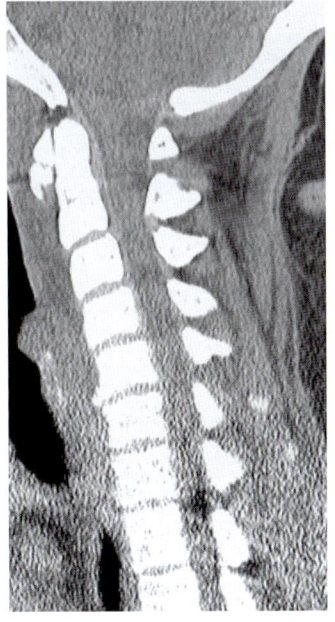 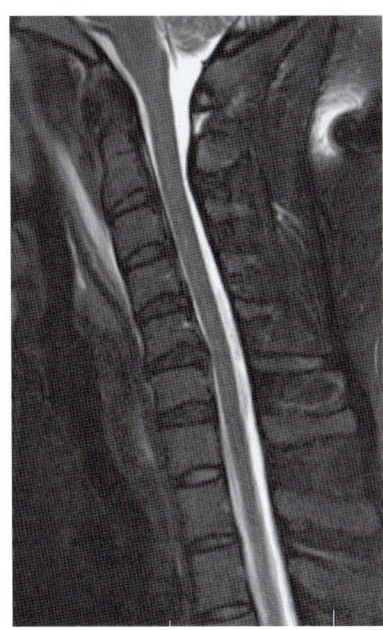

1. What are the CT and MRI findings?

2. The affected structure has three important components. Name them.

3. Which component is most commonly affected?

4. Which age group is most commonly affected?

5. What is the most appropriate treatment?

Case ranking/difficulty:

Category: Paraspinal soft tissue

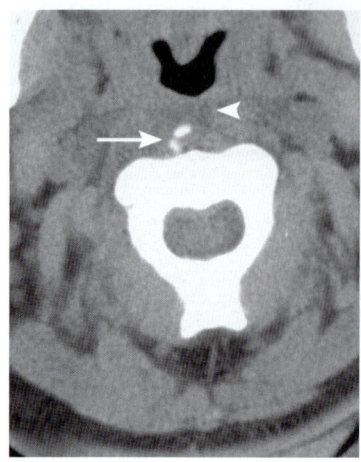

Calcium hydroxyapatite deposition in the longus colli muscle (*arrow*). Prevertebral fluid collection (*arrowhead*).

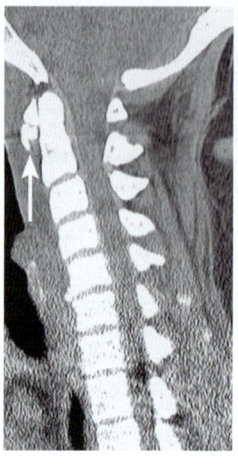

Calcium hydroxyapatite deposition in the longus colli muscle (*arrow*).

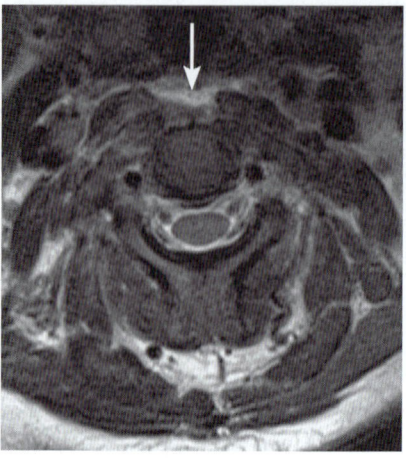

Prevertebral fluid collection.

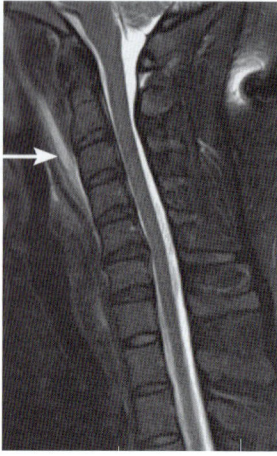

Lentiform prevertebral fluid collection.

Answers

1. There is calcification in the longus colli muscle, with a lentiform fluid collection in the prevertebral soft tissues. The findings are consistent with acute calcific tendinitis of the longus colli muscle. The differential diagnosis is retropharyngeal abscess, which can be a mimic both clinically and radiologically.

2. The longus colli muscle has three components: superior oblique, inferior oblique, and vertical.

3. The superior oblique component is most often affected in calcific tendinitis, often just inferior to the arch of C1 or at the C2-3 level.

4. Acute calcific tendinitis of the longus colli muscle is most common in the third to fifth decades, although no age group is spared.

5. Most patients respond very well to NSAIDs. Steroids are reserved for those individuals who fail to respond to NSAIDs.

- Clinical features resemble retropharyngeal abscess, with odynophagia, neck stiffness, and a low-grade fever.
- The calcification is amorphous within the muscle, and best appreciated on CT.
- The degree of calcification does not correlate with symptoms.
- MRI (and CT) often shows a lentiform prevertebral fluid collection without an enhancing wall.
- Treatment is conservative, with good response to NSAIDs.

Suggested Readings

Hall FM, Docken WP, Curtis HW. Calcific tendinitis of the longus coli: diagnosis by CT. *AJR Am J Roentgenol.*1986 Oct;147(4):742-743.

Offiah CE, Hall E. Acute calcific tendinitis of the longus colli muscle: spectrum of CT appearances and anatomical correlation. *Br J Radiol.* 2009 Jun;82(978):e117-e1121.

Silva CF, Soffia PS, Pruzzo E. Acute prevertebral calcific tendinitis: a source of non-surgical acute cervical pain. *Acta Radiol.* 2014;55(1):91-94.

Pearls

- The longus colli muscle has three important components: superior oblique, inferior oblique, and vertical.
- Calcium hydroxyapatite deposition typically occurs in the superior oblique fibers, usually just inferior to the arch of C1 or at the C2-3 levels.

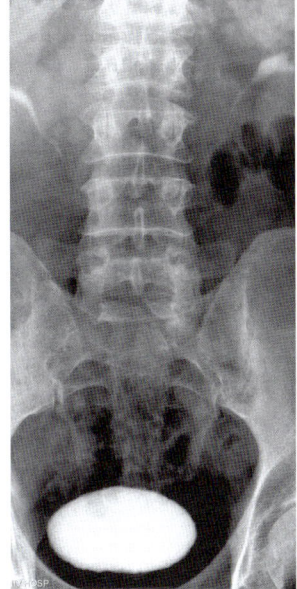
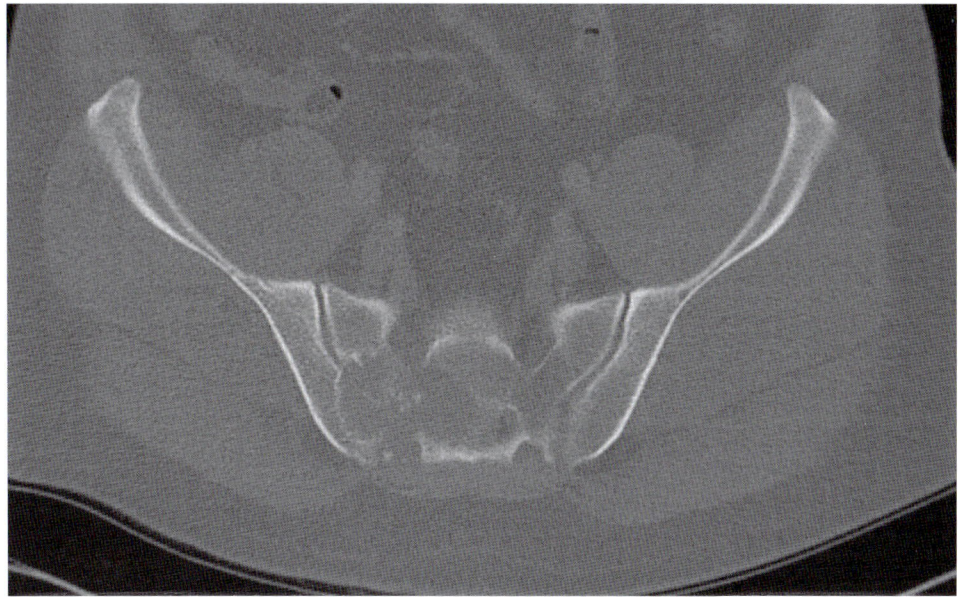

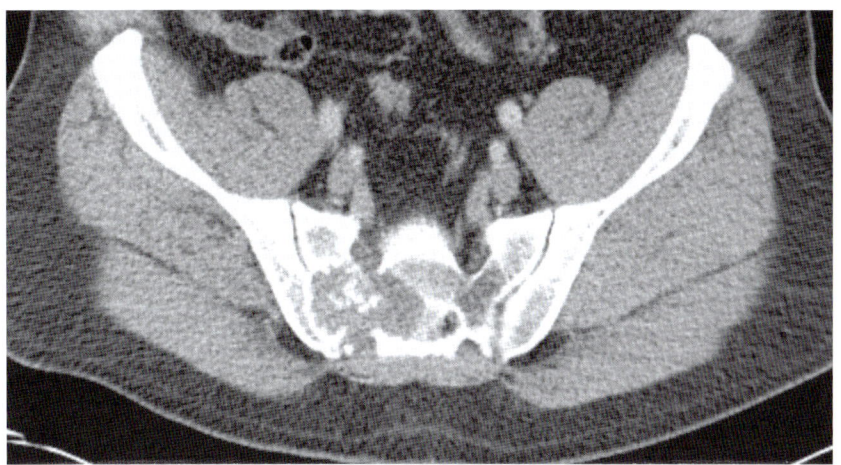

1. What are the major radiologic findings?

2. What is the differential diagnosis?

3. What is the common age group for this entity?

4. What is the appropriate initial management for this entity?

5. What syndromes are associated with an increased risk of this condition?

Case ranking/difficulty:

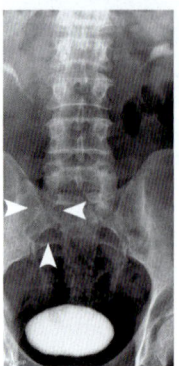

AP film of a contrast urogram shows a faint lucent lesion in the right sacrum.

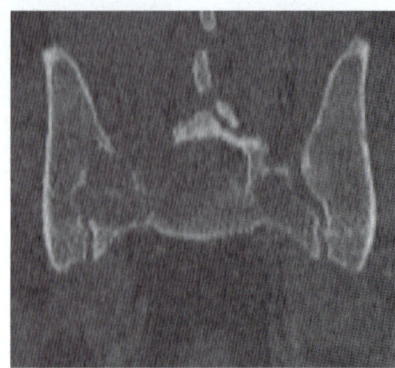

Lesion extends into the sacroiliac joint.

Answers

1. There is a lytic expansile sacral lesion with central "ring and arc" calcification, and extension into the SI joint.

2. The differential includes metastasis, chondrosarcoma, chordoma, plasmacytoma, and giant cell tumor. The presence of central calcification would exclude plasmacytoma and giant cell tumor, as well as metastases (which is also usually multifocal). Central calcification often occurs in chordoma, but not of this "ring and arc" configuration, and chordomas are usually central.

   The diagnosis is therefore chondrosarcoma.

3. Most chondrosarcomas present after the sixth decade of life. They are very rare in adolescents, unlike osteogenic sarcomas.

4. Initial management of sarcomas must be via a multidisciplinary sarcoma service for optimal patient outcome. Injudicious excisional biopsy may jeopardize future curative surgery. Discussion with a specialist surgeon is advised.

   At the appropriate time, closed image-guided core needle biopsy is performed and radical surgical excision with wide margins is the recommended treatment. Postoperative proton beam therapy may be helpful in some cases.

5. Maffucci and Ollier syndromes are associated with an increased risk of chondrosarcoma. The former is the association of multiple enchondromas with cutaneous hemangiomas, which increases the risk of chondrosarcoma by a factor as much as 20 from the normal population. Ollier disease is also associated with an increased risk of chondrosarcoma.

Pearls

- Chondrosarcoma should be in the differential diagnosis of aggressive bone lesions in middle-aged and elderly patients. It is very rare before the fourth decade.
- The characteristic features of chondrosarcoma are matrix mineralization. Thorough evaluation of the nature of the calcification is essential to narrow the differential diagnosis from other primary bone tumors, eg, osteosarcoma.
- Chondrosarcoma is commonly found in typical locations, eg, pelvis, shoulder, diametaphyseal regions of long bones and skull base, although any bone ossifying from cartilage can potentially develop a chondrosarcoma.
- It may occur by sarcomatous transformation of an enchondroma or osteochondroma. Increasing pain and an osteochondroma cartilage cap thickness greater than 2 cm warrant referral to a sarcoma center.
- A large soft tissue mass is commonly associated with chondrosarcoma, although this is also a feature of small round cell tumors and osteosarcoma.
- Syndromes are associated with an increased risk of chondrosarcoma (eg, Ollier—enchondromatosis, and Maffucci syndrome—enchondromas plus hemangiomas).

Suggested Readings

Knoeller SM, Uhl M, Gahr N, Adler CP, Herget GW. Differential diagnosis of primary malignant bone tumors in the spine and sacrum. The radiological and clinical spectrum: minireview. *Neoplasma*. 2008 Dec;55(1):16-22.

Nguyen BD, Daffner RH, Dash N, Rothfus WE, Nathan G, Toca AR. Case report 790. Mesenchymal chondrosarcoma of the sacrum. *Skeletal Radiol*. 1993;22(5):362-366.

Stuckey RM, Marco RA. Chondrosarcoma of the mobile spine and sacrum. *Sarcoma*. 2011 Jul;2011(2011):274281.

Severe neck pain after diving

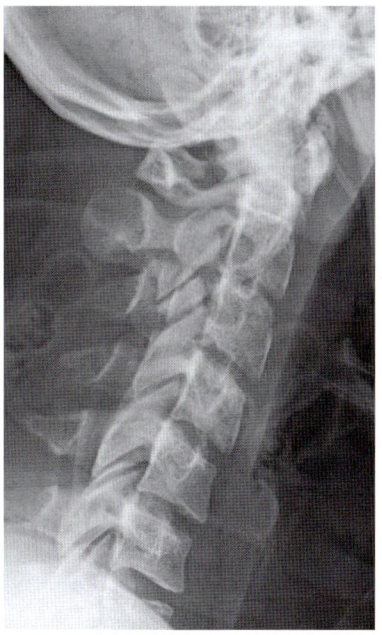 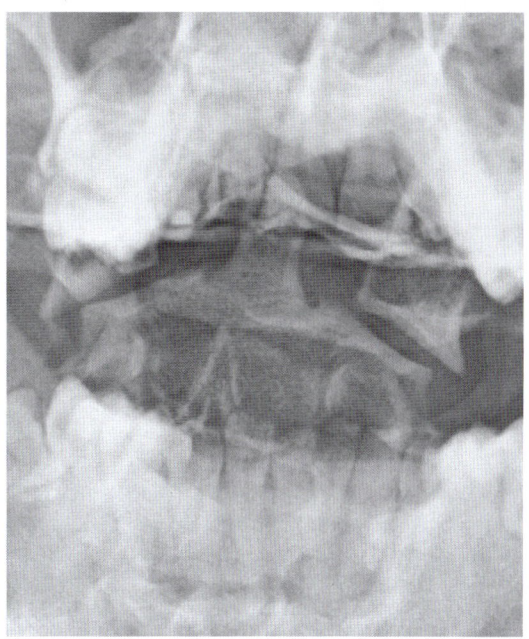

1. What is the mechanism of this injury?

2. What is used to determine the stability of the injury shown?

3. What ligament prevents posterior displacement of the odontoid peg?

4. What is the usual treatment for a stable burst fracture of C1?

5. What is the treatment required for this injury?

Case ranking/difficulty:

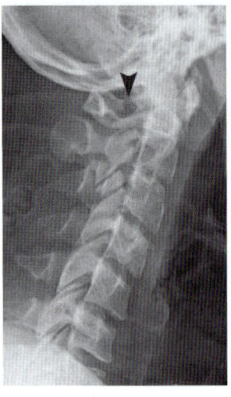

Mild widening of the predental space, break in the arch of C1 (*arrowhead*), and mild prevertebral soft tissue swelling.

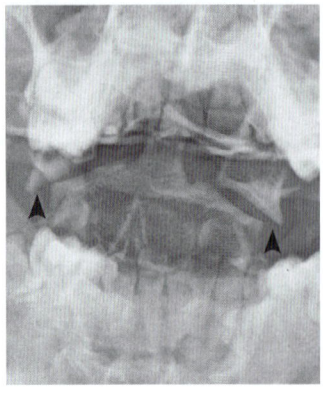

Lateral slippage of the lateral masses of C1, more than 7 mm combined, indicating transverse ligament injury and instability.

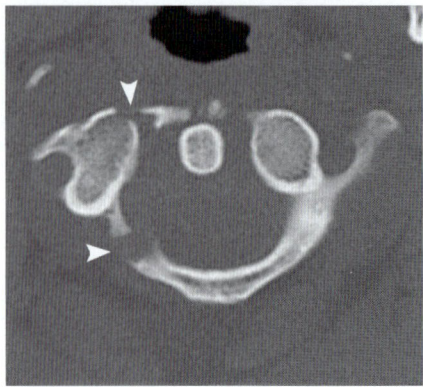

Fracture of the arch of C1 both anteriorly and posteriorly.

Answers

1. Axial loading causes most burst fractures, especially C1 Jefferson fractures. The usual mechanism is sports-related injury or diving into a shallow swimming pool.

2. If the combined lateral mass displacement with respect to the articular surfaces of the axis is greater than 7 mm, the transverse ligament is considered to be ruptured, and the fracture is inherently unstable.

3. The transverse ligament of the atlas is the only structure that prevents posterior displacement of the odontoid peg. It is a very strong ligament, the integrity of which is vital to prevent cord injury. It is at risk of rupture with Jefferson fracture, especially when the lateral masses are involved.

   If it is compromised, stability depends on the integrity of the alar ligaments.

4. The usual treatment for an undisplaced C1 fracture is a halo collar.

5. A displaced Jefferson fracture generally requires surgical stabilization of the cervical spine if the transverse ligament is ruptured, especially if associated with other cervical fractures. Many authorities will attempt nonoperative stabilization with a halo initially, depending on the severity of the injury.

Pearls

- An axial-loading injury results in a burst fracture, which includes a Jefferson (C1) fracture.

- Stability is determined by the integrity of the transverse ligament. If the transverse ligament is interrupted, stability depends on the integrity of the alar ligaments.
- If the lateral masses of C1 are displaced by a total of 7 mm relative to C2, the transverse ligament is torn; the fracture is termed unstable and may require surgical fixation.
- MRI and CT are complementary investigations in cervical spine trauma to assess the cord and bony structures respectively. CTA is also indicated to exclude vertebral artery injury.
- Initial assessment by plain films is adequate if due care and attention is paid to the open-mouth odontoid peg view for displacement of the lateral masses of C1.
- Pre-vertebral soft tissue swelling of greater than a third of the vertebral body from C1 to C3 in trauma cases should immediately trigger a CT examination to assess for an occult fracture, although the decision for a CT scan is often based on clinical parameters.

Suggested Readings

Korinth MC, Kapser A, Weinzierl MR. Jefferson fracture in a child—illustrative case report. *Pediatr Neurosurg.* 2007 Mar;43(6):526-530.

Looby S, Flanders A. Spine trauma. *Radiol Clin North Am.* 2011 Jan;49(1):129-163.

Pratt H, Davies E, King L. Traumatic injuries of the c1/c2 complex: computed tomographic imaging appearances. *Curr Probl Diagn Radiol.* 2007 Mar;37(1):26-38.

Recurrent aspiration when feeding

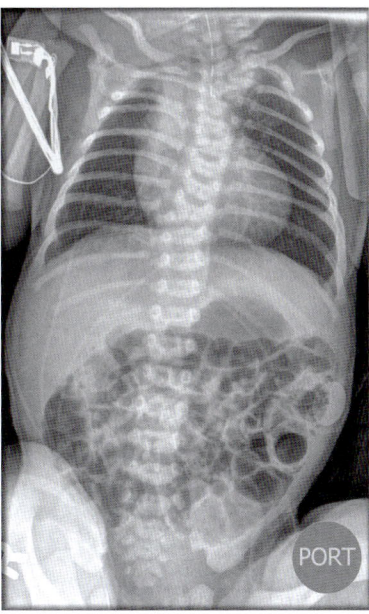

1. What are the pertinent radiographic findings?

2. What is the diagnosis?

3. What are the common cardiac conditions associated with this entity?

4. What umbilical vessel association is seen in this entity?

5. What is the association between the renal and limb abnormalities?

Case ranking/difficulty:

Category: More than one category

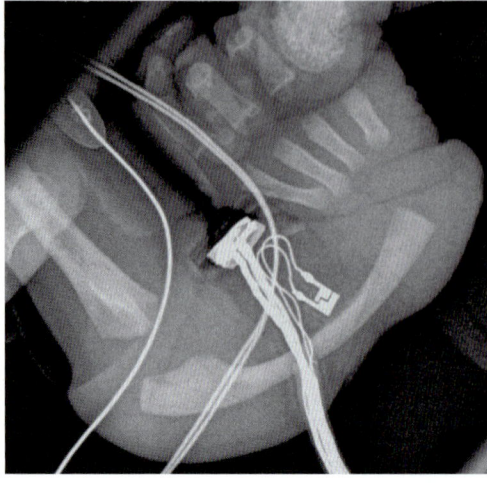

Another patient with an absent radius.

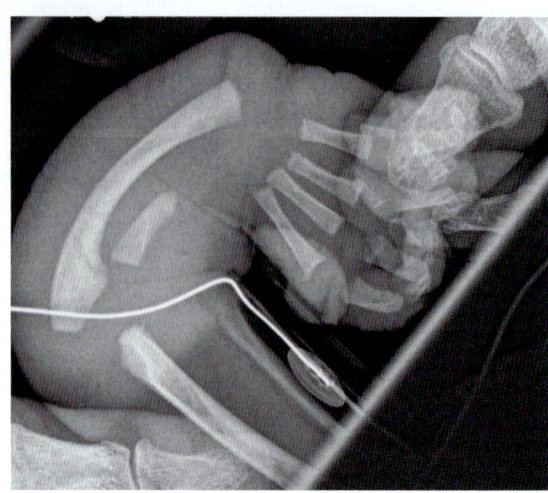

Another patient with a hypoplastic radius. All images courtesy of the Children's Hospital of Philadelphia.

Answers

1. Vertebral segmentation anomalies with synostosis of the upper right ribs are demonstrated. There is esophageal atresia, as evidenced by failure to advance a nasogastric tube.

2. The clinical and radiologic features are consistent with VACTERL syndrome.

3. Numerous cardiac anomalies are described in VACTERL, the most common being ventricular and atrial septal defects. Transposition of the great vessels, tetralogy of Fallot, and truncus arteriosus have also been described. This patient had tetralogy of Fallot and an aberrant right subclavian artery.

4. 35% of VACTERL cases have a single umbilical artery. The normal anatomy is two umbilical arteries and one vein.

5. Babies with unilateral limb abnormalities tend to have renal or urologic abnormalities on the same side. If the limb defects are bilateral, the genitourinary abnormalities are usually bilateral.

- TE: Esophageal atresia with tracheoesophageal fistula.
- R: Renal anomalies including renal malformations, UVJ obstruction, and vesicoureteric reflux.
- L: Limb anomalies including syndactyly, polydactyly, and hypoplastic thumb. Radial ray anomalies are also a feature.
- Occurrence is sporadic with no clear genetic predisposition. Infants of diabetic mothers have a somewhat higher risk.
- Treatment in the early stages includes prompt management of the gastrointestinal, cardiac, and genitourinary features.

Suggested Readings

Solomon BD, Pineda-Alvarez DE, Raam MS, et al. Analysis of component findings in 79 patients diagnosed with VACTERL association. *Am J Med Genet A*. 2010 Sep;152A(9):2236-2244.

Solomon BD. VACTERL/VATER Association. *Orphanet J Rare Dis*. 2011 Jul;6(6):56.

Pearls

- VACTERL syndrome is a nonrandom co-occurrence of numerous birth defects:
  - V: Vertebral defects, including segmentation anomalies and hypoplastic vertebrae.
  - A: Anorectal defects include anal atresia and imperforate anus.
  - C: Cardiac defects including septal defects and tetralogy of Fallot.

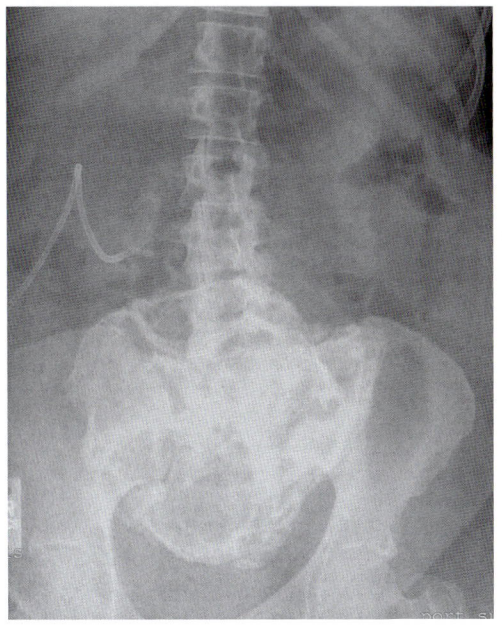 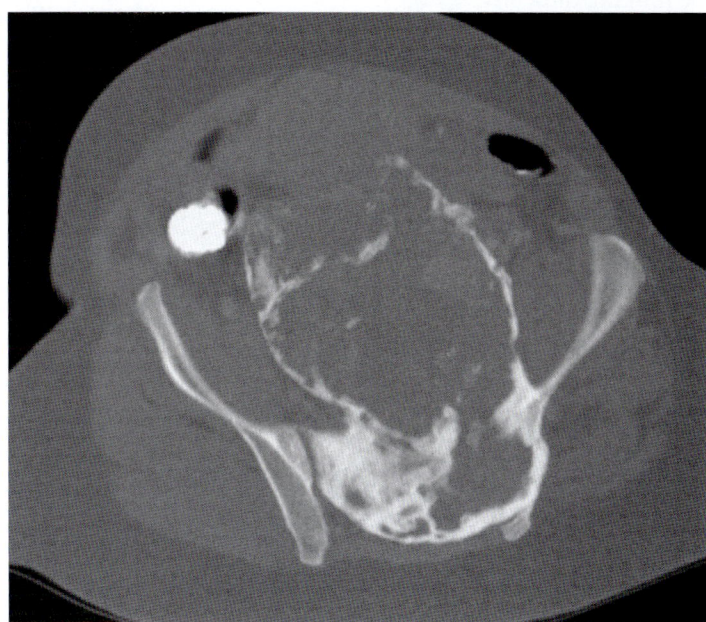

1. What are the findings on the radiograph?

2. What is the differential diagnosis?

3. What is the most likely diagnosis?

4. This entity may occur secondary to what condition?

5. What are the usual MRI signal characteristics of the lesion?

Case ranking/difficulty:

Category: Vertebral body

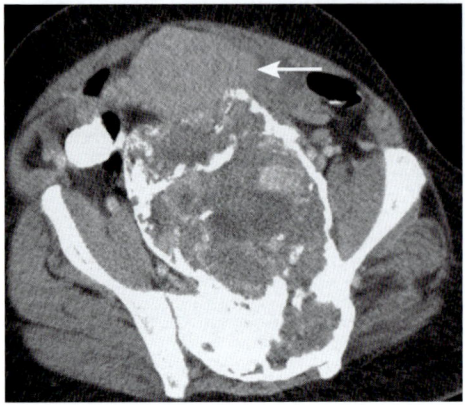

Internal necrosis and areas of hemorrhage. The uterus is displaced by the mass (*arrow*).

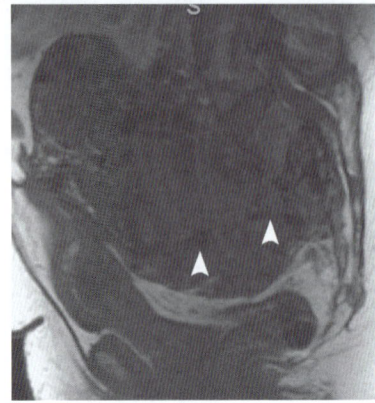

Mass arising from the sacrum. Areas of low T1 and T2 signal likely represents hemosiderin.

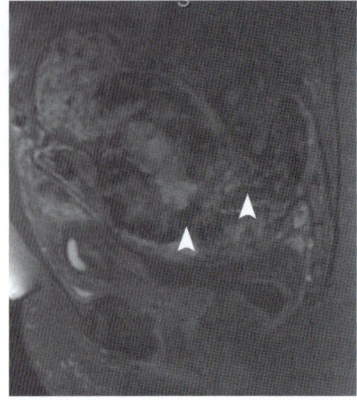

Heterogenous increased T2 signal. Areas of low T1 and T2 signal likely represents hemosiderin. There are no fluid-fluid levels in this case, although these are usually common.

Answers

1. There is a lytic expansile sacral lesion with coarse trabeculae and cortical thinning. Peripheral sclerosis is seen, which is an unusual manifestation.

2. The differential includes sacral chordoma, chondrosarcoma, metastasis, plasmacytoma, and also fibrous dysplasia. Aneurysmal bone cyst is also included in the differential.

3. The age group would make metastasis or plasmacytoma unlikely. Chordomas and chondrosarcomas typically calcify. The most likely diagnosis is giant cell tumor.

4. Giant cell tumor may occur as a rare complication of Paget disease. These typically occur in the skull and facial bones.

5. T1 hypointensity, T2 hyperintensity, and signal heterogeneity. Over 60% of cases have hemosiderin from prior hemorrhage, and will bloom on gradient echo sequences. Fluid-fluid levels are common.

Pearls

- Giant cells tumors typically occur at the end of long bones.
- The distal phalanges are also common especially in cases of multiple giant cell tumors.
- The lesions extend to the subarticular cortex, with expansion of bone and cortical thinning. Lesions are eccentric to the long axis of bone, and do not usually have a sclerotic rim.

- Uncommon locations include the vertebrae, pelvic bones, sacrum, and skull base. In the sacrum, lesions are usually central but often extend to involve the entire sacrum.
- MRI may show fluid-fluid levels, and hemosiderin in over 60% of cases.
- Recurrence is up to 50% if extended curettage is not performed, 10% if it is. Metastasis can occur in 10%-25% of patients, usually to the lungs.

Suggested Readings

Aoki J, Tanikawa H, Ishii K, et al. MR findings indicative of hemosiderin in giant-cell tumor of bone: frequency, cause, and diagnostic significance. *AJR Am J Roentgenol*.1996 Jan;166(1):145-148.

Swanger R, Maldjian C, Murali R, Tenner M. Three cases of benign giant cell tumor with unusual imaging features. *Clin Imaging*. 2008;32(5):407-410.

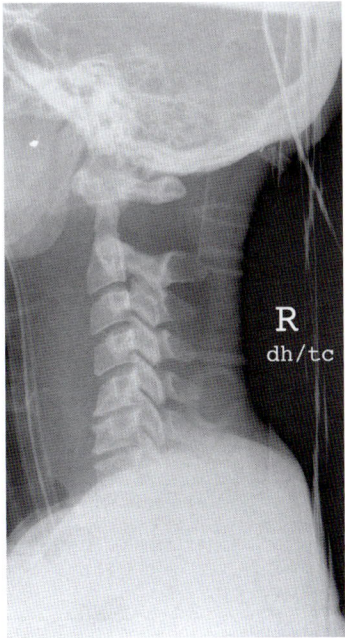 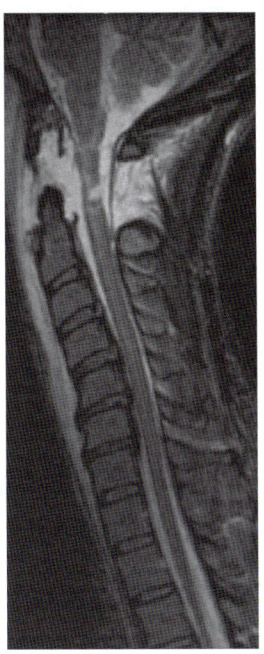

1. What are the imaging findings?

2. What are the major causes of this injury?

3. What is the normal lateral mass interval at the affected level?

4. The injury is associated with a high morbidity and mortality. True or False?

5. Adults are at greater risk of craniocervical dissociation, compared to children. True or False?

Case ranking/difficulty:

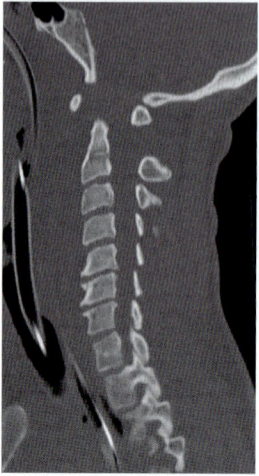

Vertical C1-C2 dissociation, predental widening.

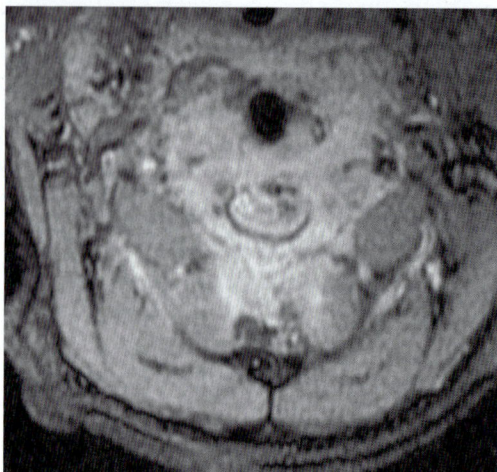

Extensive ligamentous injury and cord transection.

Answers

1. There is vertical dissociation of C1-C2, with marked prevertebral soft tissue swelling. MRI shows extensive ligamentous injury with cord transection.

2. Vertical C1-C2 dissociation occurs as a result of a high velocity injury with a distractive force, as can occur in a motor vehicle accident. Injudicious cervical halo traction can also cause or accentuate the separation.

3. The normal lateral mass interval at C2-C3 is 2.6 mm or less. An increase in this distance should raise the concern for ligamentous injury, and should trigger an MRI to assess for ligamentous injury if the patient is stable. Cervical traction must be avoided.

4. True. Associated injuries include spinal cord injury, cranial nerve palsies, and vertebrobasilar artery injuries. There is a high mortality.

5. False. Because of shallow atlantooccipital joints, lax craniocervical ligaments and relatively large head size, children are more prone to craniocervical dissociation.

Pearls

- Vertical C1-C2 dissociation is rare.
- It may occur as a result of a high-velocity injury with a distractive force, often after a motor vehicle accident. The injury may also occur, or be accentuated by, excessive cervical traction for this or other cervical spine injuries.
- Normal C1-C2 facet joint distance should measure 3 mm or less, and careful evaluation of this space is indicated when ligamentous injury is suspected.
- Lesions have a high morbidity and mortality.
- Treatment is with cessation of traction, and cervical fusion.

Suggested Readings

Botelho RV, de Souza Palma AM, Abgussen CM, Fontoura EA. Traumatic vertical atlantoaxial instability: the risk associated with skull traction. Case report and literature review. *Eur Spine J*. 2000 Oct;9(5):430-433.

Gould S, Hishmeh S, McKinney B, Stephen M. Combined traumatic occiput-C1 and C1-C2 dissociation: 2 case reports. *Am J Orthop (Belle Mead NJ)*. 2010 Aug;39(8):392-395.

Mild leg weakness

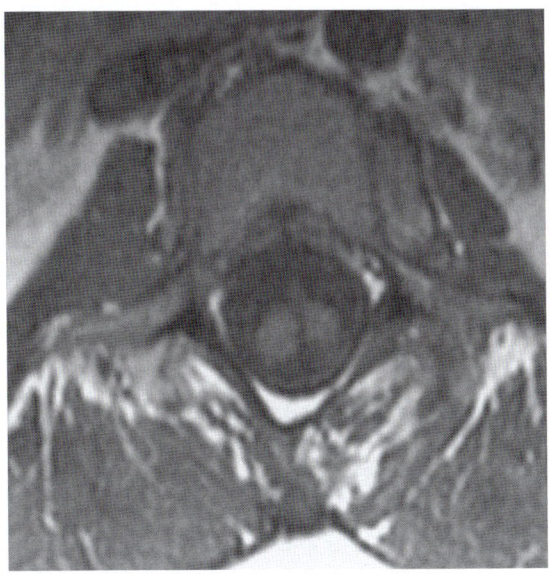 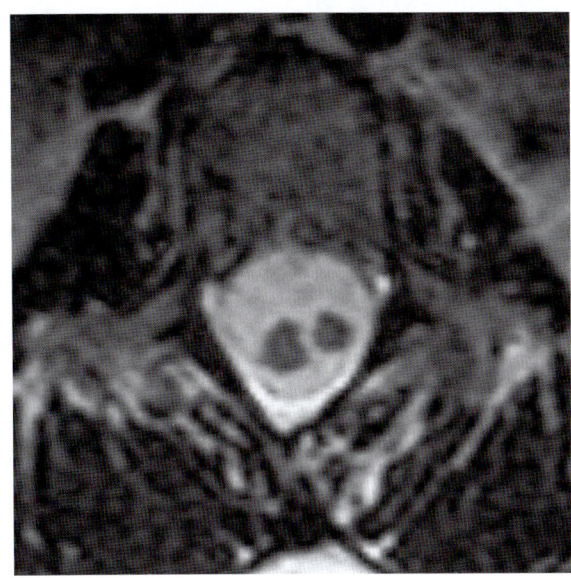

1. What are the major radiologic findings?

2. What is the diagnosis?

3. A bony septum is always demonstrated. True or False?

4. What are some of the associated clinical and radiologic findings?

5. Patients are always symptomatic. True or False?

Case ranking/difficulty: **Category:** Spinal cord

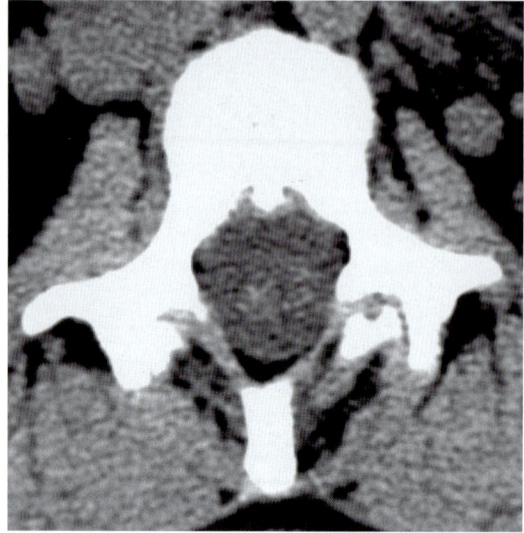

No bony or calcified septum.

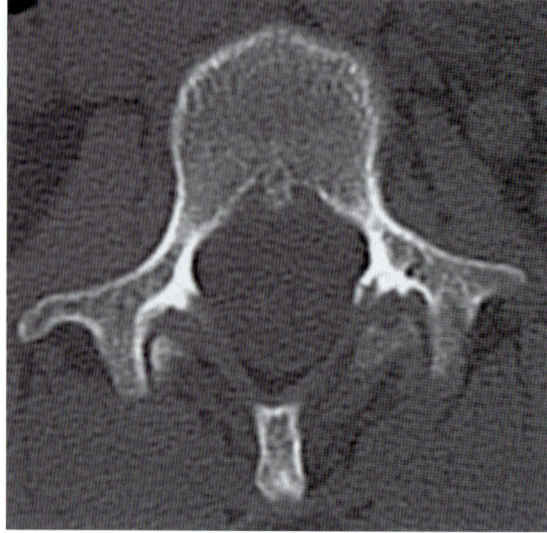

Similar findings.

Answers

1. The lower thoracic and upper lumbar spinal cord is split, with a single dural sac. No bony septum is demonstrated. The cord was tethered, although not demonstrated on these images.

2. The diagnosis is diastematomyelia, part of the split cord malformation syndrome. These fall within the category of occult spinal dysraphism.

3. False. A bony or fibrocartilaginous septum is typically seen in Type 1 SCM, but in Type 2 SCM, a fibrous septum may be seen or there may be no septum.

4. Associated features include hydromyelia, skin pigmentation, hair patches (hypertrichosis), congenital vertebral anomalies, scoliosis, as well as hemangiomas.

5. False. Patients with Type 2 SCM may have mild symptoms or may be completely asymptomatic.

Pearls

- Diastematomyelia belongs to the spectrum of split cord malformations (SCM).
- Type 1 SCM has a bony or fibrocartilaginous septum dividing the two hemicords. Type 2 has a fibrous septum or no septum can be demonstrated.
- Two dural sacs are seen in Type 1 SCM, and one in Type 2.

- Each hemicord has a single set of anterior and posterior nerve roots.
- More than 80% of cases have associated cord tethering, with fatty or thickened filum terminale. Hydromyelia is also often present.
- Clinically, Type 1 disease is more severe. 50% of the disease occurs at L1-3. 25% at T7-12.
- Treatment is with cord untethering and septum resection.

Suggested Readings

Gan YC, Sgouros S, Walsh AR, Hockley AD. Diastematomyelia in children: treatment outcome and natural history of associated syringomyelia. *Childs Nerv Syst.* 2007 May;23(5):515-519.

Rufener SL, Ibrahim M, Raybaud CA, Parmar HA. Congenital spine and spinal cord malformations—self-assessment module. *AJR Am J Roentgenol.* 2010 Mar;194(3 suppl):S38-S40.

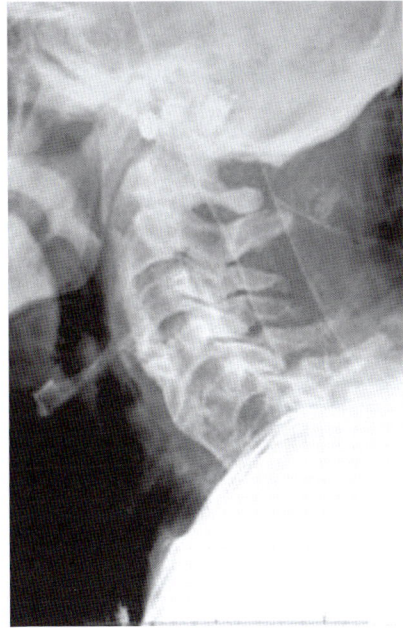 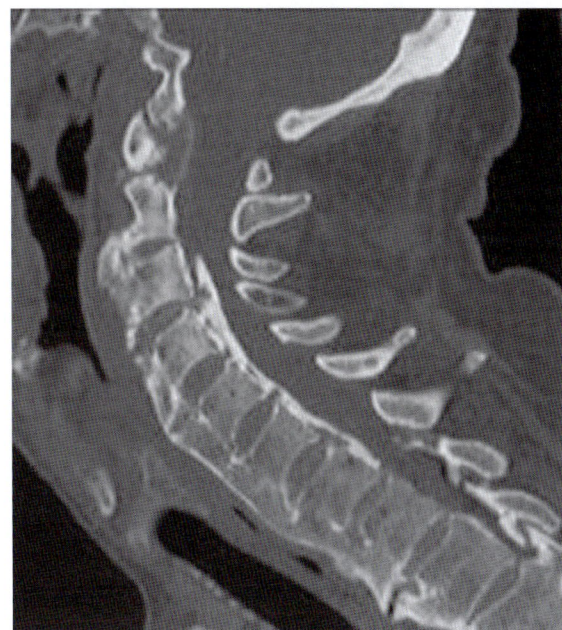

1. What are the findings on the radiographs?

2. What is the epidemiology of the findings in the spinal canal?

3. What is the natural history of the intraspinal finding?

4. What is the best imaging modality when investigating this finding?

5. What are the other associations of the intraspinal finding?

Case ranking/difficulty:

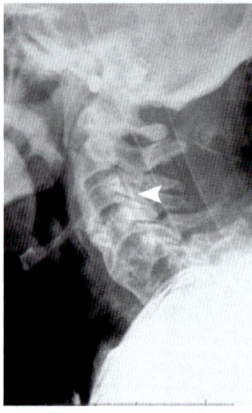

Extensive diffuse idiopathic skeletal hyperostosis (DISH) changes with ossification of the posterior longitudinal ligament (*arrowhead*).

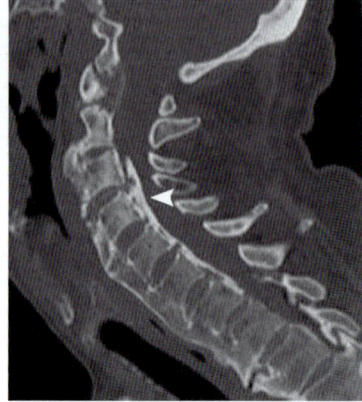

The ossification of the posterior longitudinal ligament (OPLL) is well demonstrated.

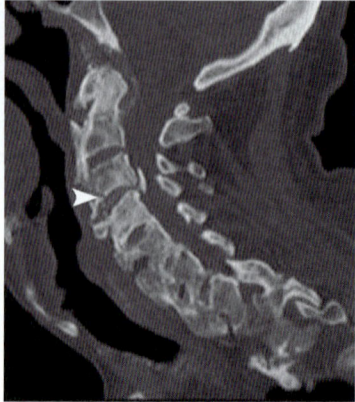

More lateral sagittal image better demonstrates a C3 fracture, the presenting event.

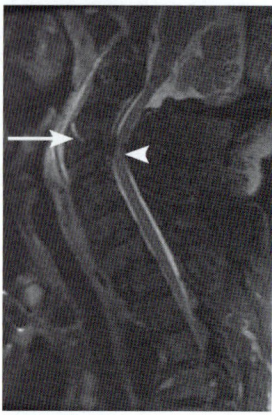

C3 body fracture (*arrow*), OPLL, and cord compression with mild cord edema (*arrowhead*) are well demonstrated.

Answers

1. There is ossification of the posterior longitudinal ligament (OPLL) and anterior paraspinal ossification consistent with DISH. The acute presenting feature was an acute traumatic fracture of the anterior inferior C3 vertebral body, not demonstrated in these radiographs.

2. Ossification of the posterior longitudinal ligament (OPLL) is most common in older Japanese males.

3. OPLL is progressive and may result in spinal stenosis.

4. MRI is the best imaging modality, as it will indicate the extent of OPLL as well as show the degree of spinal stenosis. It will also show cord changes of edema and myelomalacia.

5. 50% of patient with OPLL have DISH. There is also an association of OPLL with the spondyloarthropathies.

Pearls

- Ossification of the posterior longitudinal ligament (OPLL) occurs most commonly among Japanese.
- It may be classified as continuous if the disc is involved (either segmentally or nonsegmentally), or noncontinuous if the disc is not involved.

- The cervical spine at C3-C5 is most commonly affected (75%).
- Plain film and CT show linear ossification posterior to the vertebral bodies and possibly discs, separated by a lucent line (basivertebral venous plexus). CT will also show the degree of spinal stenosis.
- On MRI, OPLL shows T1 and T2 hypointensity with possible central T1 hyperintensity if marrow fat is present. MRI has the advantage of also showing cord changes.
- MRI will also show spinal stenosis and cord changes including cord edema and myelomalacia.

Suggested Readings

Munday TL, Johnson MH, Hayes CW, Thompson EO, Smoker WR. Musculoskeletal causes of spinal axis compromise: beyond the usual suspects. *Radiographics*. 1994 Nov;14(6):1225-145.

Widder DJ. MR imaging of ossification of the posterior longitudinal ligament. *AJR Am J Roentgenol*. 1989 Jul;153(1):194-195.

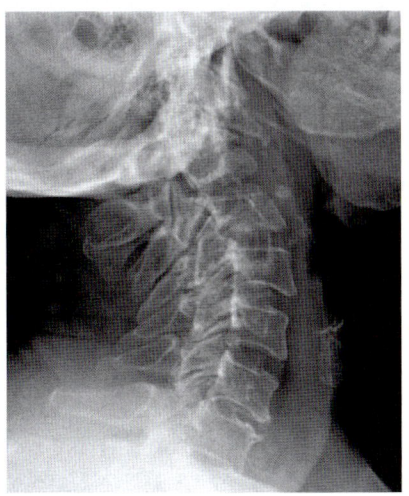
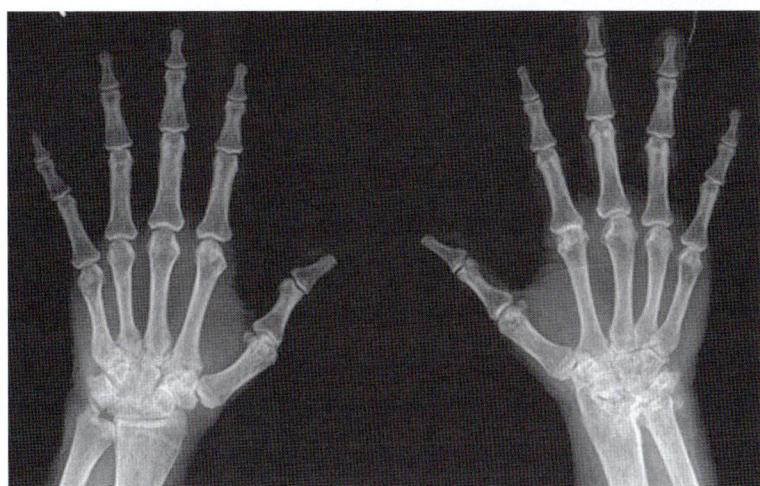

1. What are the relevant radiographic findings?

2. What is the difference between basilar impression and basilar invagination?

3. What are the most important radiological lines used in evaluating this entity?

4. What are the indications for surgery?

5. What are some of the congenital causes for this entity?

Case ranking/difficulty:

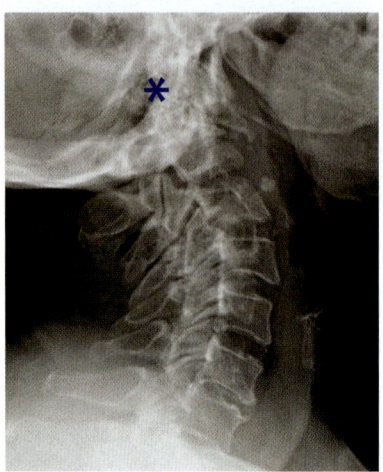

Basilar invagination, with the tip of the odontoid process (*blue asterisk*) lying above Chamberlain line. This line is drawn from the hard palate to the posterior edge of the foramen magnum and is difficult to see on these plain radiographs.

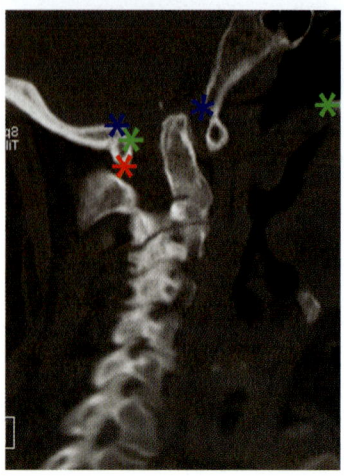

McRae line (between *blue asterisks*), Chamberlain line (between *green asterisks*), and McGregor line (between red and green hard palate *asterisks*).

Answers

1. The tip of the odontoid process projects into the foramen magnum and is consistent with basilar invagination, an acquired abnormality due to bone softening. The presence of carpal bone erosions confirms rheumatoid arthritis as the etiology.

2. Primary basilar impression is a diagnosis of exclusion, and is not a result of bone softening but is believed to be familial with an autosomal dominant inheritance pattern and incomplete penetrance. Basilar invagination is a result of bone-softening conditions such as rheumatoid arthritis and Paget disease.

3. MacGregor line is measured from the hard palate to the caudal posterior occiput curve, and the dens tip should be less than 4.5 mm below this line.

   Chamberlain line is measured from the hard palate to the foramen magnum, and the dens should be less than 6 mm below the line.

   McRae line extends from the posterior clivus to the foramen magnum, and the dens tip should be below the line although minimal protrusion may be acceptable.

   Ranawat line is measured from the center of the C2 pedicle to a line connecting the anterior and posterior arches of C1, and should be 13 mm in a female or 15 mm in a male, with reduced measurements indicating impaction.

4. Progressive neurologic compromise including signs of brainstem compression, syringomyelia or hydromyelia, apnea, and cranial nerve dysfunction.

5. Congenital causes for basilar invagination include osteogenesis imperfecta, achondroplasia, Klippel-Feil syndrome, cleidocranial dysostosis, and Schwartz-Jampel syndrome.

Pearls

- Basilar invagination occurs when the odontoid process migrates superiorly into the foramen magnum.
- It is a result of a bone softening process, including rheumatoid arthritis, Paget disease, and rickets/osteomalacia.
- Primary basilar impression is a diagnosis of exclusion, where there is no evidence of bone softening and is believed to be a familial developmental abnormality.
- Platybasia is a flattening of the skull base and may be a result of a bone-softening process, or may be congenital.
- Important lines to consider include Chamberlain line, MacGregor line, and McRae line.
- Treatment includes odontoid resection by a transoral or anterior retropharyngeal approach, or occipitocervical fusion.

Suggested Readings

Smoker WR. Craniovertebral junction: normal anatomy, craniometry, and congenital anomalies. *Radiographics*. 1994 Mar;14(2):255-277.

Smoker WR. MR imaging of the craniovertebral junction. *Magn Reson Imaging Clin N Am*. 2000 Aug;8(3):635-650.

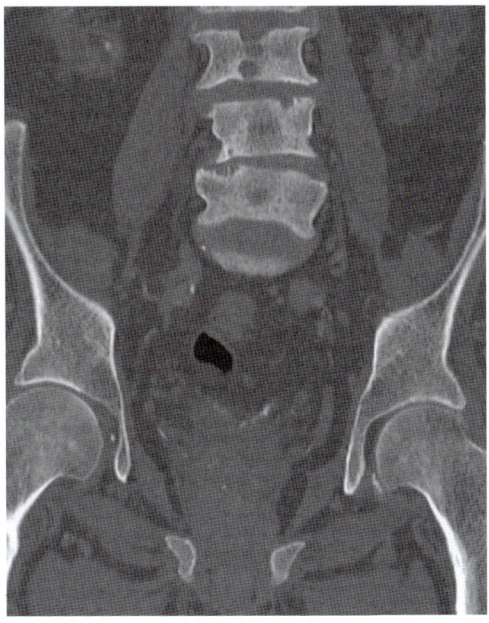 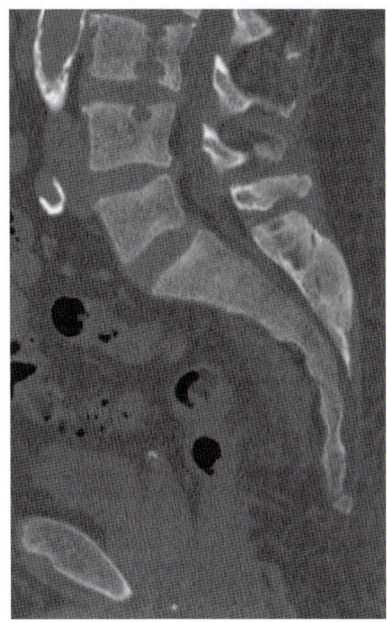

1. What are the findings in the spine?

2. What are included in the differential, and what
    is the most likely diagnosis?

3. What is the next most appropriate study?

4. Where are the common sites affected in this
    condition?

5. What are the findings to be expected on MRI?

Case ranking/difficulty:

Category: More than one category

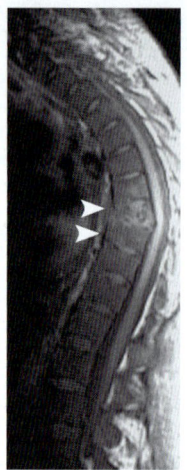

More pronounced disease in another patient, with marked destructive changes and kyphosis in the midthoracic spine.

Corresponding MRI image shows heterogenous signal at the disc. Note anterior prevertebral amyloid deposits (*arrowheads*). Note the similarity to infective spondylodiscitis.

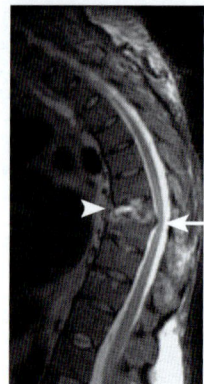

Heterogenous signal, with foci of low T2 signal in the disc and anterior prevertebral soft tissues, consistent with amyloid deposits (*arrowheads*). Note the impingement on the cord (*arrow*).

Answers

1. There is diffuse osteosclerosis, with multilevel erosions and cysts at the endplates, and mild disc space narrowing.

2. The major differentials are infective and amyloid spondylodiscitis. The diffuse osteosclerosis and multilevel involvement, along with a history of long-term dialysis, would make amyloid the most likely diagnosis.

   The presence of increased T2 signal in the disc is, however, not uncommon, often making differentiation from infection more difficult.

   Metastases and lymphoma could demonstrate osteosclerosis, but would not be expected to affect the discs.

3. An MRI would demonstrate the signal characteristics of the discs, the presence of low T2 signal amyloid, and would also show any compressive effects on the cord.

4. Amyloid spondyloarthropathy occurs predominantly, but not exclusively, in dialysis-related amyloid. The shoulders, spine (particularly the lower cervical and lower lumbar spine), wrists, hips, knees, and carpal tunnels are most commonly affected.

5. The disc change of amyloid spondyloarthropathy is typically iso- to hypointense on all pulse sequences; however, the presence of increased T2 signal in the disc is not uncommon. Hence, differentiating from infective spondylodiscitis can be difficult. Paravertebral or ligamentous soft tissue masses would show similar signal. Contrast enhancement is variable.

Pearls

- Amyloid arthropathy results from the extracellular deposition of amyloid in the joint spaces and soft tissues.
- In dialysis patients, it is related to the inability of the dialysis membrane to remove amyloid protein.
- Cervical spine and shoulders are most commonly affected.
- Plain films show cysts, erosions, and periarticular osteopenia. The joint space is preserved or widened until late in the disease.
- In the spine, there are erosions at the endplates and corners of the vertebrae, with disc space narrowing and often soft tissue masses in the prevertebral soft tissues or in the facet/interspinous ligaments. Cord compression may occur.
- Amyloid is low signal on all MR sequences with no paramagnetic effect, differentiating it from PVNS. Contrast enhancement is variable.

Suggested Readings

Cobby MJ, Adler RS, Swartz R, Martel W. Dialysis-related amyloid arthropathy: MR findings in four patients. *AJR Am J Roentgenol*. 1991 Nov;157(5):1023-1027.

Kiss E, Keusch G, Zanetti M, et al. Dialysis-related amyloidosis revisited. *AJR Am J Roentgenol*. 2005 Dec;185(6):1460-1467.

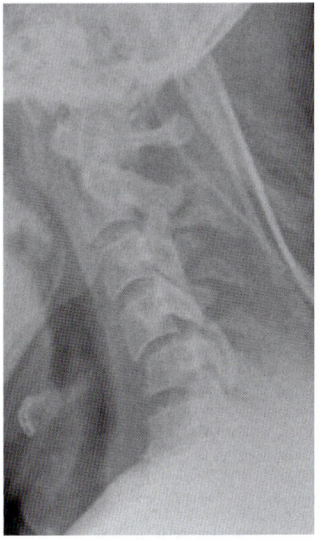 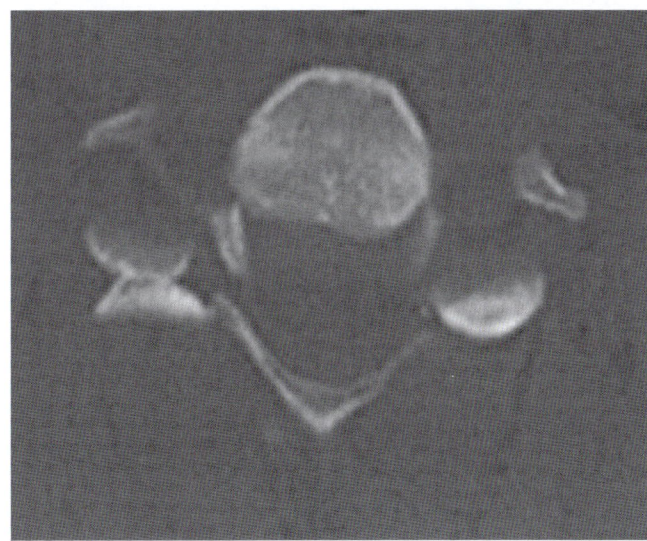

1. What are the imaging findings?

2. What is the mechanism of injury?

3. What injuries to the cervical spine are unstable?

4. In what injury is the hamburger sign seen?

5. What percentage of patients with bilateral injury have neurological compromise?

Case ranking/difficulty:

Category: Vertebral body

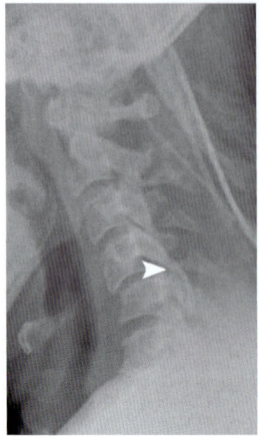

Anterolisthesis of C4 on C5, with a jumped facet (*arrowhead*) and multiple spinous process fractures.

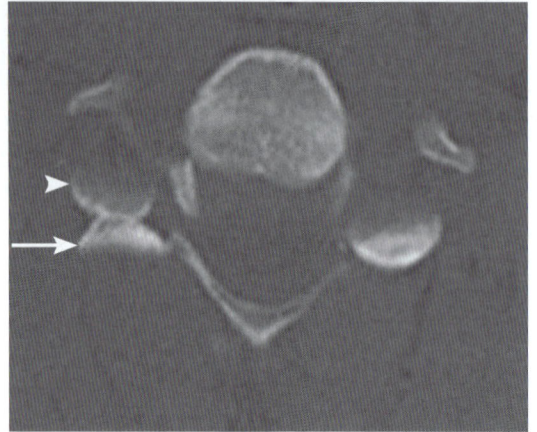

Right "hamburger" sign demonstrated. *Arrowhead* is the inferior facet of the C4 vertebra, and *arrow* the superior facet of C5.

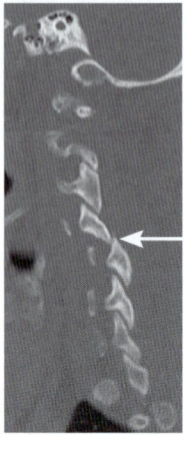

Jumped facet with an associated fracture (*arrow*).

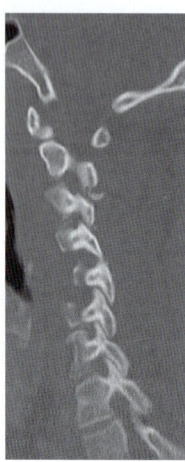

Perched facet on the left side.

Answers

1. There is a hyperflexion injury with a jumped facet, anterolisthesis of C4 on C5, and multiple spinous process fractures. The "hamburger" and "naked facet" signs are the same, and are demonstrated here.

2. The mechanism for this injury is hyperflexion. A rotary component to the injury is contributory.

3. Flexion teardrop, Jefferson and Hangman fractures, Type 2 dens fractures, and bilateral locked facets are unstable fractures. A unilateral locked facet with a fractured facet is also unstable. In addition, hyperextension dislocation is unstable.

4. A "hamburger" sign is seen in a jumped facet. On axial CT, the normal appearance of the facets is said to resemble a hamburger, with the superior articular facet of the vertebra below forming the top bun and the inferior facet of the vertebra above forming the bottom bun, and the space between the "meat." With a jumped facet, the bottom "bun" now lies anterior to the top "bun." This is known as the hamburger or naked facet sign.

5. 75% of patients with bilateral jumped facets have neurological compromise. The listhesis that occurs results in severe canal and foraminal stenosis, with cord compression or transection in severe cases.

Pearls

- A jumped facet is a result of a severe injury, usually MVA or a fall.
- The mechanism is hyperflexion rotation, and is unstable when bilateral or associated with a facet fracture.
- In bilateral jumped facets, there is typically >50% anterolisthesis and the subsequent spinal canal and neuroforaminal stenosis results in neurologic deficit in up to 75% of cases.
- Cord injury ranges from cord edema to cord transection.
- Associated fractures are common, including spinous process, facet, and a triangular corner fracture of the anterosuperior margin of the inferior involved vertebra.
- When the facets lie on to top of each other rather than overlapping, it is called a perched facet.
- The "hamburger" or "naked facet" sign is seen on axial CT images.
- Both CT and MRI are indicated: CT to define the fracture anatomy, and MRI to evaluate the cord, disc, and ligamentous structures.

Suggested Reading

Kornberg M. The computed tomographic appearance of a unilateral jumped cervical facet (the "false" facet joint sign). *Spine (Phila Pa 1976)*. 1986 Dec;11(10):1038-1040.

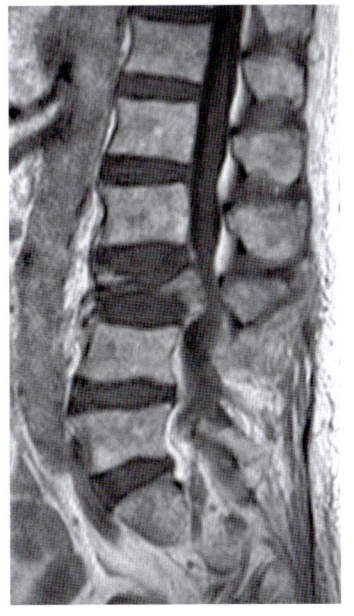 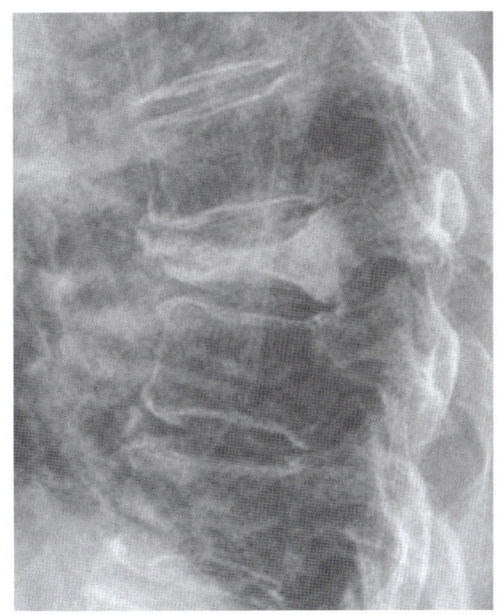

1. What are the radiographic findings?

2. What are the MRI findings?

3. What is the diagnosis?

4. What are the MR features favoring
   osteoporotic over metastatic vertebral collapse?

5. Contrast enhancement is useful in differentiating
   acute osteoporotic cord compression from
   metastatic cord compression. True or False?

Case ranking/difficulty:

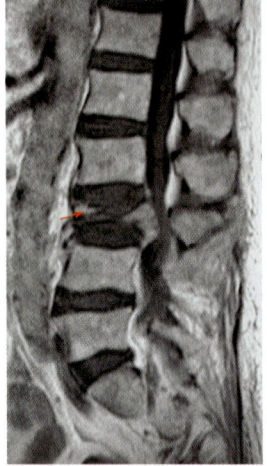

Low T2 signal band (*arrow*) is demonstrated with osteoporotic vertebral collapse.

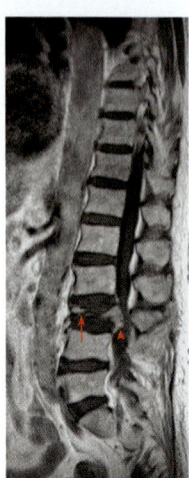

Retropulsed fragment (*arrowhead*) and low-intensity band (*arrow*).

Answers

1. Vertebral compression fracture.

2. The MRI findings are a T1 and T2 low signal intensity band, retropulsion of a posterior bone fragment, and spared marrow signal within the affected vertebral body and other bodies. There is no posterior element involvement, and no paraspinal mass.

3. The findings are suggestive of osteoporotic vertebral collapse.

4. Low signal intensity band on T1 and T2, areas of preserved bone marrow signal intensity in the affected and other vertebrae, multilevel collapse, no posterior element involvement, and no paraspinal mass. These MR features favor osteoporotic collapse.

5. True. Although it is controversial, some authors suggest heterogenous contrast enhancement in metastatic infiltration may be helpful in distinguishing this entity from cord compression secondary to osteoporotic collapse. An enhancing soft tissue mass is also not seen in osteoporosis, but can be seen in metastases.

Pearls

- Osteoporosis is a metabolic disorder affecting the modeling of bone, resulting in bone resorption. This leads to a reduction in bone mineral density.
- It is more common in females, and one in three women over the age of 65 are affected.

- Osteoporosis is one of the major causes of nontraumatic vertebral collapse, and it is important to differentiate from metastatic collapse.
- Plain x-ray and MRI are the main diagnostic tools.
- Plain x-ray: Collapsed vertebra at one or multiple levels. Decreased density of bones with vertical striations, biconcave vertebrae, Schmorl nodes, and picture framing (prominence of the cortical outline due to disproportionate trabecula resorption and peripheral trabecula reinforcement).
- MRI: Low T1 and T2 signal intensity bands, normal marrow signal intensity in other vertebrae and preserved marrow signal in the affected vertebra, posterior bone fragment retropulsion, absence of a paraspinal or epidural mass, and the presence of other compression fractures favor osteoporotic collapse over metastatic collapse.

Suggested Readings

Cuénod CA, Laredo JD, Chevret S, et al. Acute vertebral collapse due to osteoporosis or malignancy: appearance on unenhanced and gadolinium-enhanced MR images. *Radiology*. 1996 May;199(2):541-549.

Jung HS, Jee WH, McCauley TR, Ha KY, Choi KH. Discrimination of metastatic from acute osteoporotic compression spinal fractures with MR imaging. *Radiographics*. 2003;23(1):179-187.

Rumpel H, Chong Y, Porter DA, Chan LL. Benign versus metastatic vertebral compression fractures: combined diffusion-weighted MRI and MR spectroscopy aids differentiation. *Eur Radiol*. 2013 Feb;23(2):541-550. doi: 10.1007/s00330-012-2620-1. Epub 2012 Aug 18.

Sacral and coccygeal pain

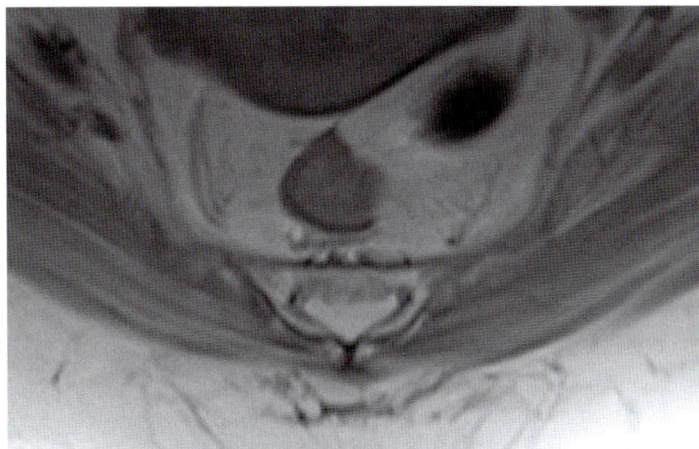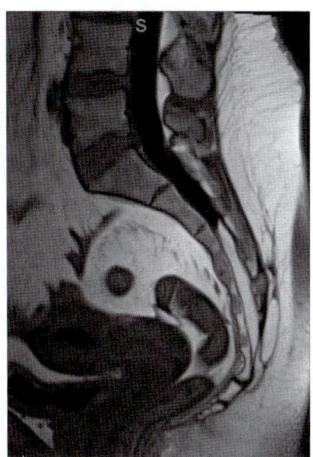

1. What are the major imaging findings?

2. What is the diagnosis?

3. What are the typical associations of intradural lipomas?

4. The lesions are neoplastic. True or False?

5. What is the typical behavior of these lesions?

Case ranking/difficulty:

Category: Spinal canal

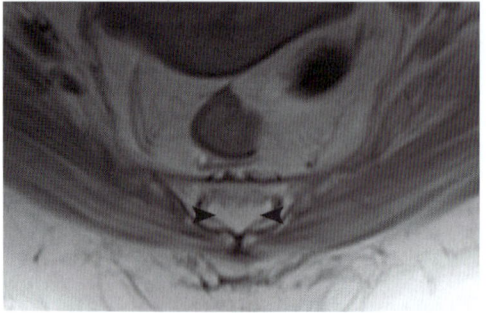

T1 hyperintense fatty mass with the sacral canal, displacing the nerve roots.

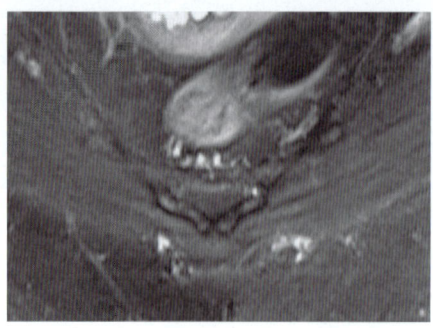

Complete fat suppression on fat-suppressed T2-weighted images.

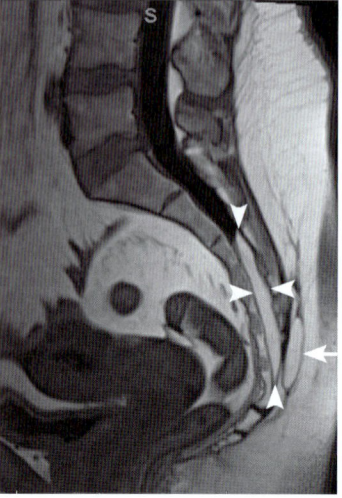

Similar findings. Note overlying subcutaneous lipoma (*arrow*) and pelvic lipomatosis.

Answers

1. There is a well-defined lentiform intraspinal fatty mass that incorporates the nerve roots anteriorly. There is associated pelvic lipomatosis and proliferation of the subcutaneous fat.

2. The presence of a fatty mass occupying the entire sacral canal is consistent with an intraspinal lipoma. There is an overlying subcutaneous lipoma and pelvic lipomatosis.

3. Intradural lipomas typically have no associated findings, unlike lipomas associated with spinal dysraphism, which may be associated with renal, vertebral, and dermal abnormalities.

4. False. Although the etiology of intraspinal lipomas is not clearly defined, most authorities believe that they are nonneoplastic and are probably hamartomatous lesions.

5. Slow growth of intradural lipomas is typical. Since the lesions are believed to be hamartomatous tissue, growth of the lesions may occur along with growth in the fat pool, hence the importance of weight control especially in patients with partial surgical decompression and recurrent or residual symptoms.

- Slow growth may occur, and symptoms are related to mass effect.
- Subcutaneous lipomas may overly the intradural lipoma.
- Incorporation of the nerve roots may occur, often resulting in the lesion appearing intramedullary at surgery.
- On MRI, the lesions completely suppress on fat-suppressed FSE T2-weighted images and there is no contrast enhancement.
- Plain radiographs may show widening of the spinal canal with thinning of the pedicles and a widened interpedicular distance.
- Treatment is with surgical decompression, although complete excision is usually not possible.

Pearls

- Intradural spinal lipomas most commonly affect the thoracic spine in adults and the cervical spine in children.
- They are not associated with dermal, vertebral, or renal abnormalities like lipomas associated with spinal dysraphism.
- The lesions are not considered neoplastic, although their etiology is poorly understood. They are probably hamartomatous tissue.

Suggested Reading

Finn MA, Walker ML. Spinal lipomas: clinical spectrum, embryology, and treatment. *Neurosurg Focus.* 2007;23(2):E10.

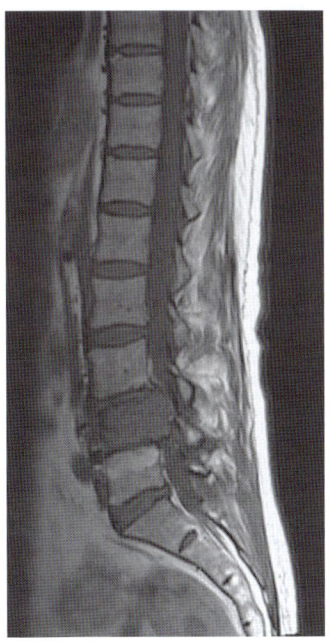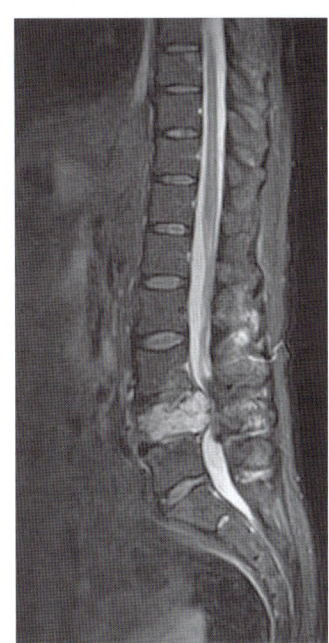

1. What are the MRI findings?

2. What are the differential diagnoses?

3. What are the specific distinguishing features of this entity on MRI?

4. T2-weighted images best to diagnose marrow replacement. True or False?

5. What sequences are not useful in demonstrating this condition?

Case ranking/difficulty:

Category: Vertebral body

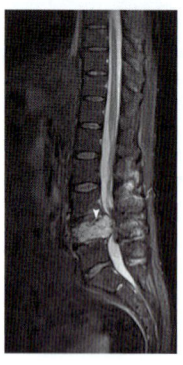

Metastatic destruction of the vertebral body with increased signal and diffuse posterior bulge, with cauda equina compression. Note subchondral low-intensity line (*arrowhead*), a feature more commonly seen in osteoporotic collapse.

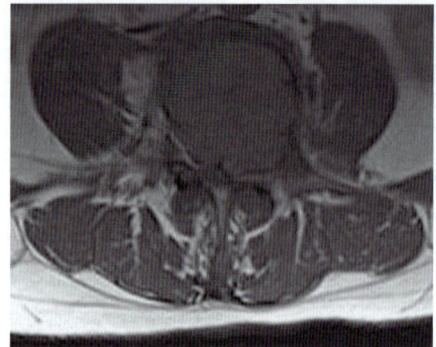

Axial image showing no room for CSF flow, and the epidural fat is compressed completely.

Contrast-enhanced image shows "sugar coating" appearance of dural metastases in another patient (*arrowheads*).

Answers

1. T1 marrow replacement, vertebral collapse and diffuse posterior wall bulge, low signal intensity band, cauda equina compression, and single-level involvement. Although a low intensity band is seen in this case, it is more commonly seen in osteoporotic compression fractures.

2. The differential diagnosis includes osteoporotic fracture, metastatic collapse, infection, posttraumatic collapse, and chordoma.

3. MRI features suggesting metastatic compression include a diffuse posterior vertebral bulge, involvement of the posterior elements, paraspinal mass, epidural mass, other spinal involvement, and "sugar coating" with contrast images (for dural metastases). T1-weighted images are useful to demonstrate multilevel marrow involvement.

4. False. T1 is the sequence of choice for evaluation of marrow replacement.

5. STIR and T2-weighted images can show increased signal in the infiltrated marrow, but it is nonspecific. Post-contrast images are useful to see dural metastases and paraspinal/epidural masses, but it is of uncertain usefulness in evaluating bony metastases. Gradient echo and proton density images are of little use.

Pearls

- Skeletal metastases are the third commonest site for metastases, and in the skeletal system, the spinal column is the most common site.
- Abnormal marrow infiltration on T1 is an important indicator. T1 diffuse marrow infiltration should also be searched for, using the disc signal as a control (marrow signal should be higher than disc on the T1-weighted images).
- The following criteria on MRI favor metastatic collapse over osteoporotic collapse: diffuse posterior bulge, paraspinal or epidural mass, involvement of the posterior elements, and multiple-level marrow involvement. A band of low T1 and T2 signal intensity is nonspecific, but favors osteoporotic collapse.
- The use of contrast is of debatable usefulness in evaluating bone metastases. However, "sugar coating" in the case of dural metastases and paraspinal or epidural masses are well demonstrated on post-contrast images.
- Urgent treatment is with cord decompression and spine stabilization. In palliative cases, vertebroplasty and kyphoplasty are offered for pain control.

Suggested Readings

Berwouts D, Remery M, Van Den Berghe T. Vertebral collapse caused by bone metastasis. *J Thorac Oncol.* 2011 Apr;6(4):823.

Jung HS, Jee WH, McCauley TR, Ha KY, Choi KH. Discrimination of metastatic from acute osteoporotic compression spinal fractures with MR imaging. *Radiographics.* 2003;23(1):179-187.

Lafforgue P, Bayle O, Massonnat J, et al. [MRI in osteoporotic and metastatic vertebral compressions: apropos of 60 cases]. *Ann Radiol (Paris).* 1991 Feb;34(3):157-166.

Gait disturbance

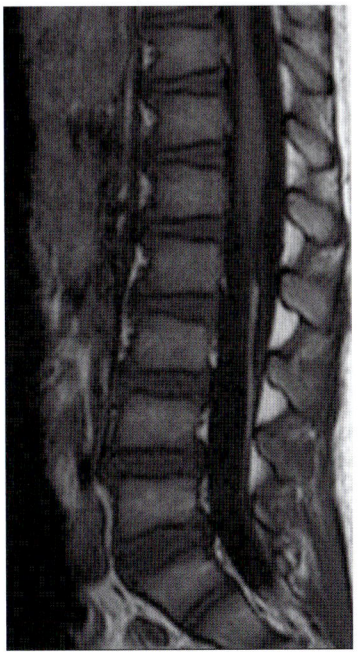 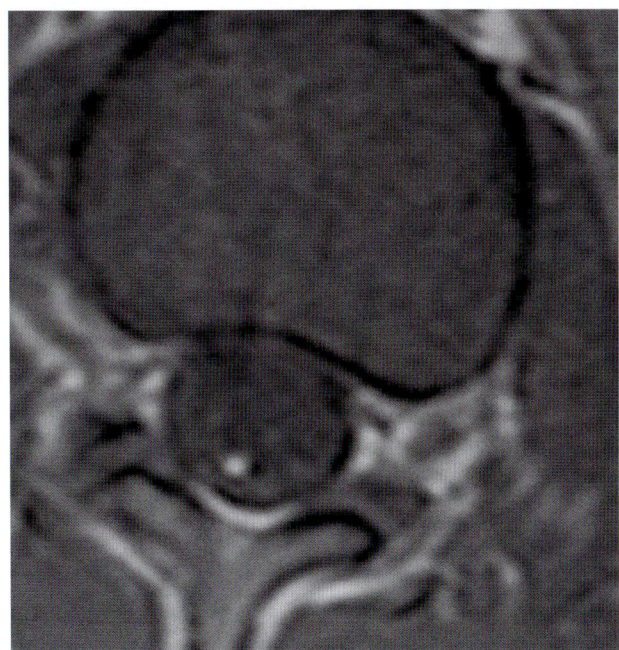

1. What is the most likely diagnosis?

2. How does the condition usually manifest?

3. Describe clinical and pathological characteristics of this entity.

4. Which imaging modality best images the condition?

5. What are the typical MR findings of this entity?

Case ranking/difficulty:

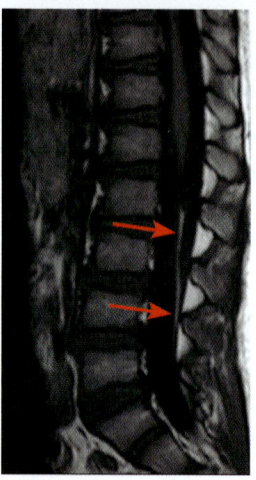

Sagittal T1-weighted sequence of the lumbar spine shows a thin cylindrical hyperintensity (*arrows*) within the filum terminale in keeping with fat. Note that the cord terminates at L1-L2. There is no evidence of associated spinal dysraphism.

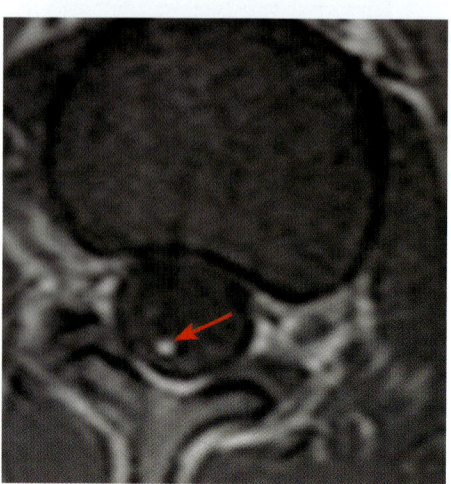

Axial T1-weighted sequence at the level of L2 vertebral body confirms the presence of fat within the filum terminale (*arrow*) in keeping with a filar lipoma.

Answers

1. Filar lipoma is a relatively common asymptomatic incidental finding and represents the most common intraspinal lipoma. Filar lipomas are secondary to persistence of caudal cells that differentiate toward fat. By definition a fatty filum that is thicker than 2 mm in cross section is classified as a filar lipoma.

2. Filar lipoma is a relatively common asymptomatic incidental finding. It may, however, be associated with tethered cord and spinal dysraphism.

3. Filar lipomas may be associated with lipomas of the caudal half of the conus medullaris, as the latter also forms by canalization and retrogressive differentiation. Fat within the filum terminale is seen in up to 5% of lumbar spine MR examinations.

   The filum terminale is thickened due to the presence of fat and appears thicker than its neighboring nerve roots. Filar lipomas may involve the intra- or extradural portion of the filum terminale or both.

   Filar lipomas may be identified on computed tomography as a cylindrical fat density within the lumbar canal. The lesional Hounsfield units may be measured, which confirm fat density (−90 to −30 HU).

   When associated with tethered cord syndrome, surgical intervention is appropriate and involves sectioning of the filum terminale.

4. MRI is the examination of choice especially when fat suppression sequences are added. The lipoma often extends over several vertebral segments and its signal follows that of fat.

5. Filar lipoma appears as a linear T1- and T2-hyperintensity within the filum terminale. Chemical shift artifact may be seen on T2* or gradient echo sequences. The lesional signal saturates following fat suppression. No enhancement of the lesion is demonstrated following contrast administration. Intradural filar lipomas are often fusiform in shape and taper down to the site where the filum pierces the dura.

Pearls

- Filar lipoma is a relatively common asymptomatic incidental finding.
- It may be associated with tethered cord and spinal dysraphism.
- Fat within the filum terminale is seen in up to 5% of lumbar spine MR examinations.
- MRI is the examination of choice especially when fat suppression sequences are added.
- When associated with tethered cord syndrome, surgical intervention is appropriate.

Suggested Readings

Lowe LH, Johanek AJ, Moore CW. Sonography of the neonatal spine: part 2, spinal disorders. *AJR Am J Roentgenol.* 2007 Mar;188(3):739-744. Review.

Park HJ, Jeon YH, Rho MH, et al. Incidental findings of the lumbar spine at MRI during herniated intervertebral disk disease evaluation. *AJR Am J Roentgenol.* 2011 May;196(5):1151-1155.

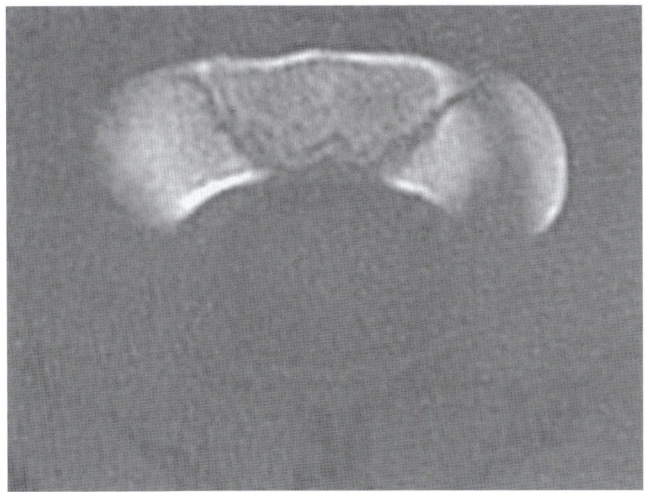

1. What should be included in the differential
   diagnosis?

2. What structures are involved?

3. Why does instability arise?

4. What are the mechanisms of injury?

5. What are the treatment options?

Case ranking/difficulty:

Category: Vertebral body

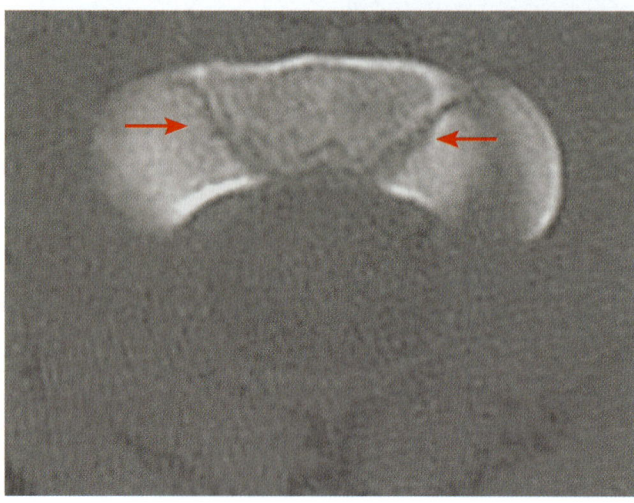

Irregular lucency through the synchondrosis, consistent with a type 3 odontoid fracture.

Answers

1. All types of C2 fractures could be considered; however, type 3 fractures extend into the vertebral body.

2. Type 3 fractures extend from the base of the dens into the vertebral body.

3. Instability in Type 3 fractures arises from the atlas and occiput moving together.

4. The mechanism is thought to be primarily from flexion with rebound extension.

5. Most patients have good union with a combination of traction and halo fixation with surgical fixation reserved for patients with nonunion.

Pearls

- Type 3 odontoid fractures extend into the vertebral body.
- These are inherently unstable fractures; however, they often heal well with immobilization.
- These fractures have a very low rate of nonunion given the involvement of cancellous bone.
- Traction may be required to maintain anatomic position and some patients may require surgical fixation.

Suggested Readings

Greene KA, Dickman CA, Marciano FF, Drabier JB, Hadley MN, Sonntag VKH. Acute axis fractures: analysis of management and outcome in 340 consecutive cases. *Spine.* 1997;22:1843-1852.

Rao SK, Wasyliw C, Nunez DB. Spectrum of imaging findings in hyperextension injuries of the neck. *Radiographics.* 2005;25:1239-1254.

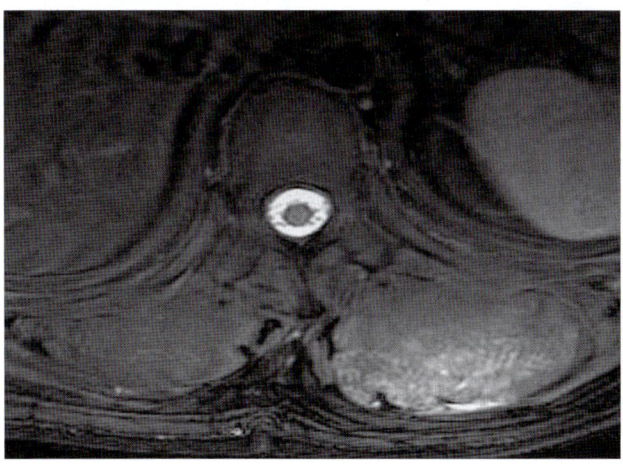
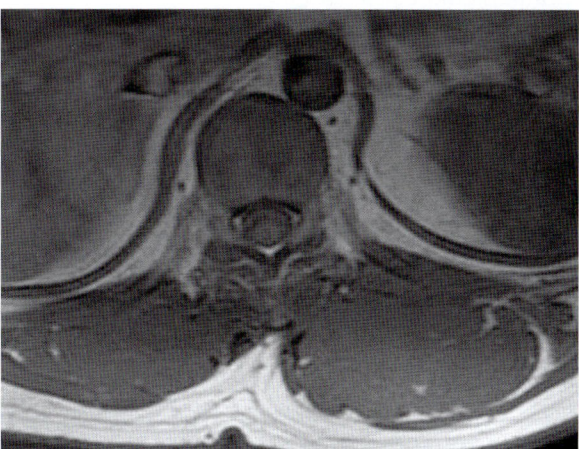

1. What should be included in the differential diagnosis?

2. What are common presenting symptoms?

3. Which syndromes are associated with osseous and soft tissue lesions?

4. What are classic imaging characteristics?

5. What are the treatment options?

Case ranking/difficulty: 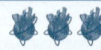   **Category:** Paraspinal soft tissue

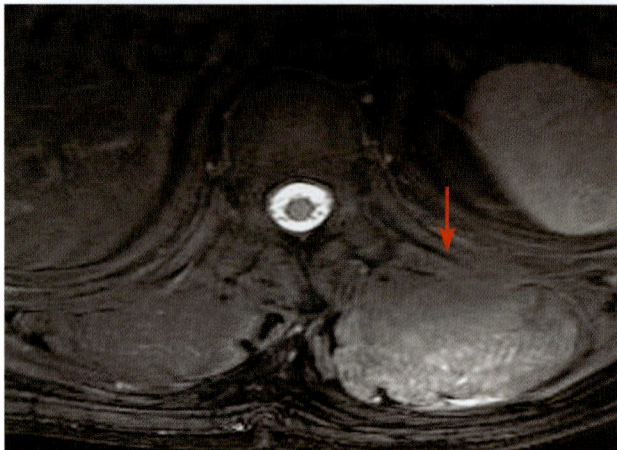

T2 image demonstrates hyperintense left paraspinal muscle enlargement.

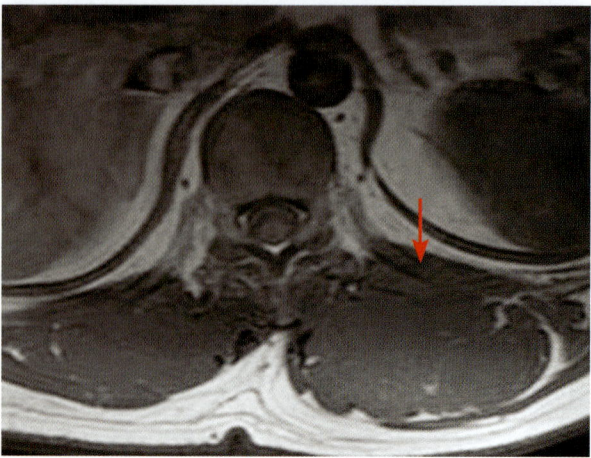

T1 image demonstrates isointense left paraspinal muscle enlargement.

Answers

1. Paraspinal muscle enlargement and T2 hyperintensity can be seen with intramuscular myxoma, soft tissue sarcoma, posttraumatic edema, myositis, and early denervation injury.

2. Myxomas may enlarge and cause restriction of movement; they are generally painless. Pathologic fracture could result from associated fibrous dysplasia.

3. Mazabraud syndrome consists of soft tissue myxomas and fibrous dysplasia. Maffucci syndrome consists of enchondromas and soft tissue hemangiomas.

4. The classic imaging appearance of myxoma are CT hypodensity, no activity on PET, T1 hypointensity, T2 hyperintensity, and no significant enhancement.

5. Symptomatic lesions may be resected; however, asymptomatic lesions require no treatment. Some argue they should be followed as there is a low risk of malignant transformation.

Pearls

- Mazabraud syndrome is a rare syndrome in which solitary or multiple intramuscular myxomas are seen in conjunction with either monostotic or polyostotic fibrous dysplasia.
- The etiology and pathophysiology of Mazabraud are unknown. There does not appear to be a genetic predilection.
- Treatment consists of surgical excision of symptomatic masses.
- Asymptomatic masses may be followed; there is a small risk of malignant transformation.

Suggested Readings

Case DB, Chapman CN, Freeman JK, Polga JP. Atypical presentation of polyostotic fibrous dysplasia with myxoma (Mazabraud syndrome). *Radiographics*. 2010;30:827-832.

Iwasko N, Steinbach LS, Disler D, et al. Imaging findings in Mazabraud's syndrome: seven new cases. *Skeletal Radiol*. 2002;31:81-87.

Chiari I malformation

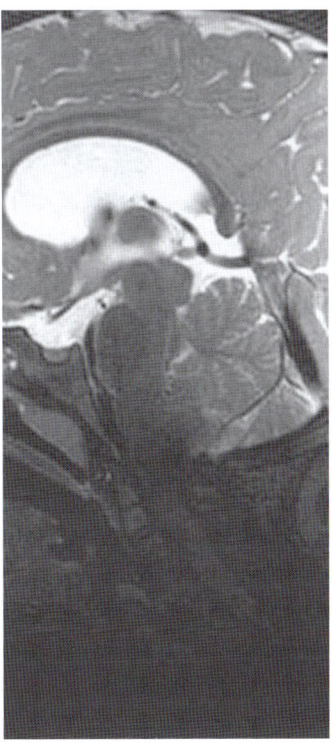

1. What are presenting symptoms?

2. Which findings indicate disruption of cerebrospinal fluid flow?

3. What are the advantages of cine phase-contrast MRI sequences?

4. What is the normal pattern of cerebrospinal fluid flow with respect to the cardiac cycle?

5. What are the treatment options?

Case ranking/difficulty: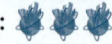

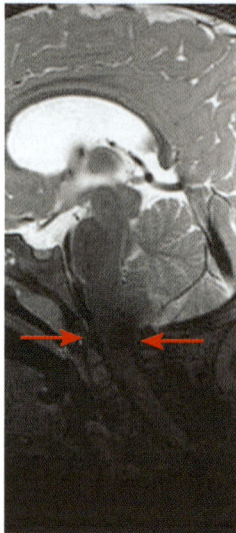

Sagittal T2 CUBE image demonstrates hypointensity at the foramen magnum, consistent with dephasing of flowing cerebrospinal fluid.

Answers

1. Classically, patients present with Valsalva-induced occipital headaches, but any kind of headache can be present. Myelopathic symptoms may occur in the setting of significant syrinx or presyrinx.

2. Spatial inhomogeneity, elevated peak velocity, simultaneous bidirectional flow, and increased cranial flow can indicate disruption of normal cerebrospinal fluid flow in the setting of Chiari I malformation.

3. Cine phase-contrast sequences do not require contrast and can be acquired in a relatively short amount of time (less than 15 minutes). The spatial resolution is good, but not as high as volumetric sequences, but the phase-contrast sequence gives additional directional and velocity information.

4. During systole, there is increased intracranial pressure secondary to inflow of blood, leading to caudal flow of cerebrospinal fluid. The reverse is true during diastole.

5. Depending on the flow studies and associated findings, suboccipital decompression, ventricular shunting, and syringosubarachnoid shunt are potential treatment options.

Pearls

- Chiari I malformation is often associated with disruption of cerebrospinal fluid flow at the craniocervical junction.
- Classically, patients present with Valsalva-induced occipital headaches, but any kind of headache can be present.
- Myelopathic symptoms may occur in the setting of significant syrinx or presyrinx.
- Cerebrospinal fluid flow studies help categorize and quantify disruption of cerebrospinal fluid flow if present.
- This can help identify patients who will benefit from suboccipital craniectomy.

Suggested Readings

Iskandar BJ, Quigley M, Haughton VM. Foramen magnum cerebrospinal fluid flow characteristics in children with Chiari I malformation before and after craniocervical decompression. *J Neurosurg.* 2004;101:169-178.

McGirt MJ, Nimjee SM, Floyd J, Bulsara KR, George TM. Correlation of cerebrospinal fluid flow dynamics and headache in Chiari I malformation. *Neurosurgery.* 2005;56:716-721.

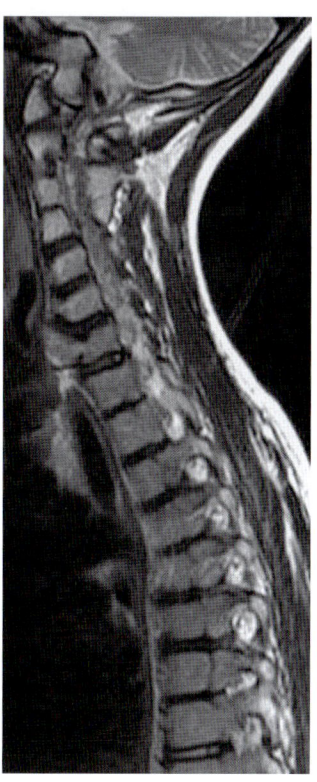

1. What should be included in the differential diagnosis?

2. What are common presenting symptoms?

3. What is the mode of transmission?

4. What portion of the spine is most commonly affected?

5. What are the treatment options?

Case ranking/difficulty:

Category: More than one category

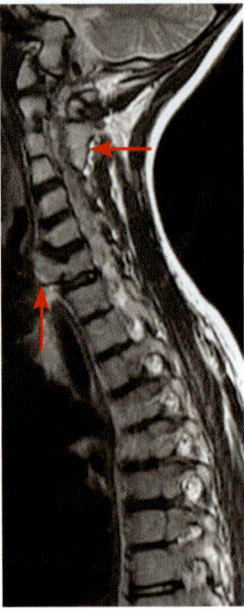

Parasagittal T2 image demonstrates osseous exostosis extending from the anterior C7 vertebral body; incidentally noted fusion of the posterior elements of C1-C3.

Answers

1. Enthesopathic changes, fibrous dysplasia, osteoma, and osteochondroma can all be included in the differential diagnosis.

2. Presenting symptoms include pain, restriction of movement, radiculopathy, and myelopathy.

3. Multiple hereditary exostoses are inherited in an autosomal dominant manner.

4. The cervical spine is most commonly affected.

5. Asymptomatic patients may be managed conservatively with consideration for imaging follow-up due to the low but real risk of malignant degeneration. Surgical resection is recommended for symptomatic lesions.

Pearls

• Multiple hereditary exostoses are characterized by multiple osteochondromas, which commonly affect the long bones.
• Most patients (approximately 2/3) will have spinal involvement, with involvement of the posterior elements and cervical spine most common.
• The disorder is inherited in an autosomal dominant manner.
• Usually these lesions are asymptomatic; however, patients may develop radicular or myelopathic symptoms depending on location.
• Continued follow-up is recommended as there is a small (<2%) risk of malignant transformation of the overlying cartilaginous cap into chondrosarcoma.

Suggested Readings

Ezra N, Tetteh B, Diament M, Jonas AJ, Dickson P. Hereditary multiple exostoses with spine involvement in a 4-year-old boy. *Am J Med Genet A*. 2010;152A:1264-1267.

Sofka CM, Saboeiro GR, Schneider R. Multiple hereditary exostoses. *HSSJ*. 2005;1:49-51.

Palpable neck mass

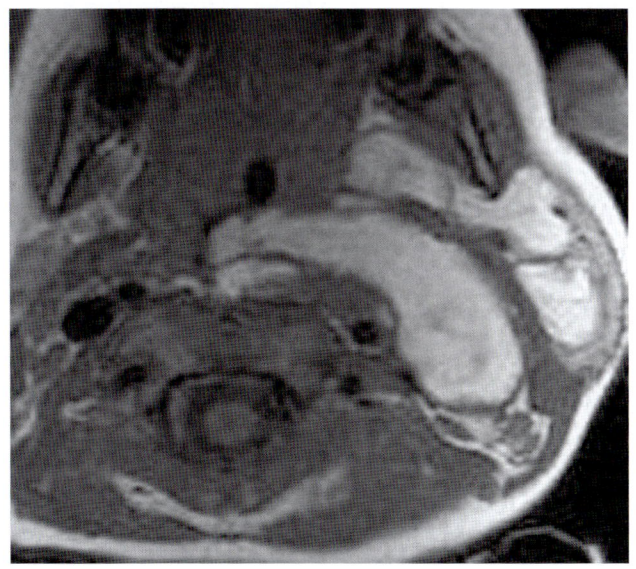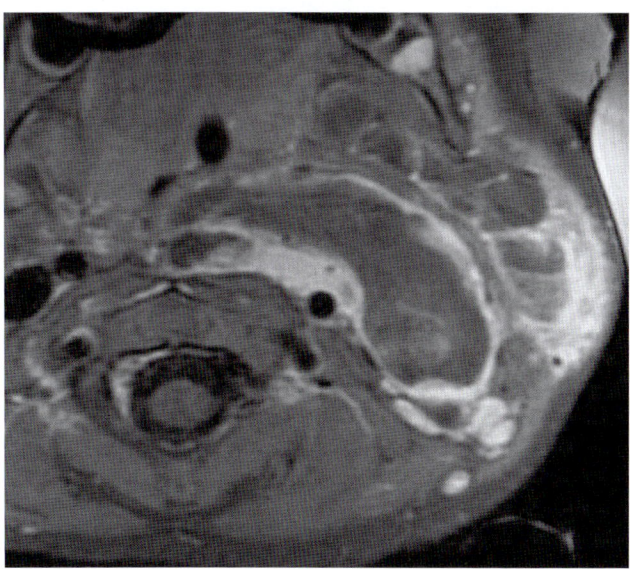

1. What should be included in the differential diagnosis?

2. What are common presenting symptoms?

3. Where do these lesions tend to occur?

4. What are the different WHO classifications of benign lipomatous tumors?

5. What are the treatment options?

Case ranking/difficulty: 

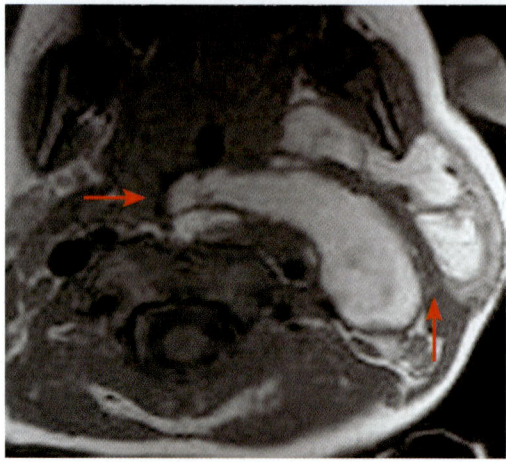

Axial T1 image demonstrates lobulated hyperintense mass within the prevertebral soft tissues, extending into the left neck.

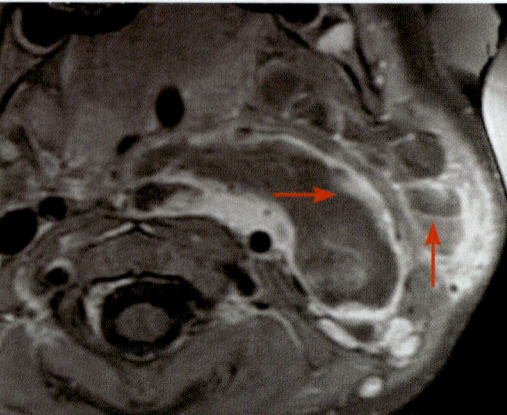

Axial T1 image following gadolinium administration, using a chemical-shift-based method to eliminate signal from fat, demonstrates enhancement of multiple septations in the prevertebral and left neck mass with loss of signal from the central portions, consistent with fat content.

Answers

1. Fat-containing lesions include lipoma, lipomatosis, lipoblastoma, lipoblastomatosis, and liposarcoma, which can be differentiated based on patient age, encapsulation, number, and cellular atypia.

2. The most common presenting symptom is a palpable or enlarging mass; depending on location, there may be associated pain or limping (if the lesion is within an extremity). Compression of the airway could cause stridor/wheezing.

3. Lipoblastomas can occur anywhere that there is fatty tissue; however, the most common location are the limbs.

4. Recognized subtypes of benign lipomatous tumors include lipoma/lipomatosis, angiolipoma, lipoblastoma/lipoblastomatosis, myolipoma, chondroid lipoma, lipomatosis of nerve, spindle cell lipoma/pleomorphic lipoma, and hibernoma.

5. For symptomatic lesions, surgical resection is recommended; however, up to one-quarter of patients will recur, necessitating further surgery. Conservative management may be appropriate for asymptomatic lesions, particularly as they have a propensity to differentiate into lipomas with increased patient age.

Pearls

- Lipoblastomas are benign fatty tumors of the soft tissues, which have a predisposition for the extremities, but also can affect the neck, mediastinum, abdomen, and retroperitoneum.
- They are almost exclusively seen in children—an important fact to remember, as they look similar to liposarcoma on imaging; however, the latter is generally a disease of adult patients.
- The classic appearance is a fat intensity mass with enhancing linear septations. There may be a prominent myxoid matrix and the lesion is usually well circumscribed; however, the lesions may be infiltrative in nature.
- Key characteristics in an imaging description include proximity to nerves and vasculature and compression of adjacent structures, such as the airway in this case.
- Treatment is surgical excision; however, these lesions have a propensity to recur and may necessitate further operative intervention.

Suggested Readings

Bancroft LW, Kransdorf MJ, Peterson JJ, O'Connor MI. Benign fatty tumors: classification, clinical course, imaging appearance and treatment. *Skeletal Radiol.* 2006;35:719-733.

Speer AL, Schofield DE, Wang KS, et al. Contemporary management of lipoblastoma. *J Ped Surg.* 2008;43: 1295-1300.

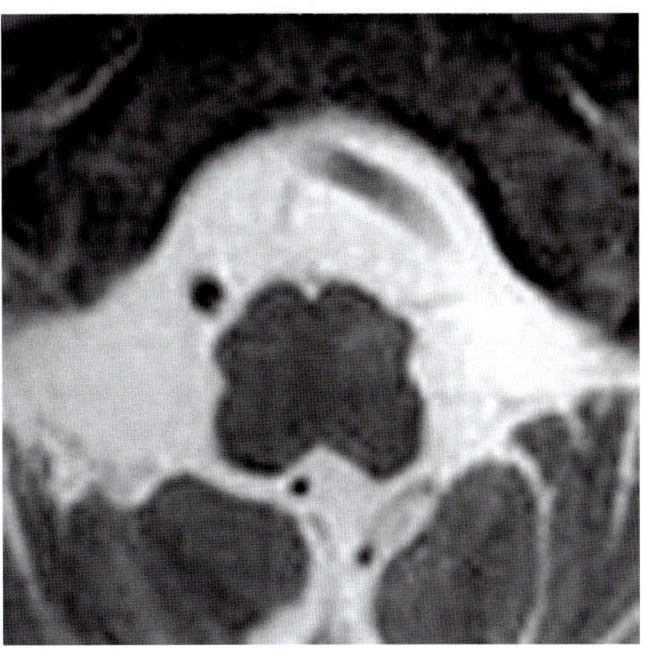

1. What should be included in the differential diagnosis?

2. Where do lesions that cause this typically occur?

3. What are common presenting symptoms?

4. What are the recognized phases?

5. What are the treatment options?

Case ranking/difficulty: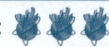

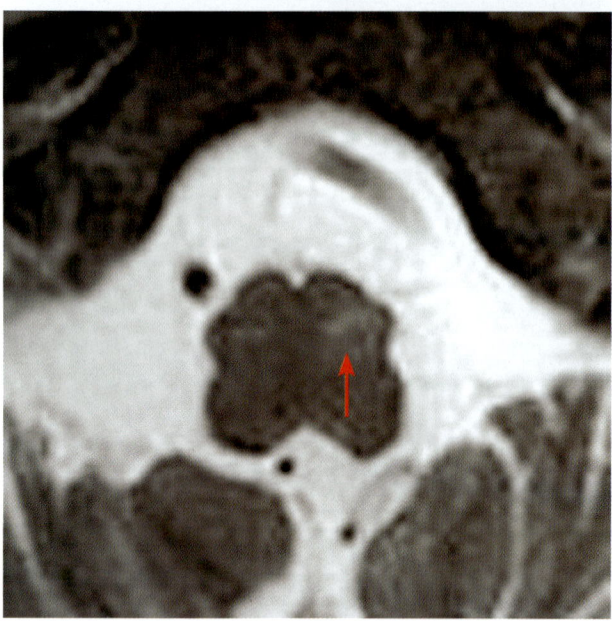

Axial T2 image demonstrates hyperintensity and expansion of the medullary olive.

Pearls

- Hypertrophic olivary degeneration is a form of transsynaptic degeneration, which can pose a diagnostic dilemma given the associated expansion instead of volume loss.
- The role of the radiologist is to correctly make the diagnosis to avoid unnecessary biopsy/workup.
- It is important to have a working knowledge of the Guillain-Mollaret triangle to assess the three patterns that can be seen:
  1. Ipsilateral hypertrophic olivary degeneration—lesion within the central tegmental tract
  2. Contralateral hypertrophic olivary degeneration—lesion within the superior cerebellar peduncle or dentate nucleus
  3. Bilateral hypertrophic olivary degeneration—lesion within the central tegmental tract and superior cerebellar peduncle

Suggested Readings

Kitajima M, Korogi Y, Shimomura O, et al. Hypertrophic olivary degeneration: MR imaging and pathologic findings. *Radiology*. 1994;192:539-543.

Shah R, Markert J, Bag AK, Cure JK. Diffusion tensor imaging in hypertrophic olivary degeneration. *AJNR*. 2010;31:1729-1731.

Answers

1. Etiologies of intramedullary T2 hyperintensity and expansion include demyelinating disease, astrocytoma, metastasis, infarction, and lymphoma.

2. Lesions within the superior cerebellar peduncle, cerebellum, dentate nucleus, and central tegmental tract can all produce hypertrophic olivary degeneration.

3. Palatal myoclonus is the most common presentation.

4. The phases of hypertrophic olivary degeneration are T2 hyperintensity, T2 hyperintensity, and hypertrophy and finally T2 hyperintensity without hypertrophy.

5. Correctly recognizing this entity eliminates the need for unnecessary workup or treatment.

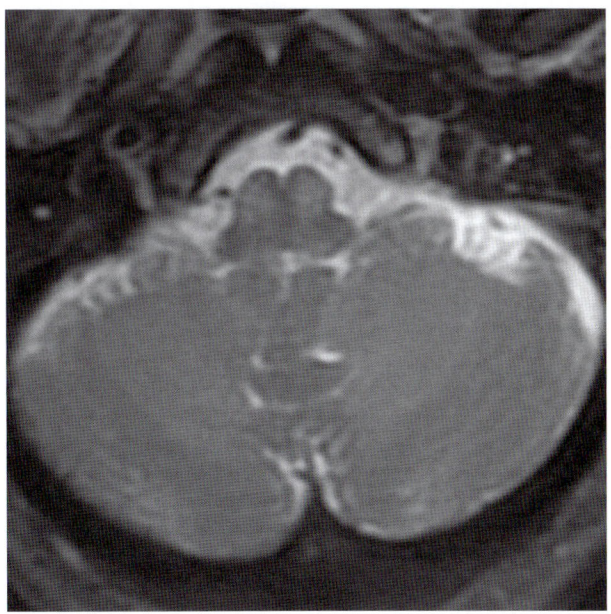

1. What should be included in the differential diagnosis?

2. What other disorders are considered to be along the same spectrum?

3. What are common presenting symptoms?

4. What are treatment options?

5. What is the prognosis and outcome for this disorder?

Case ranking/difficulty:

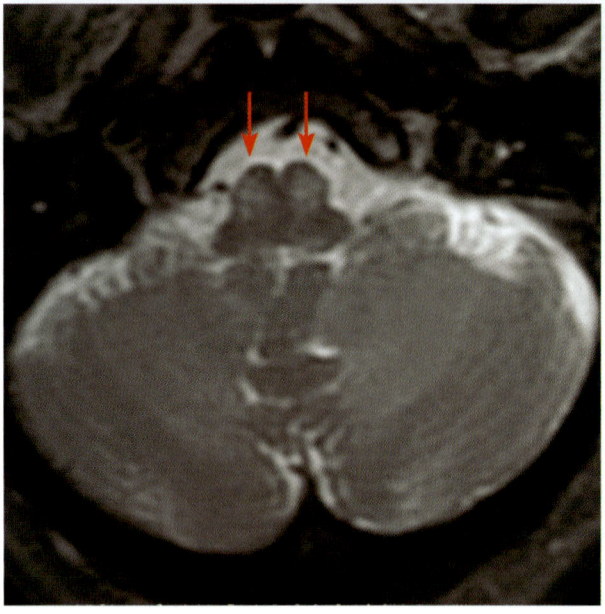

Axial T2 image demonstrates increased signal within the ventral medulla bilaterally.

Pearls

- Bickerstaff encephalitis is a rare disorder characterized by drowsiness, ophthalmoplegia, ataxia, positive Babinski sign, and hemisensory loss.
- It is along the spectrum of Guillain-Barré syndrome.
- Approximately 2/3 of patients will demonstrate a positive serum anti-GQ1b IgG antibody and treatment can be geared toward immunophoresis. In the remaining 1/3, treatment is supportive.
- The disorder generally has a monophasic course and a good outcome.
- Only 1/3 of patients demonstrate abnormalities on MRI, generally manifested as T2 hyperintensity within the brainstem.

Suggested Readings

Bickerstaff ER, Cloake PCP. Mesencephalitis and rhombencephalitis. *Br Med J*. 1951 Jul 14;77-81.

Odaka M, Yuki N, Yamada M, et al. Bickerstaff's brainstem encephalitis: clinical features of 62 cases and a subgroup associated with Guillain-Barré syndrome. *Brain*. 2003;126:2279-2290.

Answers

1. Potential etiologies include viral encephalitis, brainstem tumor, Bickerstaff encephalitis, lupus encephalitis, and paraneoplastic syndrome.

2. Bickerstaff encephalitis, Miller-Fisher syndrome, and Guillain-Barré syndrome are along a continuum and patients often present with components of multiple syndromes.

3. Bickerstaff encephalitis is composed of drowsiness, ophthalmoplegia, ataxia, positive Babinski sign, and hemisensory loss.

4. Immunophoresis directed at the anti-GQ1b IgG antibody if present is indicated; otherwise, supportive management is usually sufficient.

5. Most patients have a complete recovery; however, there is the potential for morbidity and mortality as well as some patients who develop a chronic relapsing— remitting course.

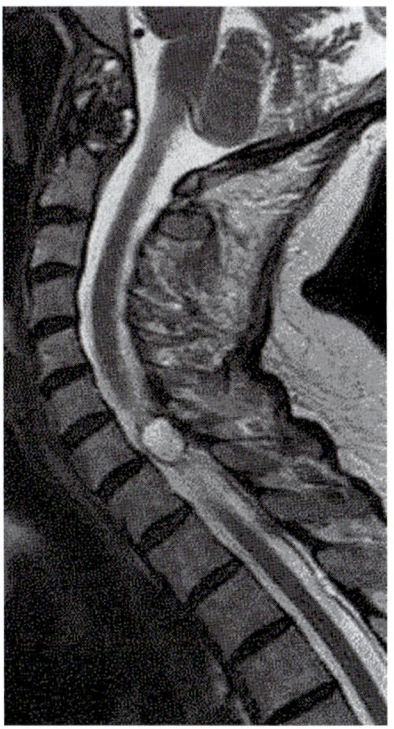 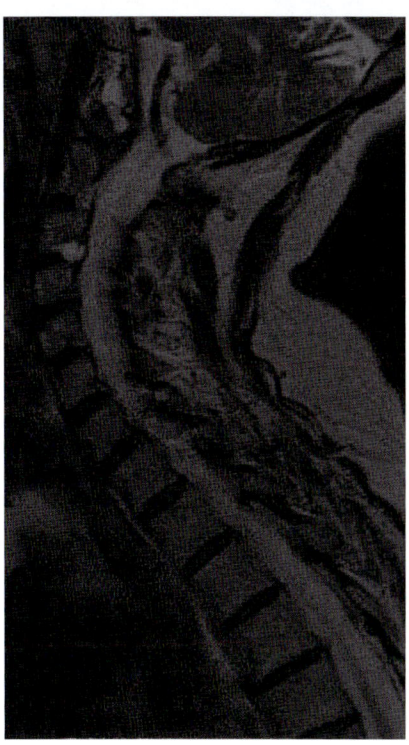

1. What should be included in the differential diagnosis?

2. What are common presenting symptoms?

3. What are potential causative factors?

4. What are the most common locations within the cervical spine?

5. What are the treatment options?

Case ranking/difficulty: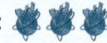

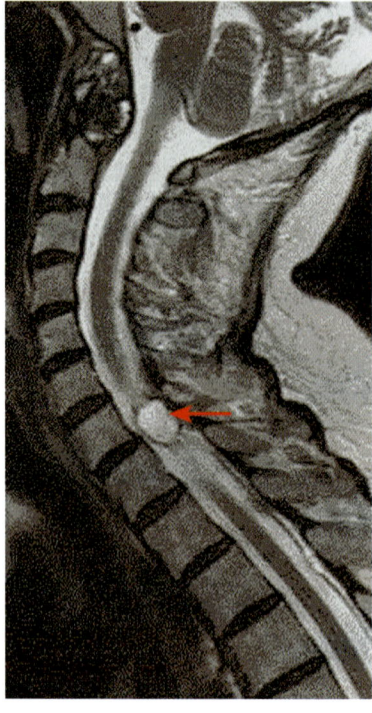

Sagittal T2 image demonstrates well-circumscribed fluid intensity mass in the dorsal spinal canal at the C7 level.

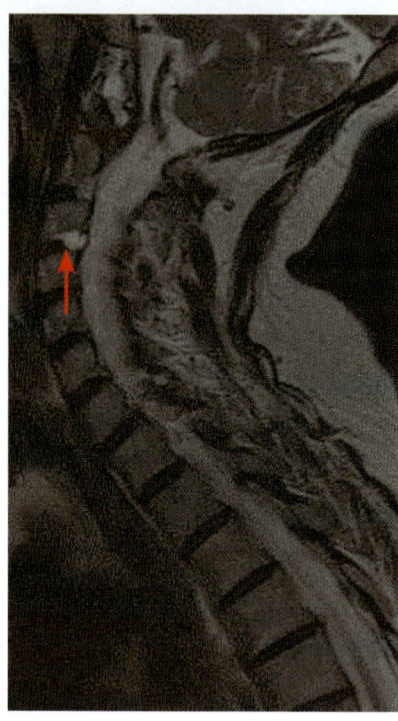

Sagittal T2 image demonstrates well-circumscribed fluid intensity mass in the ventral spinal canal at the C3-C4 level.

Answers

1. The differential for a cystic lesion include synovial cyst, ganglion cyst, ligamentum flavum cyst, and schwannoma.

2. Pain, radiculopathy, and myelopathy are the most common presenting symptoms. Synovial cysts unto themselves do not cause instability.

3. Rheumatoid arthritis, osteoarthritis, trauma, and infection can be associated with synovial cyst formation.

4. These lesions are most common at the craniocervical and cervicothoracic junction.

5. Asymptomatic lesions may be left alone; however, symptomatic lesions are best treated with resection.

Pearls

- Synovial cysts are a common cause of lumbar back pain; however, they are not commonly seen in the cervical spine.
- There is debate over the proper terminology of these lesions, which may be based on histologic characteristics.

- Synovial cysts likely arise from degenerative, traumatic, or inflammatory changes of the adjacent facet joints.
- In the cervical spine, they are most common in the atlantoaxial and cervicothoracic regions.
- Treatment is reserved for symptomatic lesions and includes resection of the cysts. Spinal fusion is generally not indicated.

Suggested Readings

Costa F, Menghetti C, Cardia A, Formari M, Ortolina A. Cervical synovial cyst: case report and review of the literature. *Eur Spine J*. 2010;19:S100-S102.

Lyons MK, Birch BD, Krauss WE, Patel NP, Nottmeier EW, Boucher OK. Subaxial cervical synovial cysts. *Spine*. 2011;36:E1285-E1289.

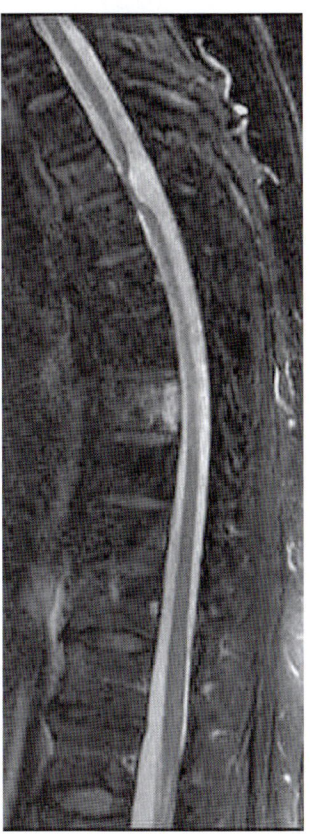

1. What should be included in the differential diagnosis?

2. What are common presenting symptoms?

3. What are the components of this syndrome?

4. What portion of the cord is most commonly affected?

5. What are the treatment options?

Case ranking/difficulty: 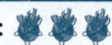

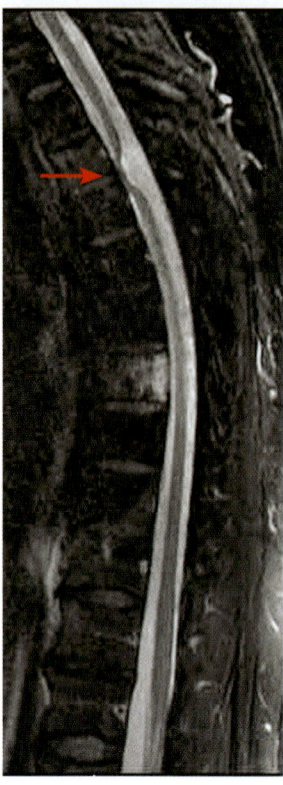

Sagittal T2 image demonstrates focal ventral displacement of the spinal cord at the T3-T4 level.

Answers

1. The differential diagnosis for displacement and thinning of the cord would include myelomalacia, postoperative adhesions, or mass effect from a cystic lesion, such as arachnoid cyst or epidermoid cyst.

2. Lower extremity paresthesia and weakness are the most common presenting symptoms, occasionally with associated spasticity. Pain and postural headache have been reported, but infrequently.

3. The components of Brown-Sequard syndrome include ipsilateral loss of motor function and touch and contralateral loss of pain and temperature sensation, resulting from a hemicord injury.

4. The thoracic cord, specifically the upper thoracic cord, is most commonly affected by transdural cord herniation.

5. Treatment consists of surgical reduction of the cord with repair of the dural defect, using grafts as necessary.

Pearls

- Transdural cord herniation is a rare abnormality, but an important etiology to differentiate from a dorsal arachnoid cyst.
- There is controversy over the factors that lead to transdural cord herniation; however, the dominant theory is that a herniated disc or osteophyte tears the dura, allowing the cord to herniate. This is supported by the data that show most of these lesions occur at a disc level, often with superimposed degenerative changes.
- Patients often present with lower extremity weakness or sensory disturbance.
- Some patients present with Brown-Sequard syndrome from hemicord injury.
- On imaging, there is ventral displacement of the spinal cord, which may be complicated by superimposed edema.
- The main differential diagnosis is a dorsal arachnoid cyst. This can be differentiated using myelography— arachnoid cysts either will not fill (if extradural) or may fill in a delayed manner (if intradural).
- Treatment is surgical with reduction of the herniation and repair of the dural defect.

Suggested Readings

Batzdorf U, Holly LT. Idiopathic thoracic spinal cord herniation: report of 10 patients and descriptions of surgical approach. *J Spinal Disord Tech*. 2012;25:157-162.

Brus-Ramer M, Dillon WP. Idiopathic thoracic spinal cord herniation: retrospective analysis supporting a mechanism of diskogenic dural injury and subsequent tamponade. *AJNR*. 2012;33:52-56.

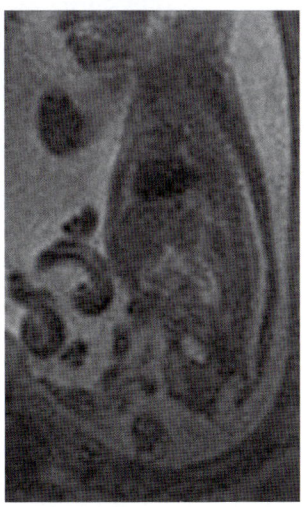 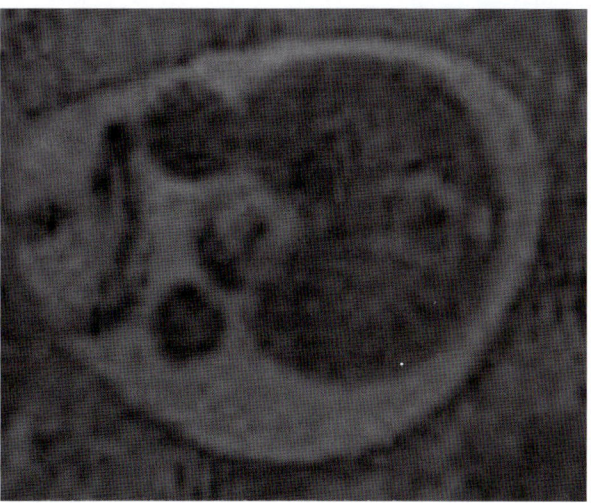

1. What should be included in the differential diagnosis?

2. What are the components of the Altman classification sequence?

3. What are potential intrauterine/obstetric complications?

4. What are the components of the Currarino triad?

5. What are the treatment options?

Case ranking/difficulty: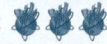

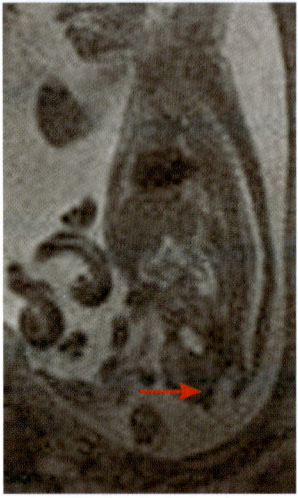

Sagittal T2 SSFSE image from a fetal MRI demonstrates a low presacral complex solid and cystic mass.

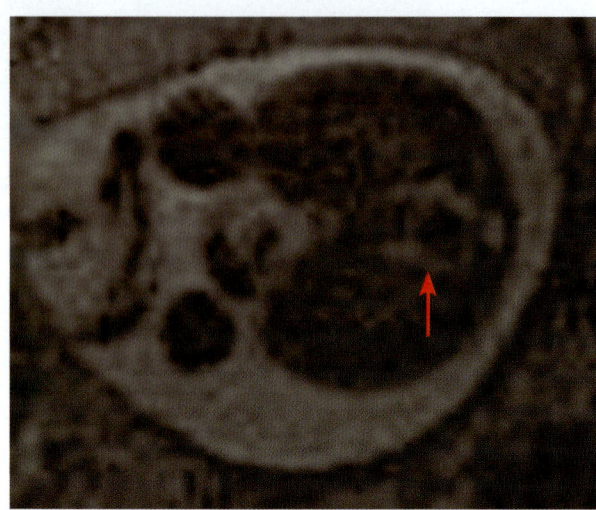

Axial T2 SSFSE image from a fetal MRI demonstrates a low presacral complex solid and cystic mass.

Answers

1. Neonatal lumbosacral masses include anterior sacral meningocele, chordoma, dermoid cyst, hemangioma, and terminal myelocystocele.

2. The Altman classification:

   Type 1—external component

   Type 2—external and small presacral components

   Type 3—internal and external components

   Type 4—internal component

   The greater the proportion of internal components, the more difficult the resection and the higher the risk of malignant degeneration.

3. Potential complications, which can be seen in three-fourths of patients carrying fetuses diagnosed with sacrococcygeal teratomas, include HELLP syndrome, hyperemesis, oligohydramnios, polyhydramnios, and preterm labor.

4. The Currarino triad includes anorectal malformation, presacral mass, and sacrococcygeal osseous defect. One-fifth of sacrococcygeal teratomas are associated with additional abnormalities.

5. Surgical resection is the treatment of choice with chemotherapy and/or radiation for malignant lesions. In utero drainage of cystic components or resection may be performed to facilitate delivery.

Pearls

- Sacrococcygeal teratomas are the most common solid tumor in neonates; two-thirds are benign.
- Classification is based on intrapelvic and extrapelvic location, which is important for surgical planning and risk of malignant degeneration.
- These are often diagnosed antenatally on ultrasound or MRI.
- Depending on lesion size, there may be implications for delivery and neonatal cardiorespiratory status.
- Surgical resection is the treatment of choice with a risk for malignant degeneration in residual tissue.

Suggested Readings

Kocaoglu M, Frush DP. Pediatric presacral masses. *Radiographics*. 2006;26:833-857.

Woodward PJ, Sohaey R, Kennedy A, Koeller KK. A comprehensive review of fetal tumors with pathologic correlation. *Radiographics*. 2005;25:215-242.

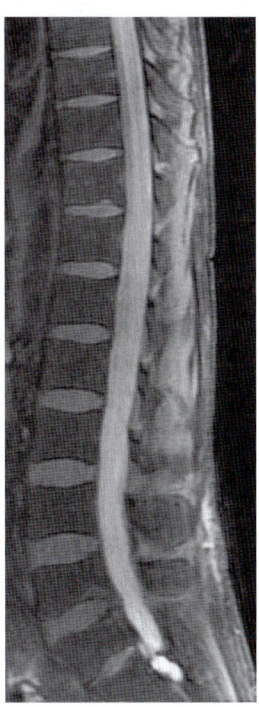

1. What should be included in the differential
   diagnosis of headache with pachymeningeal
   enhancement?

2. What imaging studies can be performed for
   further evaluation?

3. What are potential etiologies?

4. Gadolinium myelography should be performed
   with what parameters?

5. What are the treatment options?

Case ranking/difficulty: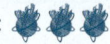

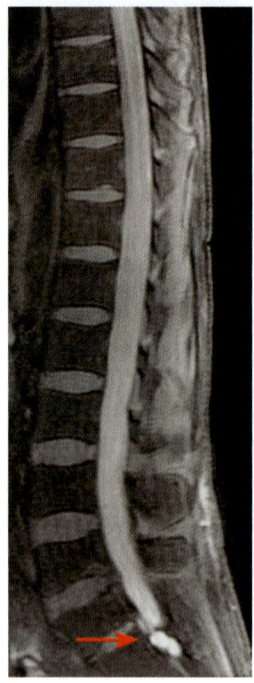

Sagittal T1 image with fat suppression following intrathecal contrast administration demonstrates multiple sacral nerve root cysts.

Answers

1. Pachymeningeal enhancement involves the dura with sparing of the leptomeninges. Etiologies include intracranial hypotension, dural metastasis, and dural lymphoma.

2. Intrathecal injection of myelographic contrast, gadolinium, and indium-111 can be performed simultaneously with acquisition of multiple images to improve diagnostic accuracy.

3. Potential causes of decreased cerebrospinal fluid pressure include trauma with dural tear, nerve root sleeve cysts, dural ectasis, lumbar puncture, and spinal surgery.

4. Imaging parameters should include T1 pre- and post-intrathecal contrast. Fat suppression is imperative for accurate evaluation of the thecal sac and nerve root sleeves; however, given the presence of potential artifact, fat suppression should also be applied before contrast administration to allow for equal comparison. Immediate and delayed imaging should be considered, as well as concurrent CT myelography.

5. Treatment options include epidural blood patch, fibrin injection, or surgical repair.

Pearls

- Spontaneous intracranial hypotension presents a diagnostic dilemma to the clinician.
- It can be easily confused with other causes of postural headache, and diagnosing the exact location of cerebrospinal fluid leak can be difficult.
- Classically, myelography was performed in association with post-contrast CT and occasionally nuclear medicine studies.
- There is new interest in the use of gadolinium myelography, which can be performed in conjunction with traditional imaging methods, as it has increased spatial resolution.

Suggested Readings

Akbar JJ, Luetmer PH, Schwartz KM, Hunt CH, Diehn FE, Eckel LJ. The role of MR myelography with intrathecal gadolinium in localization of spinal CSF leaks in patients with spontaneous intracranial hypotension. *AJNR.* 2012;33:535-540.

Kraemer N, Berlis A, Schumacher M. Intrathecal gadolinium-enhanced MR myelography showing multiple dural leakages in a patient with Marfan syndrome. *AJR.* 2005;185:92-94.

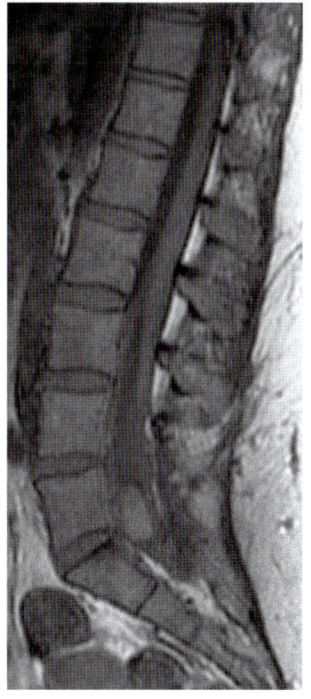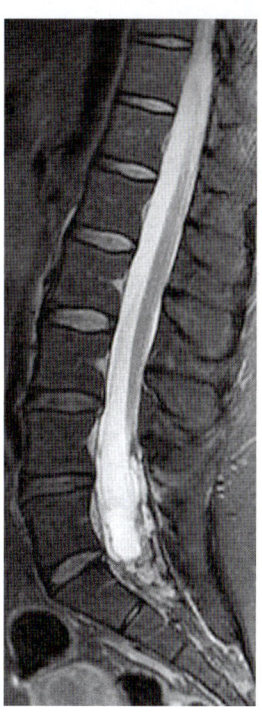

1. What should be included in the differential diagnosis?

2. What are common presenting symptoms?

3. What are associated symptoms?

4. What is the most common location within the spine?

5. What are the treatment options?

Case ranking/difficulty: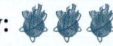

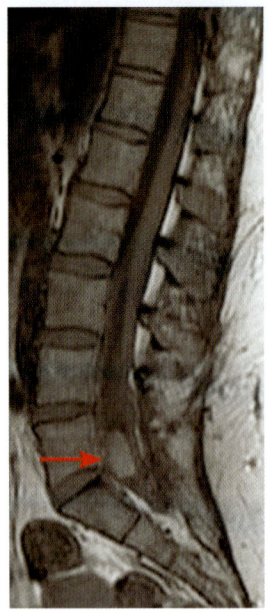

Sagittal T1 image demonstrates intradural hyperintense mass at the level of L5.

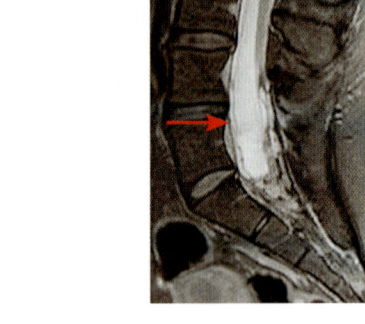

Sagittal T2 image demonstrates intradural hyperintense mass at the level of L5.

Answers

1. Lesions that tend to occur around the conus and may have complex signal characteristics include lipoma, lipomyelocele, dermoid cyst, and epidermoid cyst.

2. Common presenting symptoms include headache, back pain, radiculopathy, myelopathy, and urinary retention; however, the presence of headache raises the concern for rupture with associated chemical meningitis.

3. Acute dermoid cyst rupture can lead to secondary chemical meningitis and present with headache, nausea, vomiting, mental status changes, and coma.

4. 80% are located within the lumbosacral region or associated with the cauda equina.

5. Complete surgical resection is the optimal treatment to prevent progressive symptoms or rupture. Cysts may recur and are more likely to recur in the setting of incomplete resection.

Pearls

- Spinal dermoid cysts can be divided into two categories.
- The congenital lesions arise from residual dermal rests or from expansion of a dermal sinus.

- Acquired lesions are iatrogenic and often arise secondary to previous surgery or lumbar puncture with introduction of dermal and epidermal elements into the thecal sac.
- Patients are often asymptomatic with lesions discovered incidentally at imaging follow-up.
- Symptoms may include slowly progressive radiculopathy or myelopathy depending on the location of the dermoid.
- Rupture of a dermoid may cause chemical meningitis.
- Treatment is resection to prevent complications/ progressive symptoms.

Suggested Readings

De Maio PN, Mikulis DJ, Kiehl T-R, Guha A. Spinal conus dermoid cyst with lipid dissemination. *Radiographics*. 2012;32:1215-1221.

Liu H, Zhang J-N, Zhu T. Microsurgical treatment of spinal epidermoid and dermoid cysts in the lumbosacral region. *J Clin Neurosci.* 2012;19:712-717.

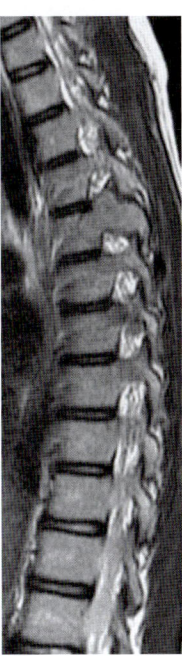

1. What should be included in the differential diagnosis for an osseous lesion?

2. What should be included in the differential diagnosis of soft tissue lesion?

3. What are common presenting symptoms?

4. What are associated findings?

5. What are the treatment options?

Case ranking/difficulty: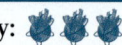

Category: Posterior elements

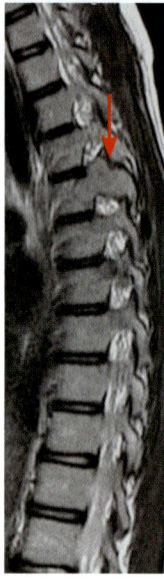

Parasagittal T2 image demonstrates expansile lesion within the posterior elements of T5. Partially visualized expansion of T7 posterior elements.

Answers

1. Etiologies for lytic osseous lesions include metastasis, lymphoma, Langerhans cell histiocytosis, infection, and giant cell tumor.

2. Soft tissue masses that must be differentiated from myofibroma include hemangiopericytoma, fibrosarcoma, leiomyoma, leiomyosarcoma, and neurofibroma.

3. Palpable mass, pain, and pathologic fracture are the most common presenting symptoms of osseous myofibromatosis.

4. Potential associated findings include lytic vertebral body lesion, epidural extension, vertebra plana, cord compression, and intramedullary extension; however, intramedullary extension has only been reported once in the literature.

5. Soft tissue lesions are usually resected for pathologic diagnosis. When there are multiple lesions and involvement of multiple organ systems, symptomatic lesions may be resected. Other treatment options, including physical therapy, bracing, and surgical fixation, may be considered if complications develop.

Pearls

- Myofibroma is the most common soft tissue tumor of infancy and the solitary form may be resected without recurrence.
- However, once patients have multiple lesions, the prognosis is slightly worse.
- Multicentric myofibromatosis may have soft tissue, osseous, and visceral involvement, with symptomatology based on system affected.
- The soft tissue tumors can be confused with benign and malignant soft tissue tumors.
- Osseous lesions are generally lytic and must be differentiated from metastases, infection, and histiocytosis.
- Lesions often demonstrate early growth followed by stabilization or regression.
- Large or symptomatic lesions can be resected; there is no other known treatment.

Suggested Readings

Green MC, Dorfman HD, Villanueva-Siles E, et al. Aggressively recurrent infantile myofibroma of the axilla and shoulder girdle. *Skeletal Radiol*. 2011;40:357-361.

Holzer-Fruehwald L, Blaser S, Roosi A, Fruehwald-Pallamar J, Thurner MM. Imaging findings in seven cases of congenital infantile myofibromatosis with cerebral, spinal or head and neck involvement. *Neuroradiology*. 2012;54:1389-1398.

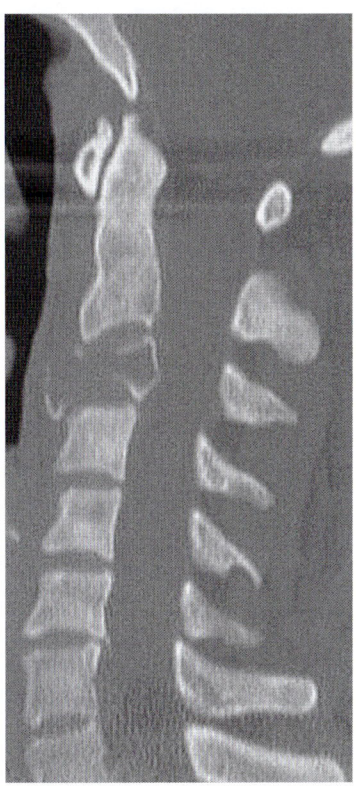

1. What should be included in the differential diagnosis?

2. What are common presenting symptoms?

3. What are the components of McCune Albright syndrome?

4. What are the components of Mazabraud syndrome?

5. What are the treatment options?

Case ranking/difficulty: 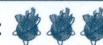   Category: More than one category

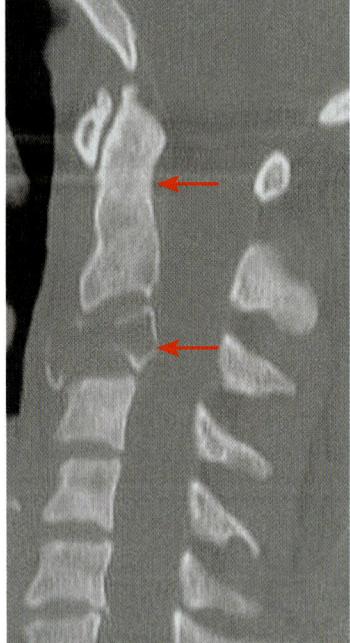

Sagittal CT image demonstrates mixed attenuation infiltration of the dens with areas of "ground glass" attenuation. Burst fracture of C3 with lytic region in the vertebral body.

Answers

1. Multiple lytic osseous lesions can be seen in infection, metastasis, Paget disease, fibrous dysplasia, and multiple myeloma.

2. Potential presenting symptoms include scoliosis, back pain, and pathologic fracture; endocrine dysfunction could be seen in McCune Albright syndrome and soft tissue mass could be seen in Mazabraud syndrome.

3. McCune Albright syndrome is composed of cafe au lait skin lesion, precocious puberty, and polyostotic fibrous dysplasia.

4. Mazabraud syndrome consists of monostotic or polyostotic fibrous dysplasia in conjunction with a single or multiple soft tissue myxomas, often intramuscular.

5. Treatment options include conservative management, bisphosphonate therapy, biopsy, surgical fixation, and curettage with packing; the decision is based on number and location of lesions and presence of complications (growth disturbance, scoliosis, pathologic fracture).

Pearls

- Fibrous dysplasia can have multiple appearances, including internal ground glass opacity and primary lytic appearance.
- The spine is generally only involved in cases of polyostotic fibrous dysplasia, which is less common than the monostotic form.
- Polyostotic fibrous dysplasia should be considered in the differential diagnosis of multiple osseous lesions.
- In the adult patient, the leading diagnosis for this case should be metastatic disease, even in the absence of a known primary.

Suggested Readings

Case DB, Chapman CN, Freeman JK, Polga JP. Atypical presentation of polyostotic fibrous dysplasia with myxoma (Mazabraud syndrome). *Radiographics*. 2010;30:827-832.

Stanton RP, Ippolito E, Springfield D, Lindaman L, Wientroub S, Leet A. The surgical management of fibrous dysplasia of bone. *Orphanet J Rare Dis*. 2012;7(suppl 1):S1.

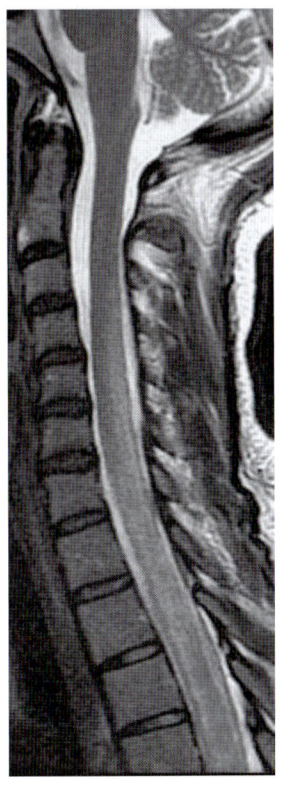
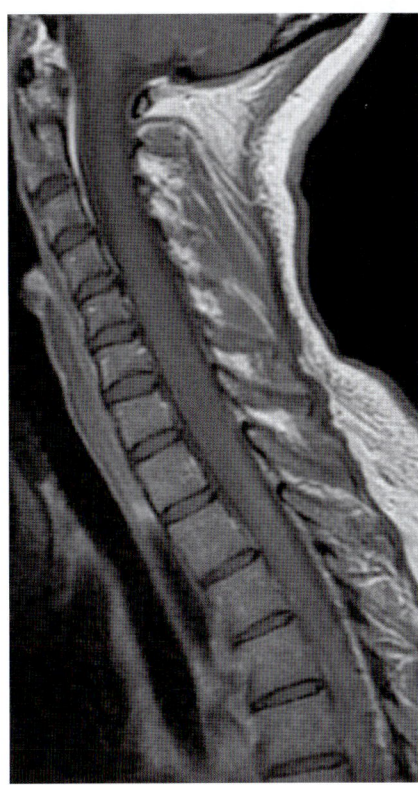

1. What should be included in the differential diagnosis?

2. What are common presenting symptoms?

3. What additional imaging findings can be seen?

4. What additional findings are necessary to make the diagnosis?

5. What are the treatment options?

Case ranking/difficulty: 🌿🌿🌿

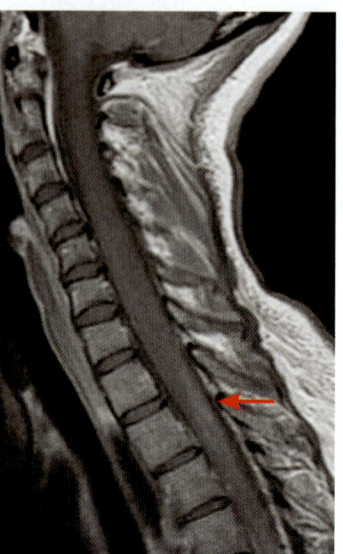

Sagittal T2 image demonstrates extensive T2 hyperintensity and expansion of the cord.

Sagittal T1 image following contrast administration demonstrates vague amorphous enhancement.

Answers

1. T2 hyperintensity and expansion of the cord can be seen in acute disseminated encephalomyelitis, infectious myelitis, multiple sclerosis, primary cord tumor, and transverse myelitis.

2. Patients often present with symptoms of optic neuritis in conjunction with variable myelopathic symptoms, including bowel and bladder dysfunction, sensory dysesthesia, and weakness.

3. Most cases (over three-quarters) will demonstrate optic nerve enhancement.

4. Cerebrospinal fluid pleocytosis is a major criterion for the diagnosis of NMO, as is negative brain imaging. NMO-IgG is not currently incorporated in the criteria; however, it is being considered.

5. First-line therapy is steroids with consideration of immunosuppression in select cases. Plasmapheresis is considered for recalcitrant cases.

Pearls

- Neuromyelitis optica (NMO) is a demyelinating disease that affects the spinal cord and optic nerves.
- It can be difficult to differentiate from other demyelinating disease but the diagnosis is based on lack of intracranial lesions, extensive T2 hyperintensity within the cord, and positive NMO-IgG titers.
- Patients often present with symptoms of optic neuritis, in conjunction with myelopathy.
- This disorder is more common in African American patients.
- Lumbar puncture may show oligoclonal bands, but cellular pleocytosis is the rule.
- Treatment is aimed at decreasing inflammation with steroids, with addition of immunosuppressive therapy after the acute attack.
- The overall prognosis of NMO tends to be worse than multiple sclerosis, with multiple relapses being the rule.

Suggested Readings

Aboul-Enein F, Krssak M, Hoftberger R, Prayer D, Kristoferitsch W. Diffuse white matter damage is absent in neuromyelitis optica. *AJNR*. 2010;31:76-79.

Wingerchuk DM, Lennon VA, Pittock SJ, Lucchinetti CF, Weinshenker BG. Revised diagnostic criteria for neuromyelitis optica. *Neurology*. 2006;66:1485-1489.

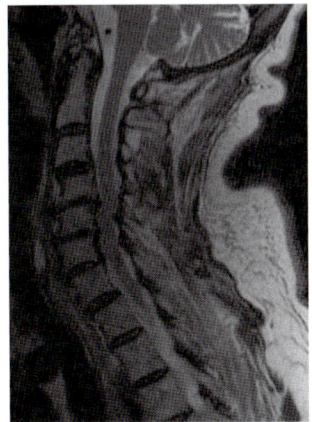
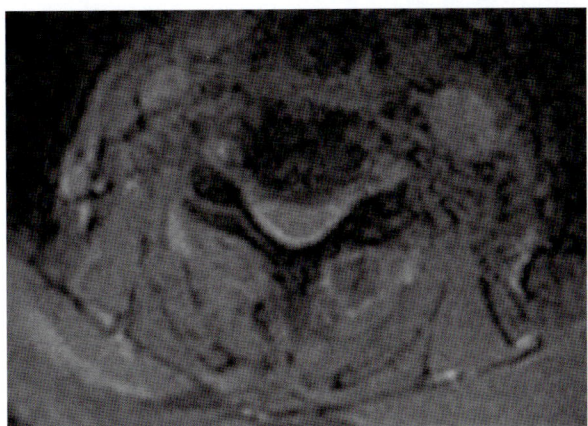
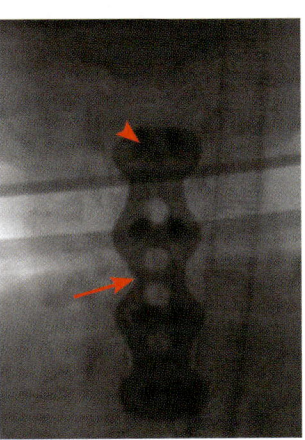
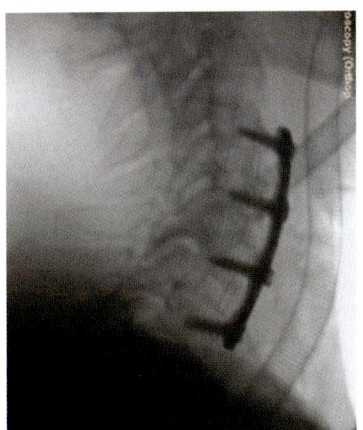

1. What is this procedure called?

2. What are the advantages of an anterior approach?

3. What is the purpose of this procedure?

4. Describe the important surgical steps of the procedure.

5. Name potential complications of this procedure.

Case ranking/difficulty: 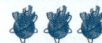   **Category:** Disc

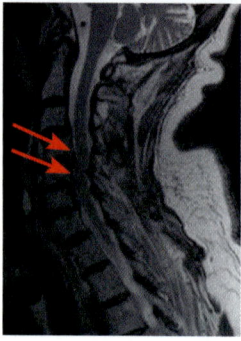

Sagittal T2-weighted sequence of the cervical spine showing multilevel disc degenerative change with disc protrusions (*arrows*) between C4 and C6. The discs abut the cervical cord anteriorly and the central canal is narrowed.

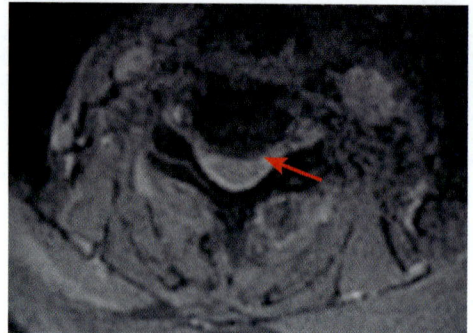

Axial T2-weighted image at the level of C5 showing a central disc protrusion (*arrow*) that impinges the cervical cord.

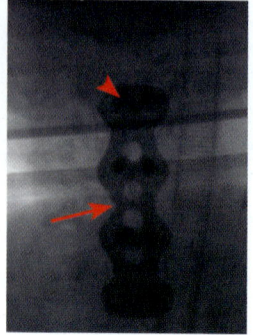

AP fluoroscopic image acquired during the procedure. A titanium plate (*arrow*) was secured using screws (*arrowheads*) following discectomy.

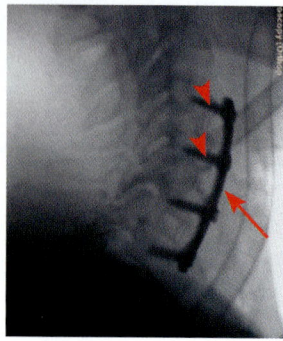

Lateral fluoroscopic image acquired during surgery. A titanium plate (*arrow*) was fixed anteriorly using screws (*arrowheads*).

Answers

1. Anterior cervical discectomy and fusion (ACDF) is a surgical procedure performed for cervical instability, painful cervical disc herniations, osteophytes compressing the nerve roots or spinal cord, and degenerative disc disease. ACDF is often performed when conservative measures have failed. This procedure is performed on the cervical spine using an anterior approach. It involves a discectomy followed by stabilization of the cervical spine.

2. The advantages of using an anterior (as opposed to a posterior) approach include a better access to the cervical spine from C2 down to the cervicothoracic junction and a significant reduction in postoperative pain as the spine can be accessed via anatomical planes.

3. The purpose of ACDF is to free the impinged nerves or spinal cord by removing the causative disc herniations or osteophytes and restore the height of the affected disc.

4. After an anterior incision the surgeon divides the platysma and then follows anatomic planes right down to the spine. The intervertebral disc and any osteophytes are then completely removed. The intervertebral foramen may also be widened in order to make more room for the exiting nerve root. The intervertebral space is then filled with bone graft to increase stability. A titanium plate may be screwed on the anterior aspect of the cervical vertebrae to ensure stability during fusion, particularly when there is more than one disc level involved. The patient may need to wear a neck brace or collar for the first few weeks to ensure proper spinal alignment.

5. ACDF is considered a fairly safe procedure and major complication occur in only about 1%-2%. Most patients will experience odyno- or dysphagia in the first few days postop due to retraction of the esophagus during the procedure. Potential complications of ACDF include injury to the larynx, laryngeal nerves, esophagus, carotid artery, spinal cord, and nerve roots. Infection and implant failure, movement, or malposition may also occur.

Pearls

- Anterior cervical discectomy and fusion (ACDF) involves a discectomy followed by stabilization of the cervical spine.
- The purpose of ACDF is to free the impinged nerves or spinal cord by removing the causative disc herniations or osteophytes and restore the height of the affected disc.
- ACDF is considered a fairly safe procedure and major complication occur in only about 1%-2%.

Suggested Readings

Fountas KN, Kapsalaki EZ, Nikolakakos LG, et al. Anterior cervical discectomy and fusion associated complications. *Spine (Phila Pa 1976)*. 2007 Oct 1;32(21):2310-2317.

Riley LH 3rd, Skolasky RL, Albert TJ, Vaccaro AR, Heller JG. Dysphagia after anterior cervical decompression and fusion: prevalence and risk factors from a longitudinal cohort study. *Spine (Phila Pa 1976)*. 2005 Nov 15;30(22):2564-2569.

Left arm and leg numbness

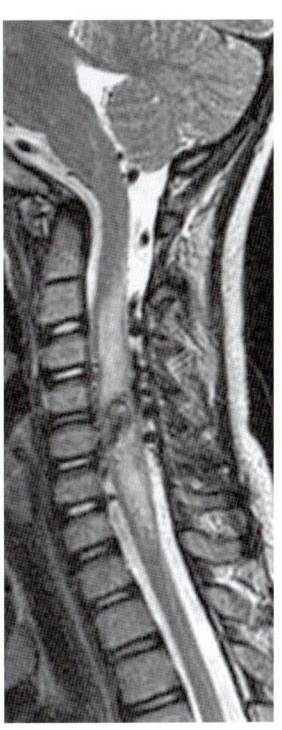

1. What should be included in the differential diagnosis?

2. What are common presenting symptoms?

3. What are components of Cobb syndrome?

4. Which part of the spine is most commonly involved?

5. What are the treatment options?

Case ranking/difficulty: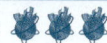

Category: More than one category

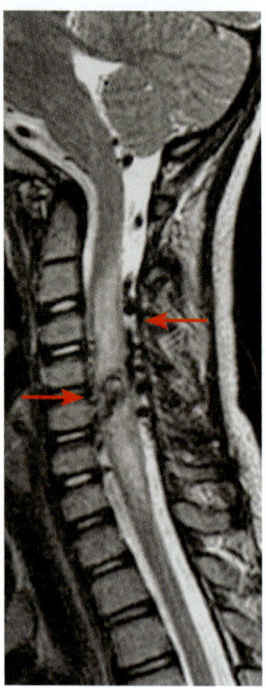

Sagittal T2 image demonstrates hyperintensity and expansion of the cord with flow voids surrounding and within the cord.

Answers

1. The differential diagnosis for intramedullary T2 hyperintensity includes astrocytoma, ependymoma, cavernoma, hemangioblastoma, type 1 juvenile arteriovenous malformation, and type 4 arteriovenous fistula.

2. Common presenting symptoms include pain, weakness, dysesthesia, bowel and bladder incontinence, and headache; headache can result from subarachnoid hemorrhage.

3. Cobb syndrome (spinal arteriovenous metameric syndrome) is characterized by osseous, cutaneous, and spinal cord vascular malformations.

4. Cervical and thoracic regions are most common; however, they can occur anywhere.

5. Embolization is the treatment of choice; partial surgical resection may be possible. However, total resection is often not technically feasible secondary to the large nidus.

Pearls

- Type 3 (juvenile) arteriovenous malformations of the spine have both intramedullary and extramedullary components.
- They may present with progressive weakness or myelopathic symptoms or subarachnoid hemorrhage.
- The diagnosis is based on seeing intramedullary and extramedullary vessels with a definable nidus.
- There are often T2 hyperintense changes within the spinal cord, which may be secondary to ischemic steal or venous hypertension.
- There may be an extraspinal component to these lesions.
- Treatment is generally performed with endovascular embolization.
- Given the diffuse nature of these lesions, complete resection is usually not possible.
- Overall prognosis is poor with progressive neurological deficits if embolization is not successful.

Suggested Readings

Niimi Y, Uchiyama N, Elijovich L, Berenstein A. Spinal arteriovenous metameric syndrome: clinical manifestations and endovascular management. *AJNR*. 2012; epub

Spetzler RF, Detwiler PW, Riina HA, Porter RW. Modified classification of spinal cord vascular lesions. *J Neurosurg*. 2002;96:145-156.

Lower extremity weakness

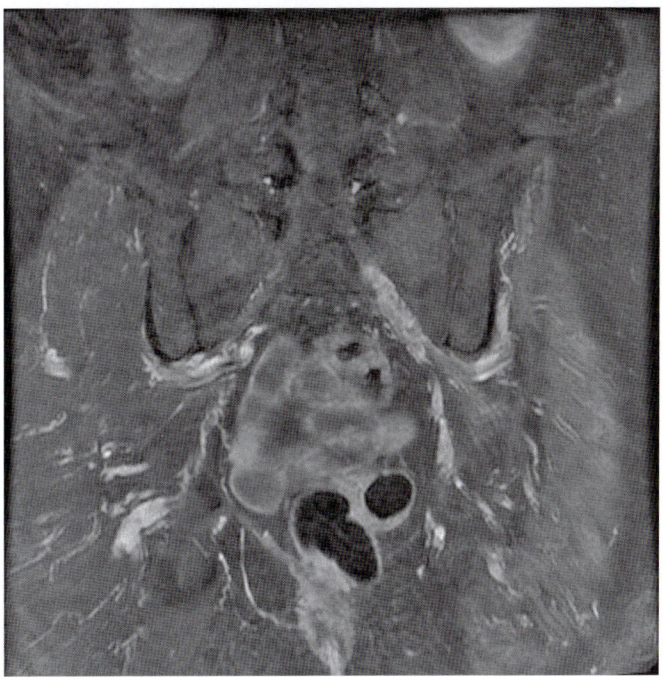

1. What nerve roots form the lumbar plexus?

2. What nerve connects the lumbar plexus and sacral plexus to form the lumbosacral plexus?

3. What is the differential diagnosis for enlargement and enhancement of the lumbosacral plexus?

4. What are common presenting symptoms?

5. What are common malignancies that infiltrate the lumbosacral plexus?

Case ranking/difficulty: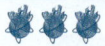

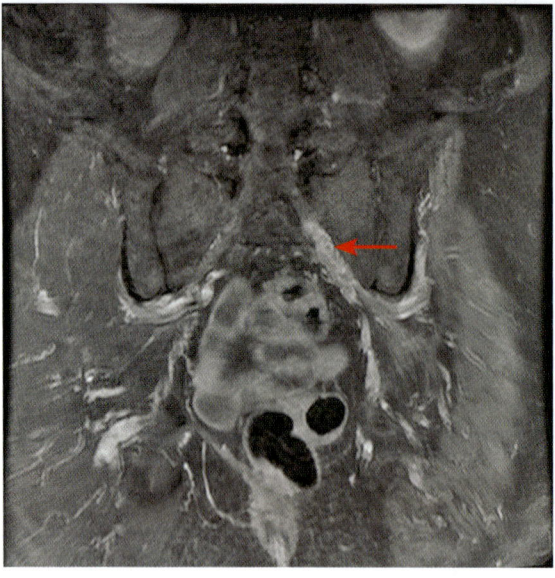

Coronal T1 image following gadolinium administration demonstrates enlargement and enhancement of the S1 and S2 nerve roots on the left.

Pearls

- Infiltration of the lumbosacral plexus most commonly occurs following direct invasion from pelvic tumors.
- Hematogenous spread can occur.
- Presenting symptoms include pain and weakness with sensory deficits. The symptoms may involve multiple nerve distributions and can be either unilateral or bilateral.
- Lumbosacral plexus infiltration generally presents as enlarged, T2 hyperintense, enhancing nerve roots.
- Treatment is directed at treating the primary malignancy.

Suggested Readings

Grisariu S, Avni B, Batchelor TT, et al. Neurolymphomatosis: an international primary CNS lymphoma collaborative group report. *Blood*. 2010;115:5005-5011.

Petchprapa CN, Rosenberg ZS, Sconfienza M, et al. MR imaging of entrapment neuropathies of the lower extremity. *Radiographics*. 2010;30:983-1000.

Answers

1. The lumbar plexus is formed from the ventral rami of L1 through L4. Thus, imaging should extend to the L1 level.

2. The lumbosacral trunk, composed primarily of the L5 nerve root with a small contribution from L4, connects the lumbar and sacral plexi to form the lumbosacral plexus.

3. Enlargement and enhancement of the lumbosacral plexus can be caused by metastatic infiltration, plexiform neurofibroma, lymphoma, or post-radiation plexopathy.

4. Presenting symptoms can include pain and sensory deficits, as well as proximal muscle weakness. Rarely patients can present with incontinence.

5. Colorectal, uterine, ovarian, and cervical carcinomas, as well as lymphoma, are common causes of lumbosacral plexus infiltration.

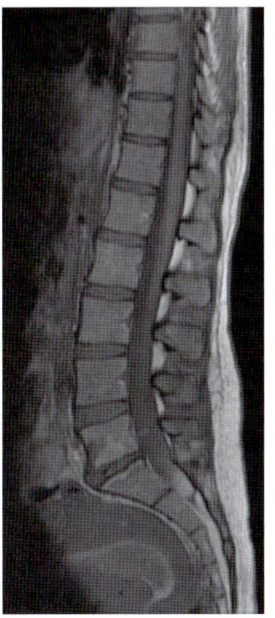 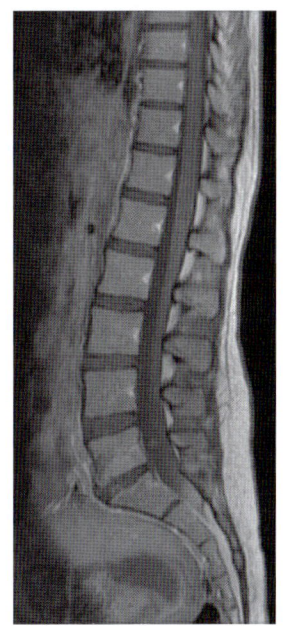

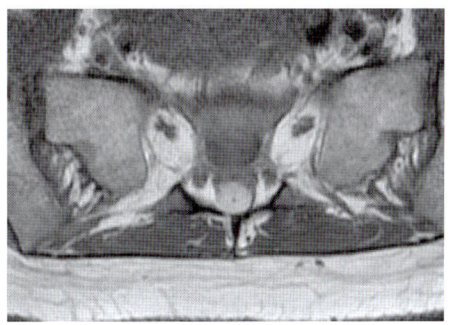

1. What is the most likely diagnosis?

2. How does the condition manifest clinically?

3. Name some causes of this condition.

4. Which imaging modality best images this condition?

5. How is this condition managed?

Case ranking/difficulty: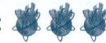

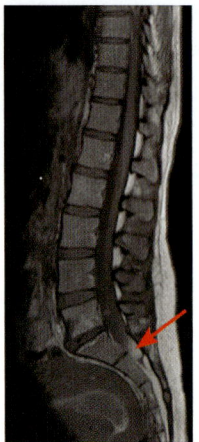

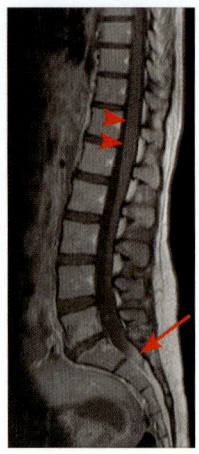

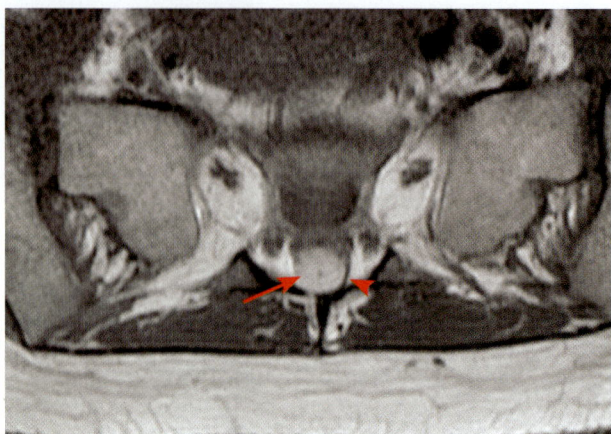

Sagittal T1-weighted sequence of the lumbar spine demonstrates a T1 hyperintense lesion (*arrow*) in the caudal aspect of the thecal sac. The lesion was isointense on T2 and is compatible with an intradural hematoma. Note is made of an enlarged uterus in keeping with recent pregnancy and delivery.

Contrast-enhanced T1-weighted sequence of the lumbar spine. The lesion does not enhance following contrast administration (*arrow*). Note abnormal leptomeningeal enhancement (*arrowheads*) likely secondary to complicating arachnoiditis.

Axial T1-weighted MRI confirms the intradural location of the hematoma (*arrow*). Note the filum terminale passing through the central part of the hematoma. The thecal sac is seen as a linear hypointensity (*arrowhead*).

Answers

1. Spinal hemorrhage is a rare entity and may be intramedullary (hematomyelia) or within the epidural, subdural, or subarachnoid spaces. Spinal subarachnoid hemorrhage (SSH) accounts for <1% of all subarachnoid hemorrhages. It is a potentially dangerous condition that may have disastrous consequences.

2. SSH presents with severe back pain or headache, which may be accompanied by acute sciatic pain, sensory disturbances, paraparesis, and sphincter disturbance.

3. SSH is often secondary to trauma (in >50% of cases), bleeding diatheses (including anticoagulant medication), underlying vascular malformations (arteriovenous malformation, spinal angioma, spinal artery, or intracranial aneurysm), neoplasia (intratumoral hemorrhage), and lumbar puncture. Rarer causes include systemic lupus erythematous, periarteritis nodosa, coarctation of the aorta, hypertension, and Behcet disease. Spinal SAH may also complicate intracranial SAH.

4. MRI is essential to determine the exact location and extent of spinal hemorrhage. It may also reveal the causative lesion or a vascular malformation. A pure subarachnoid hematoma can be easily differentiated from a subdural hematoma. SSHs are located within the thecal

sac with no evidence of an "inverted Mercedes star" sign. The latter is typical of subdural hematoma, which often has a semicircular appearance and tends to be more crescentic on axial sequences. Differentiation between subdural and subarachnoid hemorrhage may, however, be difficult, and at times, only surgical exploration will determine the exact location of the hematoma.

5. Urgent decompressive surgery remains the treatment of choice in spinal subarachnoid hemorrhage with rapidly progressive neurological findings. Conservative treatment is reserved for patients without significant neurological impairment.

Pearls

- Spinal hemorrhage is a rare entity and may be intramedullary (hematomyelia) or within the epidural, subdural, or subarachnoid spaces.
- Urgent decompressive surgery remains the treatment of choice in spinal subarachnoid hemorrhage with rapidly progressive neurological findings.

Suggested Readings

Kim JS, Lee SH. Spontaneous spinal subarachnoid hemorrhage with spontaneous resolution. *J Korean Neurosurg Soc*. 2009 Apr;45(4):253-255.

Kim YH, Cho KT, Chung CK, Kim HJ. Idiopathic spontaneous spinal subarachnoid hemorrhage. *Spinal Cord*. 2004 Sep;42(9):545-547.

Dropped head syndrome

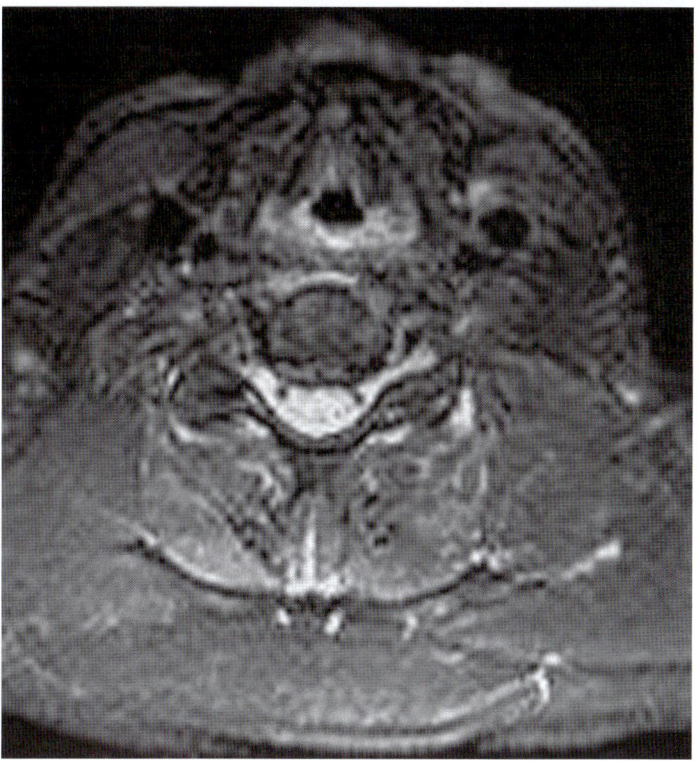

1. What are the etiologies of this abnormality?

2. What is this abnormality known as when there is no definable cause?

3. What should be included in the imaging evaluation?

4. What are common presenting symptoms?

5. What are the treatment options?

Case ranking/difficulty: 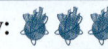 **Category:** Paraspinal soft tissue

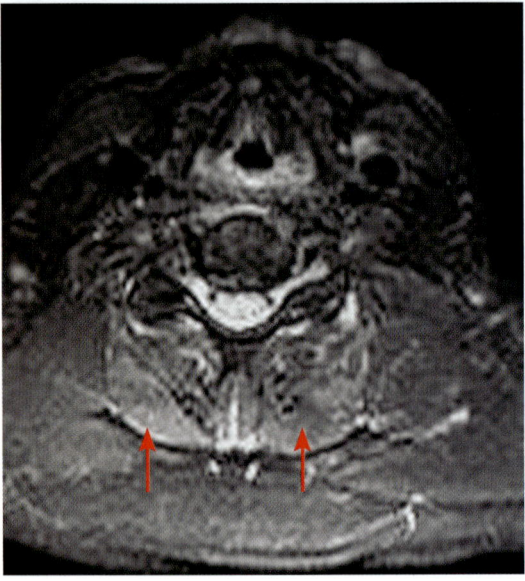

Axial T2 image demonstrates increased T2 signal within the posterior paraspinal muscles.

Answers

1. There are numerous etiologies for dropped head syndrome, including polymyositis, myasthenia, systemic sclerosis, amyotrophic lateral sclerosis, and chronic inflammatory demyelinating polyneuropathy.

2. Isolated neck extensor myopathy is a cause of dropped head syndrome and important to differentiate from other causes.

3. The evaluation of dropped head syndrome may include MRI cervical spine, electromyography, nerve conduction studies, and laboratory studies, depending on the clinical situation.

4. While the weakness is often most profound in the neck extensors, other muscle groups can be involved, including the neck flexors and shoulder abductors.

5. There is controversy over the treatment of dropped head syndrome with little evidence for efficacy of a single treatment plan. Treatment options include conservative management, steroids, intravenous immunoglobulins, plasmapheresis, and surgical fixation. Surgical fixation is reserved for refractory causes in patients who are good surgical candidates.

Pearls

- Dropped head syndrome is a general term applied to a variety of disorders that lead to focal cervical kyphosis and inability to extend one's spine against gravity.
- It can initially be difficult to differentiate from changes in alignment from the normal aging process.
- Etiologies include myasthenia gravis, chronic inflammatory demyelinating polyneuropathy, hypothyroidism, mitochondrial disease, amyotrophic lateral sclerosis, polymyositis, camptocormia, and systemic sclerosis.
- Treatment is aimed at the underlying abnormality with surgical fusion reserved for recalcitrant cases in which the patients are felt to be good surgical candidates.

Suggested Readings

Katz JS, Wolfe GI, Burns DK, Bryan WW, Fleckenstein JL, Barohn RJ. Isolated neck extensor myopathy: a common cause of dropped head syndrome. *Neurology*. 1996;46:917-921.

Rosato E, Rossi C, Salsano F. Dropped head syndrome and systemic sclerosis. *Joint Bone Spine*. 2009;76:301-303.

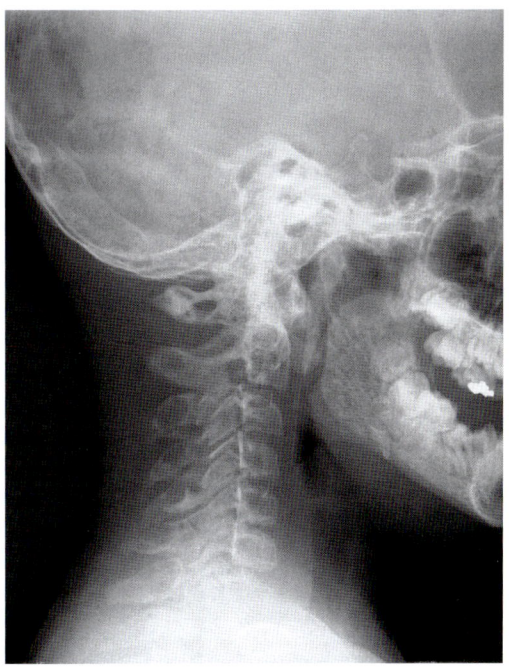

1. What should be included in the differential diagnosis?

2. What are common presenting symptoms?

3. This abnormality arises from a developmental insult prior to what age?

4. What organ systems can be involved?

5. What are the treatment options?

Case ranking/difficulty:

Category: More than one category

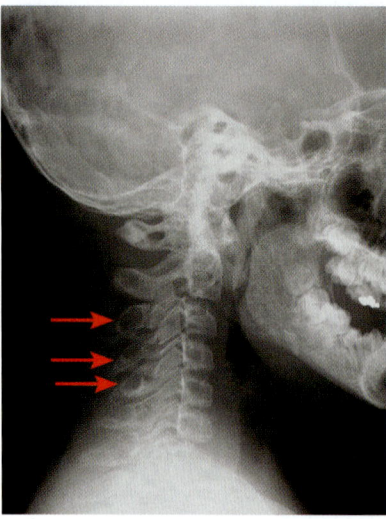

Lateral radiograph demonstrates multiple lucent lesions throughout the osseous structures; alignment is maintained.

Answers

1. The differential for multiple lytic osseous lesions includes metastases, infection, Langerhans cell histiocytosis, and lymphangiomatosis. Letterer-Siwe disease is the previous name for multifocal multisystem Langerhans cell histiocytosis.

2. In the setting of primary osseous involvement, pain and pathologic fracture are the most common presenting symptoms; other symptoms include palpable mass and chylous pleural effusion.

3. The insult is felt to likely occur between 14 and 20 weeks.

4. Lymphangiomatosis can involve any organ system.

5. Treatment options include conservative management, surgical fixation, radiation, bisphosphonate therapy, and interferon therapy. While these are all potential treatment options, there is no set successful treatment algorithm.

Pearls

- Lymphangiomatosis is a rare cause of multiple osseous lytic lesions.
- It can also present with visceral and mediastinal involvement.
- Lymphangiomatosis is usually diagnosed in childhood.
- There is no known etiology; however, it is associated with persistent dilation of lymphatics secondary to disrupted development in utero.
- Patients should be monitored for the development of pain, which may signify pathological fracture.
- If extensive lesions threaten osseous stability, prophylactic surgical fixation may be performed.

Suggested Readings

Kwag E, Shim SS, Kim Y, Chang JH, Kim KC. CT features of generalized lymphangiomatosis in adult patients. *Clin Imag.* 2013;37(4):723-727.

Wunderbaldinger P, Paya K, Partik B, et al. CT and MR imaging of generalized cystic lympangiomatosis in pediatric patients. *AJR.* 2000;174:827-832.

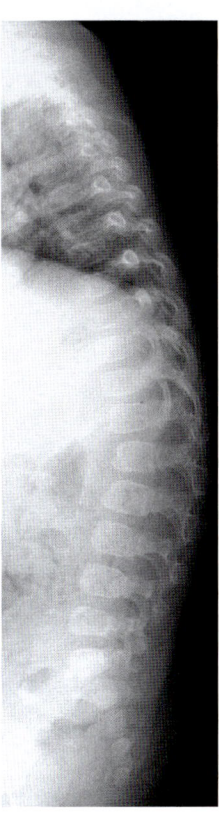

1. What should be included in the differential diagnosis?

2. When performing radiographs for evaluation of skeletal dysplasia, what are the spinal parameters that should be reported?

3. What are the imaging findings?

4. What are the treatment options?

5. What should be considered in the timing of potential surgical correction?

Case ranking/difficulty: 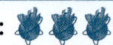   **Category:** Spinal canal

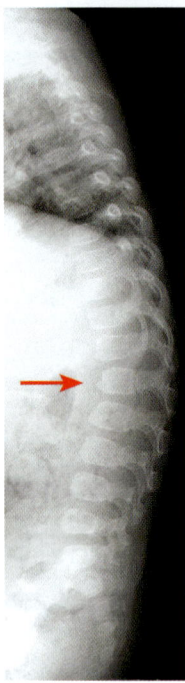

Lateral radiograph demonstrates focal thoracolumbar kyphosis with mild anterior beaking of the T12 vertebral body.

Answers

1. Gibbus deformity is most commonly associated with mucopolysaccharidoses; other etiologies include Scheuermann disease, idiopathic scoliosis, achondroplasia, and spondyloepiphyseal dysplasia. Gibbus deformity may also be acquired eg, in tuberculosis.

2. Alignment, pedicular length, vertebral body shape, and fusion or segmentation anomalies should all be reported.

3. Findings that can be seen in mucopolysaccharidoses include hypoplasia of the dens, platyspondyly, dural thickening, and foramen magnum stenosis.

4. External bracing has not been shown to change the outcome. However, surgery is generally reserved for high-degree kyphosis or scoliosis.

5. Generally delaying surgical fusion as long as possible is ideal to allow maximum growth and make the surgery technically easier. Other factors include rate of progression of kyphosis/scoliosis and myelopathic symptoms.

Pearls

• Gibbus deformity is an unusual radiographic finding that should prompt an evaluation for underlying mucopolysaccharidosis.
• The kyphosis should be measured with radiographic follow-up to document progression.
• Kyphosis greater than 40° is more likely to progress.
• Progressive kyphosis may necessitate surgical fusion.

Suggested Readings

Parnell SE, Phillips GS. Neonatal skeletal dysplasias. *Pediatr Radiol.* 2012;42:S150-S157.
White KK. Orthopaedic aspects of mucopolysaccharidoses. *Rheumatology.* 2011;50:v26-v33.

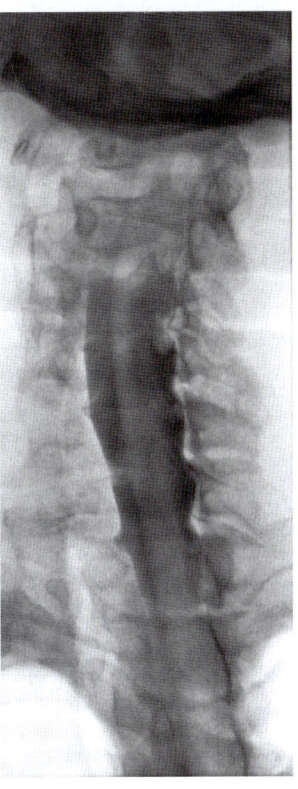

1. Which is the correct order of the brachial plexus components from proximal to distal?

2. What are common presenting symptoms?

3. Where are the components of the brachial plexus located with respect to osseous and soft tissue landmarks?

4. What imaging studies can be used in the evaluation of brachial plexus injuries?

5. What are the treatment options?

Case ranking/difficulty: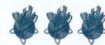

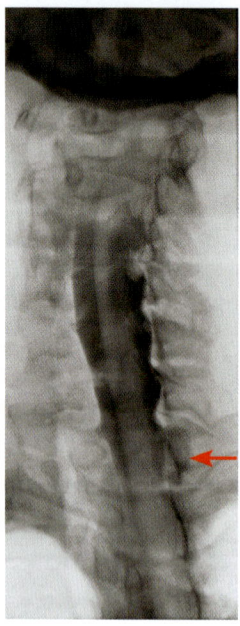

AP image of the cervical spine following intrathecal contrast administration demonstrates focal outpouching of contrast at the level of the left T1 and T2 nerve roots.

Answers

1. The correct order from proximal to distal is roots, trunks, divisions, cords, and branches.

2. The brachial plexus has both motor and sensory components and both can be affected by injury. Horner syndrome can occur from injury to the infraclavicular plexus. Diaphragmatic paralysis can occur from injuries involving the C3, C4, and C5 nerve roots.

3. Roots are located in the neural foramina; trunks are located between the scalene muscles; divisions are located posterior to the clavicle; cords are located inferior to the clavicle. Knowing the anatomic location is important for identifying abnormalities.

4. CT myelography and MRI are equivalent for diagnosis. While myelography is invasive, discussion with the ordering provider regarding their preference is important. Chest radiographs can be helpful; if diaphragmatic paralysis is present, this generally implies a permanent deficit.

5. Treatment options include physical therapy and surgical exploration for either reanastomosis or grafting. Immobilization is contraindicated and may lead to a frozen joint.

Pearls

- Brachial plexopathy symptoms tend to be vague and nonspecific.
- Cases of neuropraxic (stretching) injuries and avulsions tend to present with motor symptoms.
- Brachial plexus injuries can occur during delivery, particularly in the setting of shoulder dystocia.
- A radiologist should attempt to define the gap distance between the avulsed nerve segments, which can be important information for a surgeon planning potential reanastomosis.
- Additionally, evaluation for associated injuries, including to the spinal cord should be performed.

Suggested Readings

Castillo M. Imaging the anatomy of the brachial plexus: review and self-assessment module. *AJR.* 2005;185:S196-S204.

Sureka J, Cherian RA, Alexander M, Thomas BP. MRI of brachial plexopathies. *Clin Radiol.* 2009;64:208-218.

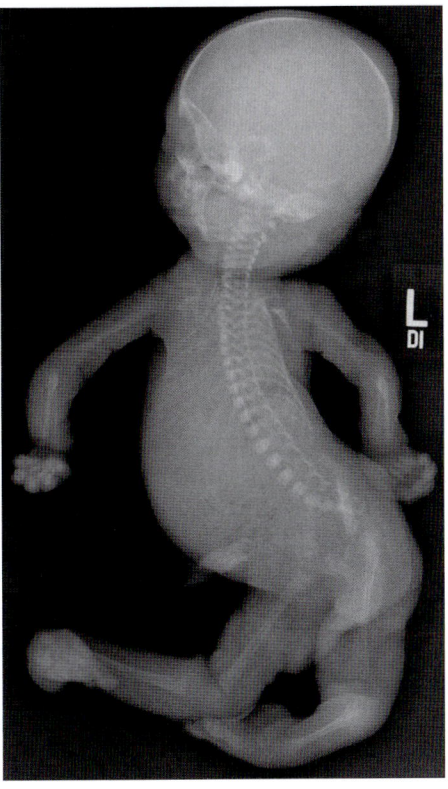

1. What should be considered in the differential diagnosis for neonatal scoliosis?

2. What are the etiologies?

3. What are prenatal ultrasound findings?

4. What are associated neuropathic abnormalities?

5. What are the treatment options?

Case ranking/difficulty: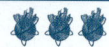

Category: Spinal canal

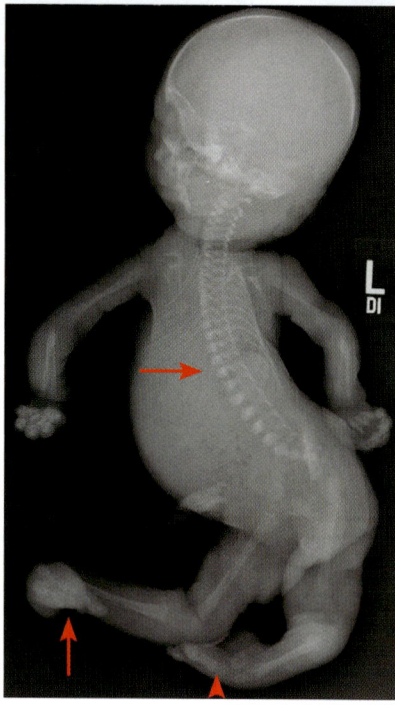

AP radiograph demonstrates C-shaped scoliosis and multiple joint contractures.

Answers

1. The differential diagnosis for neonatal scoliosis includes hemivertebra, vertebral bar, neuromuscular scoliosis, and paraspinal mass.

2. The primary abnormality is felt to be impaired intrauterine fetal movement, which can arise from multiple causes, including neurologic abnormalities, intrauterine space compromise, placental insufficiency, teratogenic exposure, and muscle abnormalities. Additionally, connective tissue abnormalities, maternal disease (such as diabetes mellitus, myotonic dystrophy, myasthenia gravis, and multiple sclerosis), and infection have been implicated.

3. Prenatal ultrasound findings include fixed flexion deformities, intrauterine growth retardation, increased nuchal translucency, and scoliosis.

4. The neuropathic abnormalities seen in arthrogryposis are varied and can include cerebellar hypoplasia, anterior horn cell loss, dorsal column degeneration, pyramidal tract degeneration, and peripheral neuropathy. Additional abnormalities include cortical frontal atrophy, neuronal migration abnormalities, and olivopontocerebellar degeneration.

5. Therapy and splinting are the mainstays of treatment with adjunct orthopedic surgery. Spinal cord stimulation and ventriculoperitoneal shunt placement may be considered in select patients.

Pearls

- Arthrogryposis is a rare disorder that causes multiple joint contractures.
- It is multifactorial and may be secondary to neurological disorders in the neonate or causes of restricted intrauterine movement.
- It should be considered in the evaluation of the neonate with scoliosis.
- Treatment is geared at orthopedic abnormalities and includes fixation/surgical intervention as indicated, as well as physical and occupational therapy.

Suggested Readings

Gordon N. Arthrogryposis multiplex congenita. *Brain Dev*.1998;30:507-511.

Jacobsen HG, Herbert EA, Poppel MH. Arthrogryposis multiplex congenita. *Radiology*. 1955;65:8-18.

Kalampokas E, Kalampokas T, Sofoudis C, Deligeoroglou E, Bostis D. Diagnosing arthrogryposis multiplex congenita: a review. *ISRN Obstet Gynecol*. 2012; Article ID 264198, 6 pages.

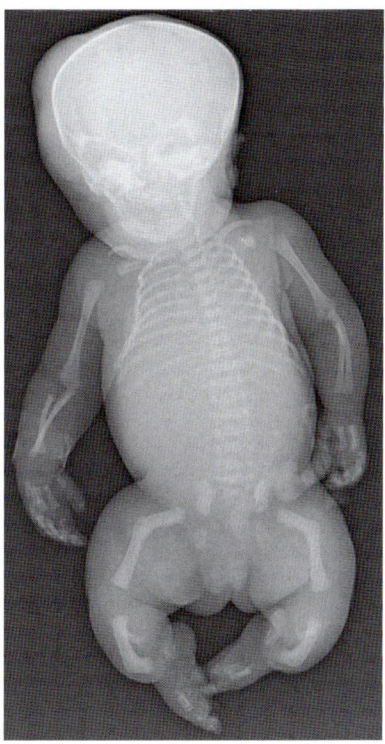

1. What are the major differential diagnoses?

2. What is the likely diagnosis, and what are the major features that suggest this diagnosis?

3. What is the typical lifespan?

4. What are some of the nonskeletal-associated features?

5. What is the presumed etiology of this entity?

Case ranking/difficulty:    **Category:** More than one category

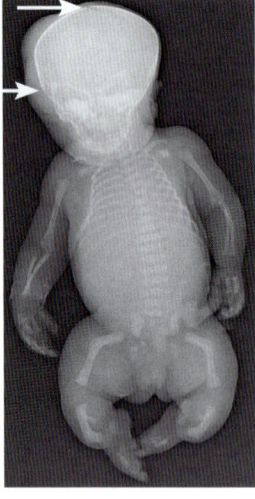

Absent pedicle T1-10, angular bowing of lower extremities. Short ribs and hypoplastic scapulae. Skull fractures (*arrows*) with cephalohematoma due to hydrocephalus and traumatic birth. The acetabulae and iliac bones are dysplastic.

Absent pedicles from T1-10, with hypoplastic vertebrae.

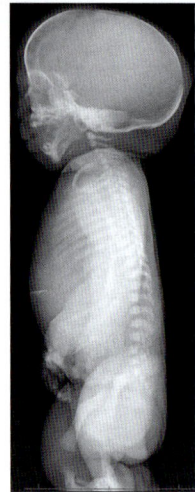

Note the "flat face" appearance and hydrocephalus.

Answers

1. The differential includes any dwarfism, including thanatophoric and diastrophic dwarfism, achondroplasia, osteogenesis imperfecta, and campomelic dwarfism.

2. The hypoplastic scapulae, vertical iliac bones, and hypoplastic vertebrae are characteristic of campomelic dwarfism.

3. The severe respiratory insufficiency that is a result of the hypoplastic ribs, laryngotracheomalacia, and abnormal thorax typically results in death within the first year of life.

4. Associated features include hearing loss, congenital heart disease, hydronephrosis, hydrocephalus, and laryngotracheomalacia. The latter, along with the hypoplastic ribs, results in the severe respiratory compromise that is typically fatal.

5. Campomelic dysplasia is caused by an alteration in the *SOX9* gene. This gene is responsible for both bone formation and testes development. This may result in sex reversal and occurs in 66% of genetic males, with ambiguous genitalia. It is also the primary reason for the marked skeletal abnormalities.

Pearls

- Campomelic dysplasia is a rare dwarfism with an autosomal dominant inheritance pattern.
- Characteristic radiologic features include:
  - 11 short ribs
  - Absent thoracic pedicles and vertebral hypoplasia
  - Angular bowing of the femora and tibiae
  - Hypoplastic fibulae
  - Hypoplastic scapulae
  - Dysplastic iliac bones and acetabulae with dislocated hips
  - "Flat" facies
- Associated features include:
  - Congenital heart disease
  - Hydrocephalus
  - Hydronephrosis
- Death is usually due to respiratory insufficiency, often in the first year of life.

Suggested Readings

Dahdaleh NS, Albert GW, Hasan DM. Campomelic dysplasia: a rare cause of congenital spinal deformity. *J Clin Neurosci.* 2010 May;17(5):664-666.

Gimovsky M, Rosa E, Tolbert T, Guzman G, Nazir M, Koscica K. Campomelic dysplasia: case report and review. *J Perinatol.* 2008 Jan;28(1):71-73.

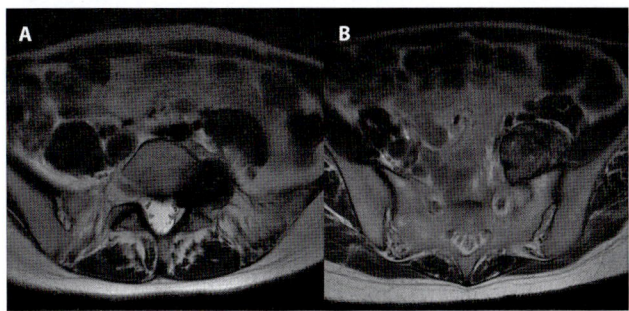

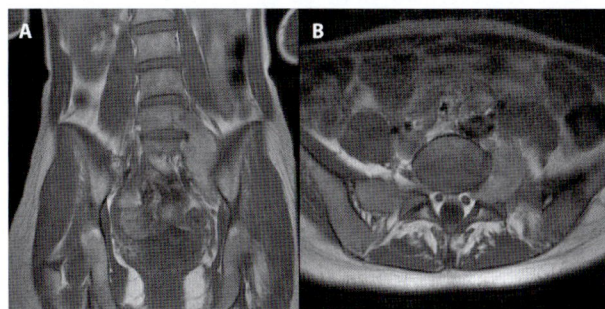

1. What is the most likely diagnosis?

2. How do these lesions usually behave?

3. What should be included in the differential diagnosis?

4. Which of the following modalities best image the condition?

5. How is the diagnosis confirmed?

Case ranking/difficulty: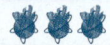

Category: Nerve roots/Nerve plexus/Peripheral nerves

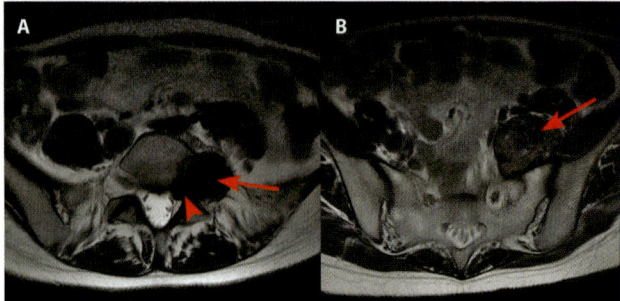

Axial T2-weighted images at the level of L5 vertebra (panel A) and the sacroiliac joints (panel B). A hypointense heterogeneous lesion with a "dumbbell" shape is seen to arise from the left exiting L5 nerve root (*arrow*, panel A) and extends caudally along the anterior surface of the left sacral ala (*arrow*, panel B). The lesion causes expansion of the left intervertebral foramen (*arrowhead*, panel A).

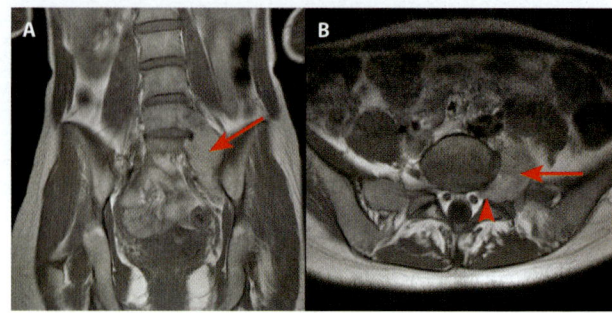

Coronal (Panel A) and axial (Panel B) T1-weighted images show a T1-hyperintense lesion (*arrows*, panels A and B) extending from the left L5 intervertebral foramen (*arrowhead*, panel B) along the left sacral ala.

Answers

1. Melanocytic schwannomas are very rare tumors derived from the neural crest that arise in the spinal nerve roots but may also originate from the central nervous system and in soft tissues.

2. Tumor behavior is difficult to predict, but they are often locally aggressive and have the capacity to metastasize. The clinical outcomes are often disappointing and local recurrence and invasion tend to occur despite surgery and radiotherapy.

   It is thought that melanin is acquired by the Schwann cells from nearby nonneoplastic melanocytes via a process called *cytocrine injection*. Alternatively, Schwann cells may phagocytize melanin.

3. Differential diagnosis includes other melanocytic neoplasms, ganglioneuroblastoma, melanotic medulloblastoma, pigmented neurofibroma, pigmented neuroblastoma, melanotic neuroendocrine carcinomas, carcinoids, and neurotropic melanoma.

4. Melanocytic schwannomas cannot be distinguished from other neurogenic tumors on CT as it does not show any characteristic features. MRI is the imaging investigation of choice and characteristically shows intrinsic high signal intensity on T1-weighted images due to the presence of melanin. Melanin shortens both T1 and T2 relaxation times.

5. A percutaneous biopsy is often needed for definite diagnosis.

Pearls

- Melanocytic schwannomas are very rare tumors derived from the neural crest, which often arise in the spinal nerve roots.
- The clinical outcomes are often disappointing, and local recurrence and invasion tend to occur despite surgery and radiotherapy.
- MRI is the imaging investigation of choice and shows characteristic intrinsic high signal intensity on T1-weighted images due to the presence of melanin.
- A percutaneous biopsy is often needed for definite diagnosis.

Suggested Readings

Killeen RM, Davy CL, Bauserman SC. Melanocytic schwannoma. *Cancer*. 1988 Jul 1;62(1):174-183.

Liessi G, Barbazza R, Sartori F, Sabbadin P, Scapinello A. CT and MR imaging of melanocytic schwannomas; report of three cases. *Eur J Radiol*. 1990 Sep-Oct;11(2):138-142.

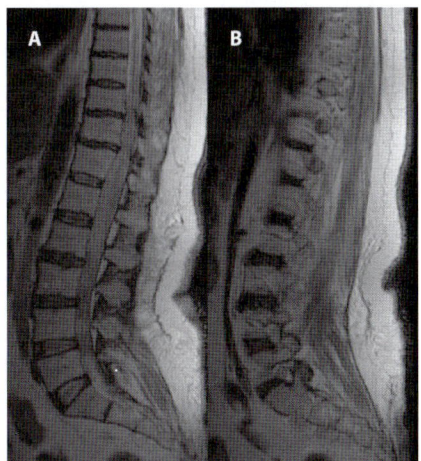
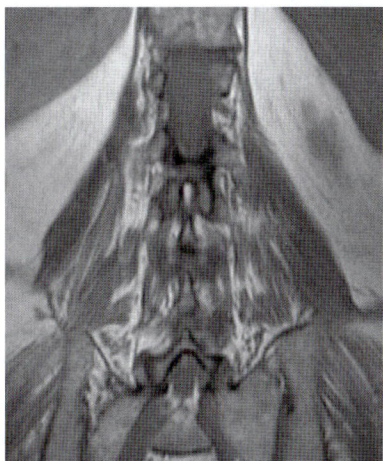
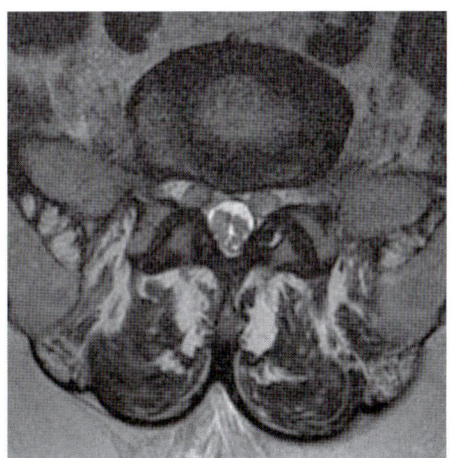

1. What is the most likely diagnosis?

2. What should be included in the differential diagnosis?

3. Which symptoms are encountered in this condition?

4. Which imaging modality best images this condition?

5. Which treatments may be beneficial?

Case ranking/difficulty: 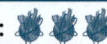   **Category:** Nerve roots/Nerve plexus/Peripheral nerves

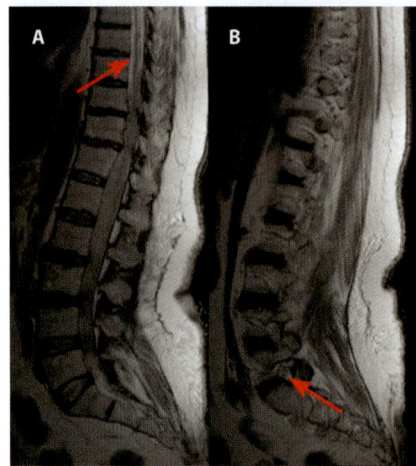

Sagittal T2-weighted sequence of the lumbar spine. Note that the CSF (*arrow*, panel A) is completely effaced in the lumbar canal due to hypertrophy of the cauda equina roots. The left L5 exiting nerve root is also hypertrophied (*arrow*, panel B).

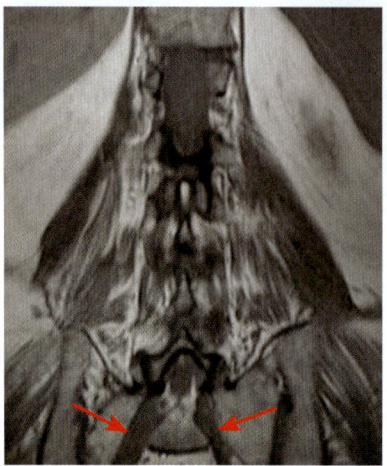

Coronal T1-weighted sequence of the lumbar spine demonstrates bilateral hypertrophied S1 exiting nerve roots (*arrows*). Note is also made of splenomegaly.

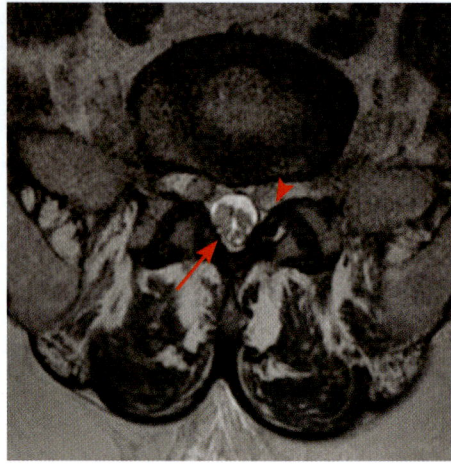

Axial T2-weighted image of the lumbar spine. There is clumping of the hypertrophied cauda equina roots (*arrow*). Note the increased cross-sectional diameter of the exiting nerve roots (*arrowhead*).

Answers

1. Chronic inflammatory demyelinating polyneuropathy (CIDP) is a chronic progressive or relapsing symmetric sensory-motor disorder.

   It is considered the chronic counterpart of Guillain-Barre syndrome.

2. Differential diagnosis include acute inflammatory demyelinating polyradiculoneuropathy, inclusion body myositis, cervical myelopathy, dermatomyositis, polymyositis, HIV-1–associated progressive polyradiculopathy, Lambert-Eaton myasthenic syndrome, diabetic neuropathy, amyotrophic lateral sclerosis, myasthenia gravis, syringomyelia, metabolic myopathies, neurosarcoidosis, and nutritional neuropathies.

3. Affected individuals may present with motor, sensory, or autonomic disturbances. Symptoms include initial proximal and distal limb weakness, paresthesia (characteristically in a stocking-glove distribution), gait disturbances, fatigue, and orthostatic dizziness.

4. MRI demonstrates abnormal hypertrophy of the nerve roots (in the cauda equina, brachial, and lumbosacral plexuses) which is likely secondary to repeated demyelination and remyelination. Clumping of the nerve roots is also seen. Abnormal contrast enhancement of the roots may be seen particularly in active disease.

5. Treatment includes the administration of corticosteroids, which may be prescribed alone or in combination with immunosuppressant drugs.

   Physical therapy also has an important role and improves muscle strength, function, and mobility.

Pearls

- Chronic inflammatory demyelinating polyneuropathy (CIDP) is a chronic progressive or relapsing symmetric sensory-motor disorder.
- MRI demonstrates abnormal hypertrophy and clumping of the nerve roots and pathological contrast enhancement.

Suggested Readings

Kale HA, Sklar E. Magnetic resonance imaging findings in chronic inflammatory demyelinating polyneuropathy with intracranial findings and enhancing, thickened cranial and spinal nerves. *Australas Radiol.* 2007 Oct;51 Spec No. B21-4.

Kitakule MM, McNeal A. Massive nerve root hypertrophy in chronic inflammatory demyelinating polyradiculoneuropathy. *J Assoc Acad Minor Phys.* 1997;8(3):55-57.

Sudden loss of power of neck extensor musculature

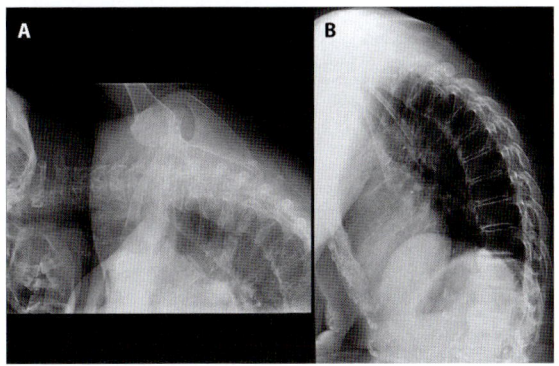

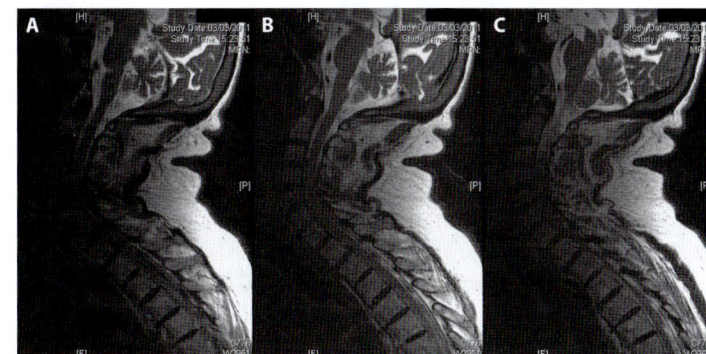

1. What is the most likely diagnosis?

2. What should be included in the differential diagnosis?

3. Which treatments have proved to be beneficial?

4. Describe clinical and pathological characteristics of this condition.

5. Which investigations may aid diagnosis?

Case ranking/difficulty:    **Category:** Miscellaneous

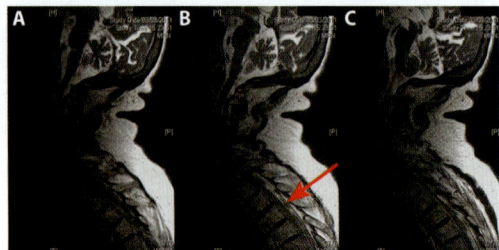

Stacked sagittal T2-weighted MR images of the cervicothoracic spine. Exaggerated thoracic kyphosis with compensatory cervical lordosis is seen, although the changes are less dramatic compared to plain radiography as the patient was scanned in the supine position. The vertebrae have normal heights and marrow signal. Prominent CSF flow artifacts in the upper thoracic spine (*arrow*, image B) reflect altered CSF flow dynamics. There are no significant intervertebral disc protrusions or spinal canal stenosis.

Answers

1. Inclusion body myositis (IBM) is an inflammatory muscle disease characterized by slowly progressive weakness and wasting of both distal and proximal muscles, mostly apparent in the musculature of the upper and lower extremities.

   The condition manifests itself in two different ways: sporadic inclusion body myositis and hereditary inclusion body myopathy. The histopathological changes in IBM were first described in the mid-1960s, although the disorder was not distinguished from polymyositis and named until 1971.

2. Dropped head syndrome results from neck extensor muscle weakness and has been described in a number of neurological disorders. These include amyotrophic lateral sclerosis, multiple sclerosis, and extensor myopathy. Radiotherapy and cervical cord injury have also been implicated.

3. In contrast to other inflammatory myopathies such as dermatomyositis and polymyositis, IBM is relatively resistant to standard immunosuppressive therapy, with muscle strength improving minimally if at all to corticosteroids and other agents.

   Some studies have reported a partial response to corticosteroids with either mild improvement in or stabilization of muscle strength. Serum creatine kinase levels often fall and may even normalize.

4. Patients with inclusion body myositis usually present after several years of gradually worsening muscle weakness. Age of presentation is an important prognostic predictor. The older the age of onset of the disease, the more rapid is the loss of strength and function. By 15 years, most patients will require assistance to cope with basic activities of daily living and some become

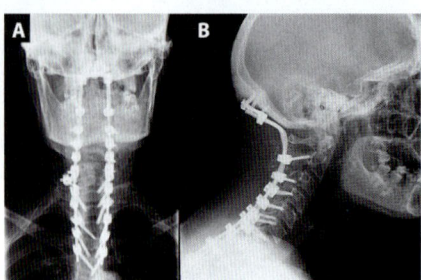

Postoperative frontal (image A) and lateral (image B) radiographs show posterior instrumented fixation of the cervical spine, using a double rod and screw construct.

wheelchair bound or bedridden. IBM can be an indirect cause of death due to respiratory failure or infection.

5. Elevated (up to 10 times the normal range) creatine kinase levels are typical of inclusion body myositis but patients can also present with normal CK levels. Electromyographic studies often display abnormalities. Inclusion body myositis is a pathological challenge and even with a biopsy, the diagnosis can be ambiguous.

Pearls

- Inclusion body myositis (IBM) is an inflammatory muscle disease characterized by slowly progressive weakness and wasting of both distal and proximal muscles.
- It has been described in a number of neurological disorders.
- The condition manifests itself in two different ways: sporadic inclusion body myositis and hereditary inclusion body myopathy.
- Age of presentation is an important prognostic predictor.
- IBM is relatively resistant to standard immunosuppressive therapy.
- IBM can be an indirect cause of death due to respiratory failure or infection.

Suggested Readings

Peng A, Koffman BM, Malley JD, Dalakas MC. Disease progression in sporadic inclusion body myositis: observations in 78 patients. *Neurology*. 2000;55:296.

Phillips BA, Zilko PJ, Mastaglia FL. Prevalence of sporadic inclusion body myositis in Western Australia. *Muscle Nerve*. 2000;23:970.

Wilson FC, Ytterberg SR, St Sauver JL, Reed AM. Epidemiology of sporadic inclusion body myositis and polymyositis in Olmsted County, Minnesota. *J Rheumatol*. 2008;35:445.

Chronic low back pain

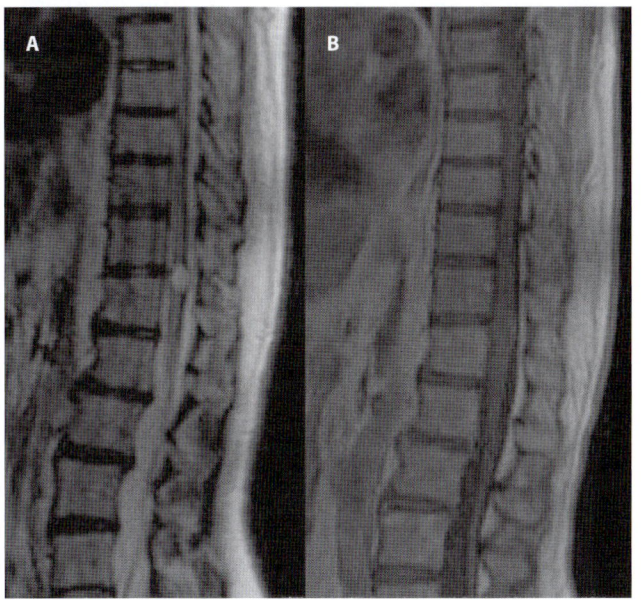

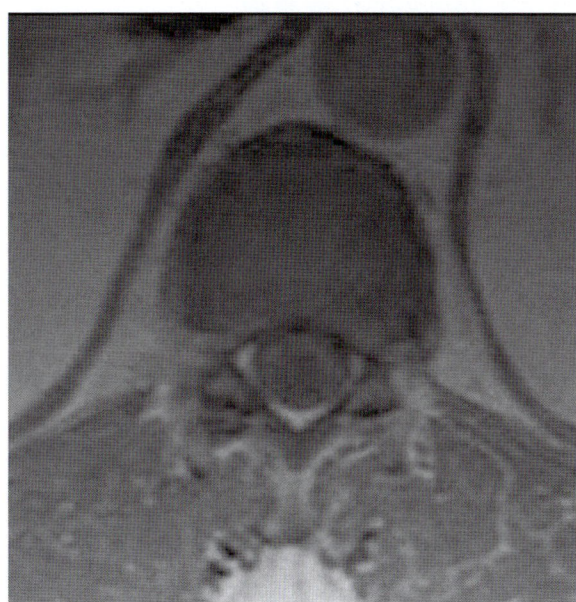

1. What is the most likely diagnosis?

2. What should be included in the differential diagnosis?

3. Where are these lesions most commonly encountered?

4. Which vertebral anomalies are associated with the condition?

5. Which conditions from part of the bronchopulmonary foregut malformations?

Case ranking/difficulty: 🌸🌸🌸

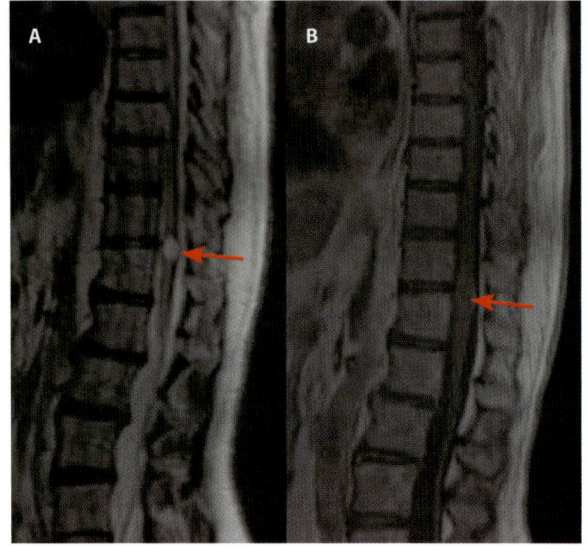

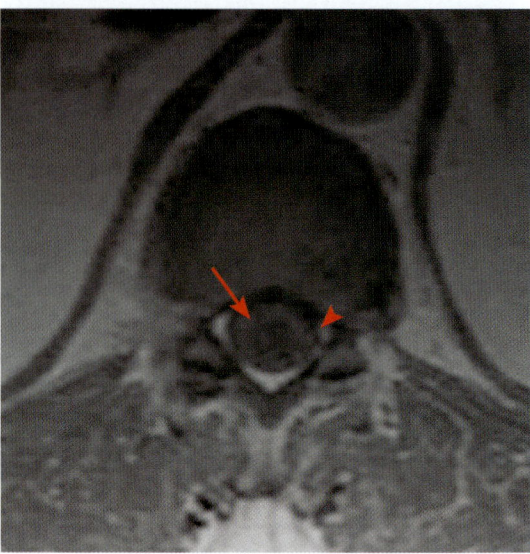

Sagittal T2- (Panel A) and T1- (Panel B) weighted MRI of the lower thoracic and lumbar spine. There is a well-defined intramedullary cyst at the level of T11-T12. The cyst is thin walled and follows fluid signal on both T1 and T2 sequences.

Axial T1-weighted sequence at the level of T12 vertebral body shows a well-defined intramedullary cyst causing slight expansion of the spinal cord (*arrow*). The thecal sac is marked with an *arrowhead*.

Answers

1. Enterogenous cysts of the central nervous system account for 0.7%-1.3% of spinal cord tumors. They are cystic lesions of endodermal origin lined by a single epithelial layer that resembles cells of the alimentary canal. They result from incomplete separation of the foregut and notochord during the third week of embryonic development resulting in the persistence of the canal of Kovalevski, which joins the yolk sac to the notochord.

2. The main differential diagnoses are a posttraumatic cyst, a demyelinating plaque, and syrinx.

3. They are generally located in the intradural extramedullary compartment with occasional intramedullary involvement.

4. Neurenteric cysts occur primarily in children and young adults where they are often associated with other congenital spinal abnormalities. Such abnormalities include anterior and posterior spina bifida, hemivertebrae, absent vertebrae, scoliosis, fused vertebrae, butterfly vertebrae, and diastematomyelia.

5. Neurenteric cysts represent the rarest form of bronchopulmonary foregut malformations, which also include pulmonary sequestrations, bronchogenic cysts, and enteric cysts.

Pearls

- Neurenteric cysts are cystic lesions of endodermal origin lined by a single epithelial layer.
- They represent the rarest form of bronchopulmonary foregut malformations.
- Occur primarily in children and young adults when they are often associated with other congenital spinal abnormalities.
- Most frequently encountered in the spinal canal, particularly at the cervicothoracic region.
- Generally located in the intradural extramedullary compartment with occasional intramedullary involvement.

Suggested Readings

Rotondo M, D'Avanzo R, Natale M, et al. Intramedullary neurenteric cysts of the spine. Report of three cases. *J Neurosurg Spine*. 2005 Mar;2(3):372-376.

Savage JJ, Casey JN, McNeill IT, Sherman JH. Neurenteric cysts of the spine. J *Craniovertebr Junction Spine*. 2010 Jan;1(1):58-63.

Singhal BS, Parekh HN, Ursekar M, Deopujari CE, Manghani DK. Intramedullary neurenteric cyst in mid thoracic spine in an adult: a case report. *Neurol India*. 2001 Sep;49(3):302-304.

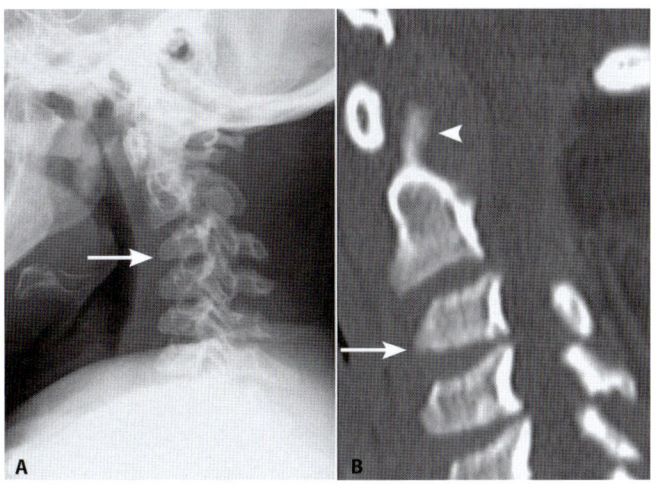

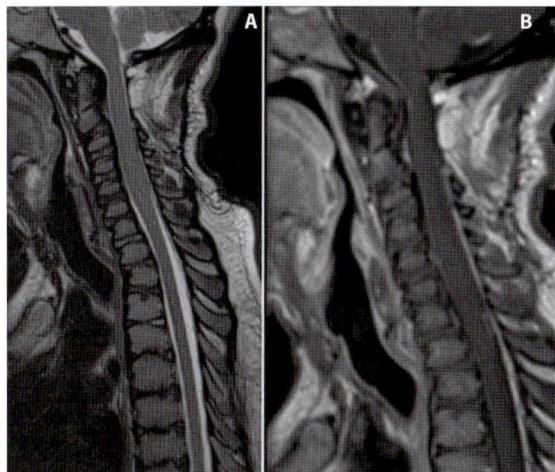

1. What is the most likely diagnosis?

2. Which conditions are also part of the "mucopolysaccharidosis" spectrum?

3. Name some manifestations of this syndrome.

4. Describe clinical and pathological characteristics of this condition.

5. In which conditions is inferior vertebral beaking seen?

Case ranking/difficulty:

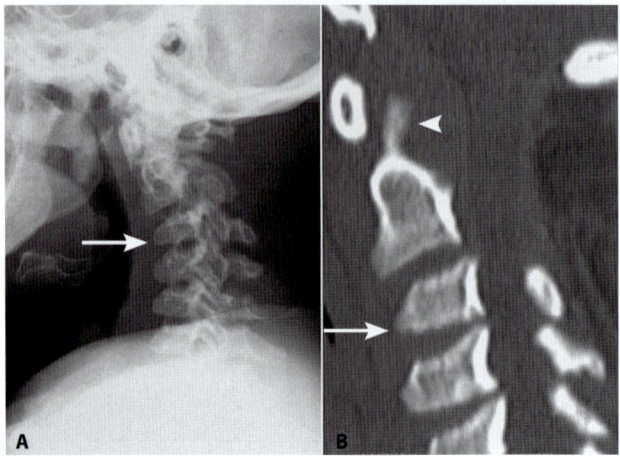

Lateral radiograph (A) and sagittal CT (B) show hypoplastic cervical vertebrae with pathognomonic "inferior beaking" (*arrows*). Previous posterior cervical decompression and characteristic hypoplasia of the odontoid process (*arrowhead*) is seen.

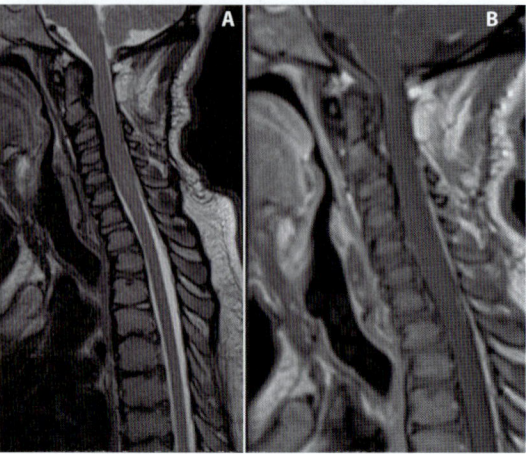

Sagittal T2 (A) and contrast-enhanced T1 (B) sequences show expansion of the cervical cord, with no identifiable mass lesion or syrinx.

Answers

1. Hurler syndrome is a rare lysosomal storage disorder with a prevalence of 1 in 100 000. It is caused by a defective IDUA gene that codes for α-L-iduronidase and has an autosomal recessive inheritance. Enzyme deficiency results in accumulation of dermatan and heparan sulfate in multiple tissues, which leads to progressive deterioration and eventual death.

2. Seven distinct clinical types and numerous subtypes of mucopolysaccharidoses have been identified. They are a group of metabolic disorders, which include Hunter syndrome, Sly syndrome, Sanfilippo syndrome, and Scheie syndrome.

3. Clinical manifestations of Hurler syndrome include profound intellectual disability, cardiac disease, corneal clouding, coarse facial features, and a low nasal bridge. Characteristic musculoskeletal manifestations, cervical myelopathy, and excessive hair growth may also be encountered.

4. Hurler syndrome is an autosomal recessive condition. Affected individuals often succumb to the condition in the first decade, from respiratory and cardiac complications.

5. Inferior vertebral beaks are seen in achondroplasia, pseudoachondroplasia, trisomy 21, and congenital hypothyroidism.

   The vertebral body beaks in Morquio syndrome arise from the central part (middle third) of the anterior vertebral body.

Pearls

- Hurler syndrome is a rare autosomal recessive, lysosomal storage disorder.
- Affected individuals demonstrate typical clinical manifestations, and the diagnosis is confirmed by demonstrating α-L-iduronidase deficiency.
- Characteristic radiological findings include inferior vertebral beaking and odontoid hypoplasia.

Suggested Readings

Belani KG, Krivit W, Carpenter BL, et al. Children with mucopolysaccharidosis: perioperative care, morbidity, mortality, and new findings. *J Pediatr Surg.* 1993;28:403-408.

Kachur E, Del Maestro R. Mucopolysaccharidoses and spinal cord compression: case report and review of the literature with implications of bone marrow transplantation. *Neurosurgery-Baltimore.* 2000;47:223-229.

Kirkpatrick K, Ellwood J, Walker RW. Mucopolysaccharidosis type 1 (Hurler syndrome) and anesthesia: the impact of bone marrow transplantation, enzyme replacement therapy, and fiberoptic intubation on airway management. *Paediatr Anaesth.* 2012;22:745-751.

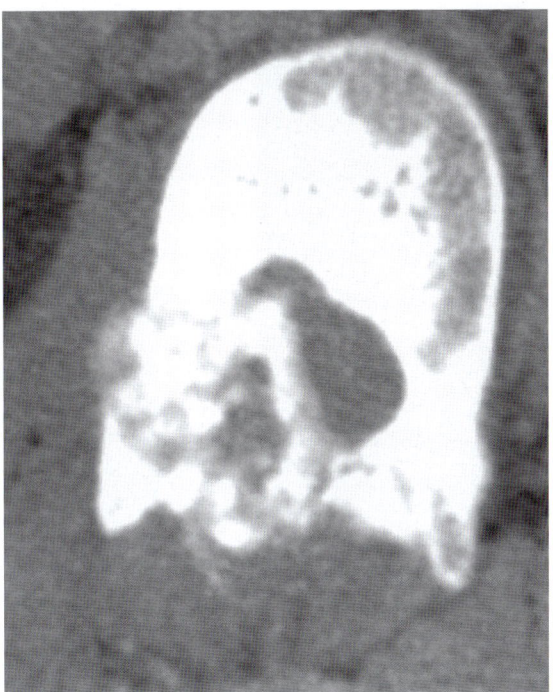 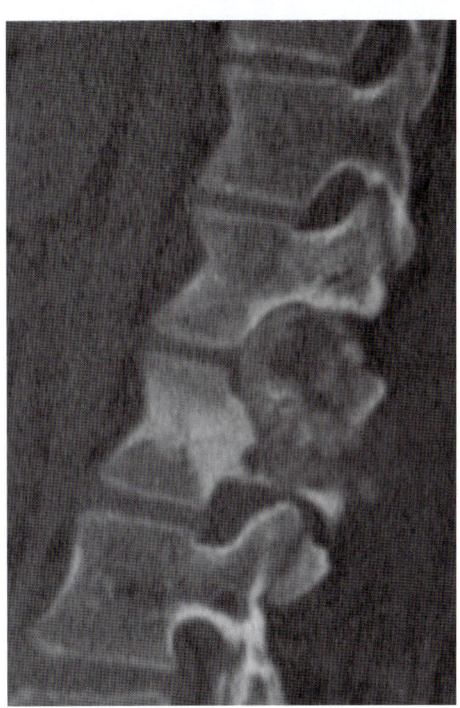

1. What are the findings on CT?

2. What is the differential diagnosis, and what is the most likely etiology?

3. What are common locations for this lesion?

4. What differentiates the aggressive form of this lesion from the nonaggressive form?

5. What is the management for these lesions?

Case ranking/difficulty: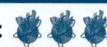

Category: Vertebral Body

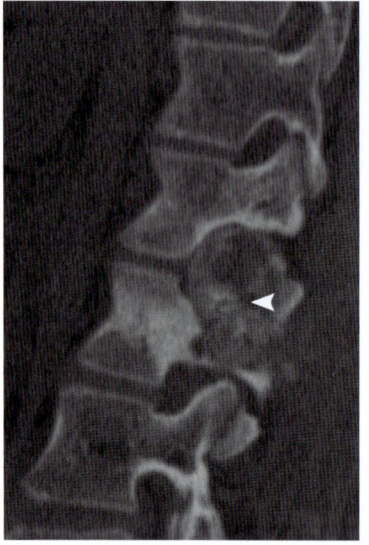

Expansile posterior element lesion with a central mineralized matrix, cortical expansion, and breakthrough with adjacent vertebral sclerosis.

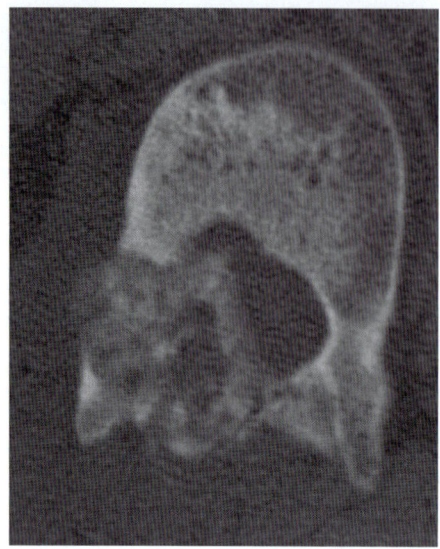

Similar findings.

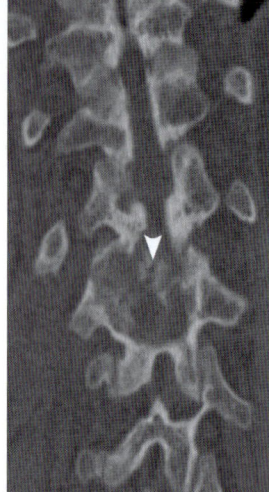

Coronal reformatted images show the highly mineralized matrix and bone expansion.

Answers

1. Lucent expansile lesion with central mineralization located in the posterior elements, and with cortical breakthrough. Sclerosis is seen in the vertebral body with bony remodeling.

2. Differential includes osteoblastoma, aneurysmal bone cyst, giant cell tumor, and a low-grade osteosarcoma. Given the age of the patient, size of lesion, and bony expansion, aggressive osteoblastoma is the favored diagnosis. Osteoid osteoma is not expansile.

3. Osteoblastomas typically occur in the posterior elements of the spine or the diaphysis of long bones. The metaphysis is less common.

4. An aggressive osteoblastoma is characterized by bony expansion, cortical breakthrough, and soft tissue infiltration, as shown in this case. Tumor recurrence is common. Metastasis is extremely uncommon and usually occurs if there is malignant transformation to an osteosarcoma, following radiation therapy.

5. Aggressive osteoblastomas usually require surgical excision, but unfortunately there is a high recurrence rate of up to 50%.

   In surgically unresectable tumors, radiation therapy and chemotherapy have been tried, but there is the risk of post-radiation sarcoma.

Pearls

- Osteoblastomas are histologically similar to osteoid osteoma.
- They are, however, larger, greater than 2 cm in size.
- Nocturnal pain and relief with aspirin, as seen in an osteoid osteoma, are not typical features.
- The lesion is commonly located in the posterior elements of the spine and the diaphysis of long bones.
- Lesions are lucent, and may have central mineralization. There can be mild expansion, especially in the spine, with surrounding sclerosis. Variable central mineralization is present.
- An aggressive osteoblastoma with cortical expansion and breakthrough and infiltration of the soft tissues has been described. These aggressive lesions can recur, but have no metastatic potential.
- Aggressive osteoblastomas are usually greater than 3 cm.
- MRI shows isointensity to hypointensity on T1-weighted images, with variable T2 signal.

Suggested Readings

Abramovici L, Kenan S, Hytiroglou P, Rafii M, Steiner GC. Osteoblastoma-like osteosarcoma of the distal tibia. *Skeletal Radiol.* 2002 Mar;31(3):179-182.

Ramirez JA, Sandoz JC, Kaakaji Y, Nietzschman HR. Case 3: Aggressive osteoblastoma. *AJR Am J Roentgenol.* 1998 Sep;171(3):863, 867-868.

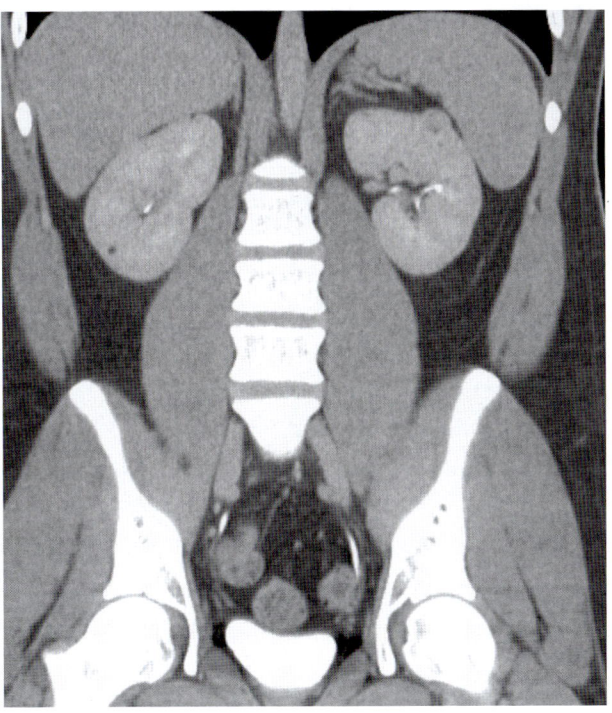
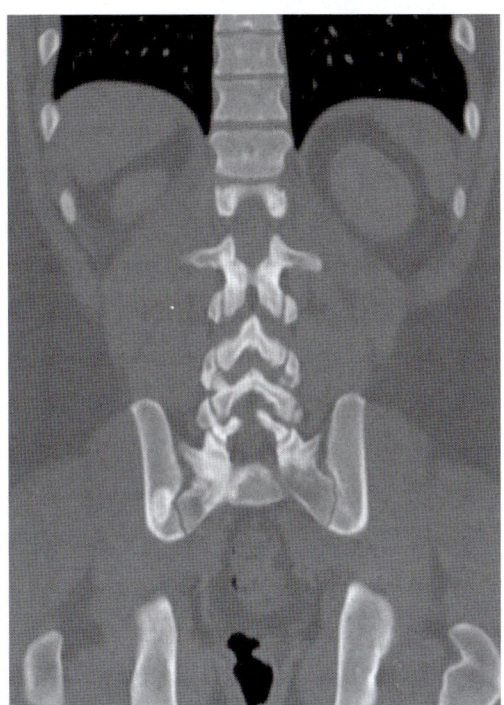

1. What are the major radiologic findings?

2. What is the likely diagnosis?

3. What are the classic osseous manifestations of this entity?

4. What are two rare osseous manifestations of this entity?

5. What are the expected radionuclide bone scan findings?

Case ranking/difficulty: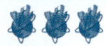

Category: Miscellanous

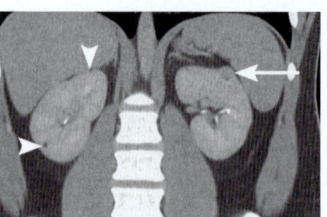

Multiple fat attenuating renal angiomyolipomas (*arrowheads*), and a complicated cyst (*arrow*).

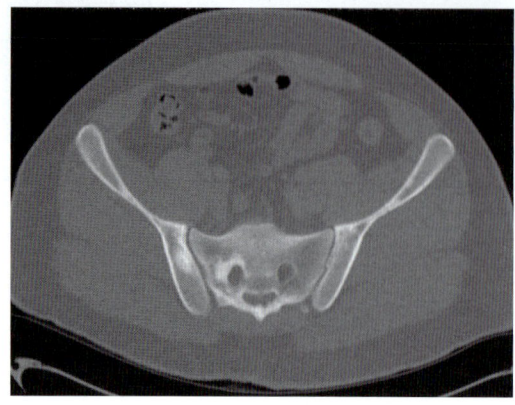

Multiple sclerotic lesions.

Radionuclide bone scan shows the sclerotic lesions have normal uptake.

Answers

1. There are multiple fat-containing renal lesions consistent with angiomyolipomas, as well as multiple sclerotic lesions. A hyperdense left renal lesion was a complex cyst.

2. The combination of renal angiomyolipomas, renal cysts, and sclerotic bone lesions is consistent with tuberous sclerosis.

3. TSC bone lesions included dense sclerosis due to calvarial thickening and periosteal thickening in the long bones. Multiple bones cysts can occur, especially in the metacarpals and phalanges, which, in combination with pulmonary disease, can lead to a misdiagnosis of neurofibromatosis or sarcoid. Erosions of the terminal tufts of the phalanges from subungual angiofibromas may occur.

   Dysplasia of the body of the sphenoid in patients with retinal hamartomas can be seen (unlike the sphenoid wing dysplasia in neurofibromatosis).

4. There are case reports of a clivus chordoma in a child with TSC, and of occipital thinning in the bone overlying a cortical tuber.

5. The radionuclide bone scan appearance is variable. However, the scan is usually normal, as seen in this patient.

Pearls

- Tuberous sclerosis (TSC) is a multisystem disorder that is a result of a spontaneous mutation of two genes, *TSC1* and *TSC2*, which code for the proteins hamartin and tuberin, respectively. These proteins act as tumor growth suppressors.

- The manifestations are protean. They include
  - Cutaneous: adenoma sebaceum
  - Neurologic: subependymal tubers and giant cell astrocytomas, cortical tubers
  - Cardiac: rhabdomyomas
  - Ophthalmic: retinal astrocytomas
  - Pulmonary: cystic pulmonary abnormalities
  - Renal: cysts, angiomyolipomas (AMLs), renal cell carcinomas
  - Dental: pitting of the enamel, gingival fibromas
  - Gastrointestinal: hamartomas and polyposis
  - Hepatic: cysts and hepatic AMLs
  - Skeletal: densely sclerotic lesions with calvarial and periosteal bone thickening, occasional cysts. The differential for the skeletal lesions includes osteopoikilosis or metastatic disease, depending on the patient's age.
- If the osseous sclerotic lesions are combined with bone cysts and pulmonary lesions, the differential will include sarcoid and neurofibromatosis.

Suggested Readings

Evans JC, Curtis J. The radiological appearances of tuberous sclerosis. *Br J Radiol*. 2000 Jan;73(865):91-98.

Schroeder BA, Wells RG, Starshak RJ, Sty JR. Clivus chordoma in a child with tuberous sclerosis: CT and MR demonstration. *J Comput Assist Tomogr*. 1987;11(1):195-196.

Terada T, Nakai E, Moriwaki H, Hayashi S, Komai N. Tuberous sclerosis with an atypical radiological skull change: case report. *Neurosurgery*. 1985 Jun;16(6):804-807.

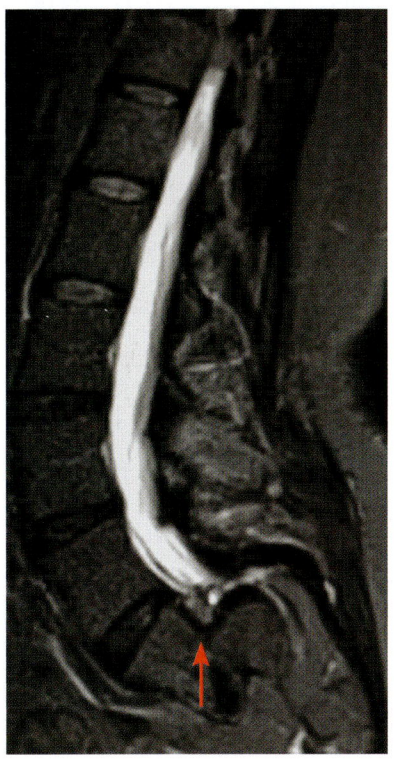 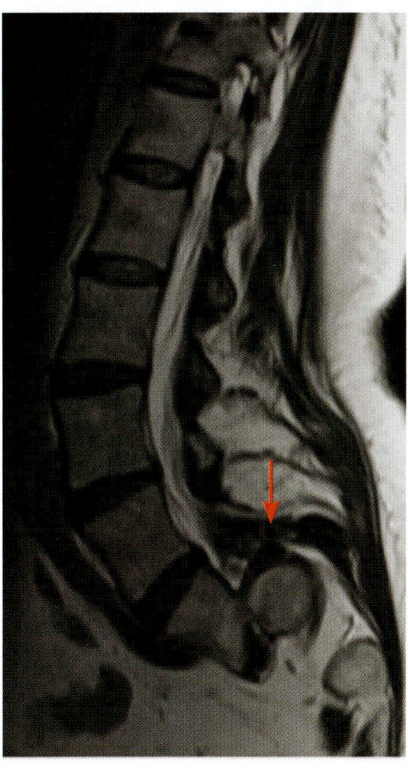

1. What is the diagnosis?

2. What are the common patient demographics for this condition?

3. Deficiency of which structure is usually responsible for this specific entity?

4. What are the usual complications of this condition?

5. What is the treatment of choice for progressive deformity/complications?

Case ranking/difficulty: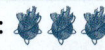

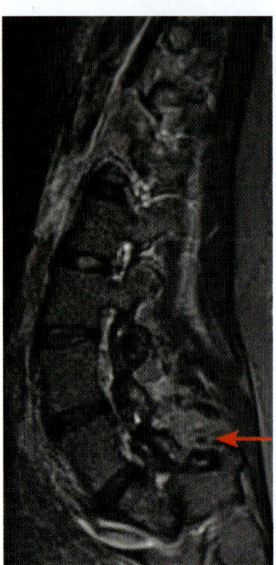

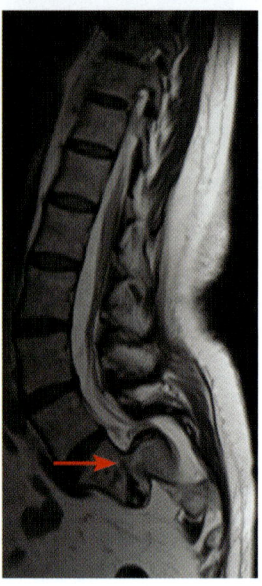

The dysplastic (horizontal) superior articular facets of S1 are well demonstrated on the sagittal images.

There is a diminutive fused L5/S1 articulation and compensatory lumbar hyperlordosis.

Answers

1. Dysplastic spondylolisthesis is a common cause of slips identified in adolescents and young adults. It relates to congenital dysplasia of the posterior elements, usually superior articular facets of S1.

2. Dysplastic spondylolisthesis is congenital, more common in women and found more frequently in Caucasians.

3. Dysplastic spondylolisthesis usually results from a congenitally malformed superior articular facet of S1.

4. Severe deformity leads to a hyperlordotic lumbar spine. There is usually L5/S1 disc degeneration. As the slip progresses, there may be severe central canal and lateral recess stenosis.

5. As slips progress, they may require surgical intervention. A posterior decompression with fusion in situ is the preferred approach, as it allows the central canal to be decompressed, and fixation prevents further progression of the slip and deformity.

Pearls

- Dysplastic spondylolisthesis is a common cause of a slip in an adolescent or young adult at L5/S1.
- The key distinction between an isthmic and a dysplastic cause is the spinal canal, which is widened

as a result of pars defects, and narrowed as a result of facet joint dysplasia and subluxation.

- The identification of a dysplastic (horizontal) superior horizontal articular facet of S1 is virtually pathognomic of this condition, although other dysplastic etiologies include abnormal vertically oriented facet joints.
- Spondyloptosis (100% slip) is probably only commonly seen in cases of dysplastic spondylolisthesis; hence, if this degree of slip is noted, a congenital dysplastic etiology should be considered.
- The L5/S1 articulation is often partly fused and diminutive in this type of spondylolisthesis.
- Regular follow-up is advised for consideration of surgery as high-grade dysplastic spondylolisthesis may have severe central canal stenosis and deformity.

Suggested Readings

Pucher A, Jankowski R, Szulc A, Stryczyński P, Strzyzewski W. Surgical treatment of dysplastic and isthmic spondylolisthesis. *Ortop Traumatol Rehabil.* 2005 Dec;7(6):639-645.

Vialle R, Dauzac C, Khouri N, Wicart P, Glorion C, Guigui P. Sacral and lumbar-pelvic morphology in high-grade spondylolisthesis. *Orthopedics.* 2007 Aug;30(8):642-649.

Acute on chronic back pain with sudden loss of bladder and bowel function. History of prior spine surgery

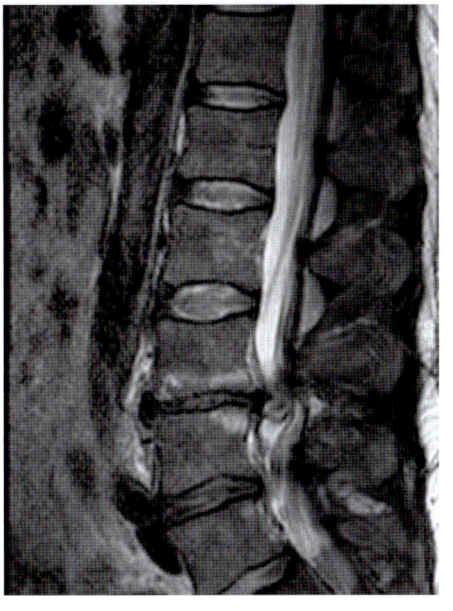
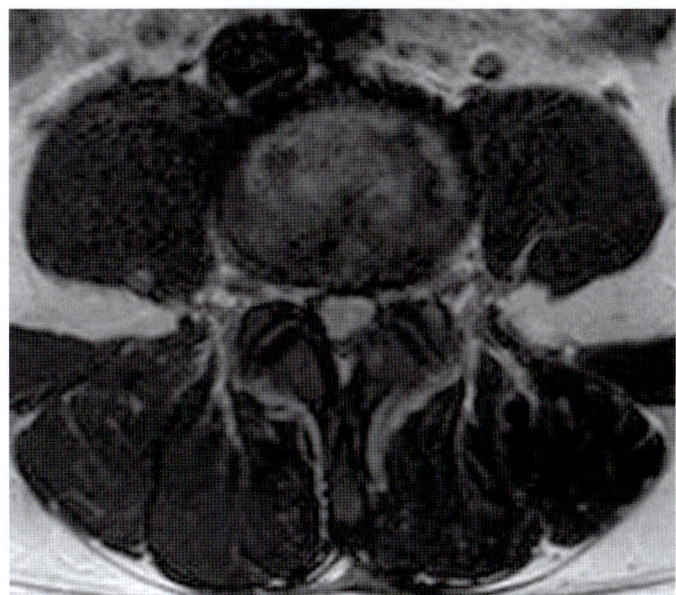

1. What are the MRI findings?

2. What is the differential diagnosis of intradural, extramedullary lesions?

3. What is the diagnosis?

4. What makes the diagnosis challenging?

5. How are these lesions classified?

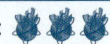

Case ranking/difficulty: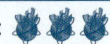

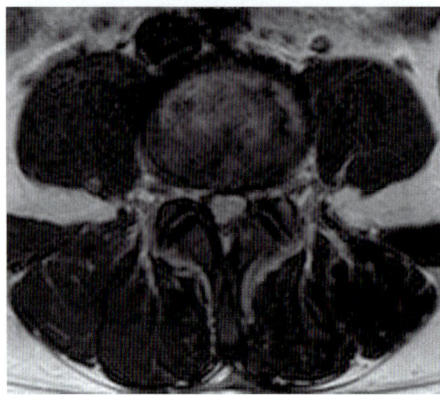

Central canal is obscured by cystic disc material, and the normal nerve roots are displaced peripherally.

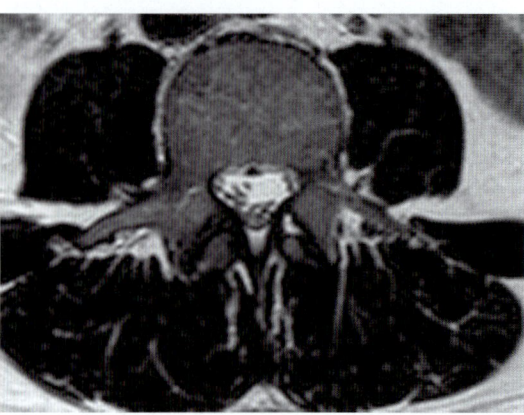

Normal nerve roots for comparison.

Answers

1. Intradural and extramedullary lesion that is T2 hyperintense, peripherally displacing nerve roots.

2. The differential diagnosis includes herniated intradural disc material, meningioma, neurofibroma, and metastasis.

3. Cystic disc material is seen displacing the normal nerve roots peripherally, consistent with herniated intradural disc material.

4. The diagnosis can be made challenging by the presence of cystic changes and calcification of the disc suggesting other etiologies. In this case, the cystic disc material resembles CSF, and the nerve roots are displaced peripherally. The postoperative status of a patient, and the presence of congenital adhesions and a constitutionally narrow spinal canal can also make the diagnosis difficult.

5. Type A: Herniation of the disc into the dural sac.

   Type B: Herniation of the disc into the dural sheath in the preganglionic region.

Pearls

- Intradural herniated disc is a rare cause of cord or cauda equina compression.
- It accounts for 0.26% or 0.3% of all herniated disc cases, most commonly in the lumbar region, usually at L4/5.
- Congenital adhesion between the ventral surface of the thecal sac and posterior longitudinal ligament acts as a predisposing factor.

- They can be difficult to diagnose especially when they undergo cystic or calcified changes.
- According to Mut et al, they can be classified into two types:
  - Type A: Herniation of a disc material into the dural sac.
  - Type B: Herniation into the dural sheath in the pre-ganglionic region.
- MRI is the investigation of choice. Contrast-enhanced MRI is used to differentiate from intradural and extramedullary lesions such as neurofibroma and meningioma, and also from intradural lesions such as epidermoid and dermoid. Disc material does not enhance immediately after administration of contrast.
- Treatment usually involves urgent removal of the disc, especially when causing compressive symptoms.

Suggested Readings

Arnold PM, Wakwaya YT. Intradural disk herniation at L1-L2: report of two cases. *J Spinal Cord Med.* 2011;34(3):312-314.

Singh PK, Shrivastava S, Dulani R, Banode P, Gupta S. Dorsal herniation of cauda equina due to sequestrated intradural disc. *Asian Spine J.* 2012 Jun;6(2):145-147.

Mut M, Berker M, Palaoğlu S. Intraradicular disc herniations in the lumbar spine and a new classification of intradural disc herniations. *Spinal Cord.* 2001 Oct;39(10):545-548.

Subject Index

Note: Numbers in parentheses refer to Case IDs.

Chapter Index

Note: Numbers in parentheses refer to Case IDs.

Subchapter Index

Note: Numbers in parentheses refer to Case IDs.

Difficulty Level Index

Note: Numbers in parentheses refer to Case IDs.

Author Index

Note: Numbers in parentheses refer to Case IDs.

Acknowledgment Index

Note: Numbers in parentheses refer to Case IDs.